Sialendoscopy and Lithotripsy

Guest Editor

MICHAEL H. FRITSCH, MD

OTOLARYNGOLOGIC CLINICS OF NORTH AMERICA

www.oto.theclinics.com

December 2009 • Volume 42 • Number 6

SAUNDERS an imprint of ELSEVIER, Inc.

W.B. SAUNDERS COMPANY

A Division of Elsevier Inc.

1600 John F. Kennedy Boulevard • Suite 1800 • Philadelphia, Pennsylvania 19103-2899

http://www.theclinics.com

OTOLARYNGOLOGIC CLINICS OF NORTH AMERICA Volume 42, Number 6
December 2009 ISSN 0030-6665, ISBN-13: 978-1-4377-1254-4, ISBN-10: 1-4377-1254-1

Editor: Joanne Husovski

Otolaryngologic Clinics of North America (ISSN 0030-6665) is published bimonthly by Elsevier, Inc., 360 Park Avenue South, New York, NY 10010-1710. Months of issue are February, April, June, August, October, and December. Business and Editorial Offices: 1600 John F. Kennedy Blvd., Suite 1800, Philadelphia, PA 19103-2899. Customer Service Office: 6277 Sea Harbor Drive, Orlando, FL 32887-4800. Periodicals postage paid at New York, NY and additional mailing offices. Subscription prices is $290.00 per year (US individuals), $527.00 per year (US institutions), $142.00 per year (US student/resident), $382.00 per year (Canadian individuals), $662.00 per year (Canadian institutions), $429.00 per year (international individuals), $662.00 per year (international institutions), $219.00 per year (international & Canadian student/resident). Foreign air speed delivery is included in all *Clinics*' subscription prices. All prices are subject to change without notice. **POSTMASTER:** Send address changes to *Otolaryngologic Clinics of North America*, Elsevier Health Sciences Division, Subscription Customer Service, 3251 Riverport Lane, Maryland Heights, MO 63043. **Telephone: 1-800-654-2452 (U.S. and Canada); 314-447-8871 (outside U.S. and Canada). Fax: 314-447-8029. E-mail: journalscustomerservice-usa@elsevier.com (for print support); journalsonlinesupport-usa@elsevier.com (for online support).**

Reprints. For copies of 100 or more of articles in this publication, please contact the Commercial Reprints Department, Elsevier Inc., 360 Park Avenue South, New York, NY 10010-1710. Tel.: 212-633-3812; Fax: 212-462-1935; E-mail: reprints@elsevier.com.

Otolaryngologic Clinics of North America is also published in Spanish by McGraw-Hill Interamericana Editores S.A., P.O. Box 5-237, 06500 Mexico D.F., Mexico.

Otolaryngologic Clinics of North America is covered in *MEDLINE/PubMed (Index Medicus), Current Contents/Clinical Medicine, Excerpta Medica, BIOSIS, Science Citation Index,* and *ISI/BIOMED.*

Printed and bound by CPI Group (UK) Ltd, Croydon, CR0 4YY

Transferred to Digital Print 2011

Contributors

GUEST EDITOR

MICHAEL H. FRITSCH, MD, FACS
Professor, Department of Otolaryngology-Head and Neck Surgery, Indiana University School of Medicine, Indiana University Medical Center, Indianapolis, Indiana

AUTHORS

JACKIE BROWN, BDS, MSc, FDSRCPS, DDRRCR
Consultant in Dentomaxillofacial Radiology, Department of Dentomaxillofacial Radiology, King's College, London, Dental Institute of Guy's, King's College, St Thomas' Hospitals, London, United Kingdom

PASQUALE CAPACCIO, MD
Aggregate Professor of Otolaryngology, Department of Specialist Surgical Sciences, Fondazione I.R.C.C.S. Ospedale Maggiore Policlinico, Mangiagalli e Regina Elena, University of Milan, Milano, Italy

MICHAEL H. FRITSCH, MD, FACS
Professor, Department of Otolaryngology-Head and Neck Surgery, Indiana University School of Medicine, Indiana University Medical Center, Indianapolis, Indiana

URBAN W. GEISTHOFF, Priv.-Doz. Dr. med
Medical Faculty, University of the Saarland, Homburg/Saar, Germany; Department of Otorhinolaryngology, Holweide Hospital, Hospitals of the City of Cologne, Cologne, Germany

AGNÈS GUERRE, MD
Clinician, Salivary Glands Functional Explorations Institut, Paris, France

JOHN D. HARRISON, PhD, FDSRCSEng, FRCPath
Reader and Consultant, Department of Oral Pathology, King's College London, Dental Institute at Guy's, King's College and St Thomas' Hospital, London, United Kingdom

DANA M. HARTL, MD, PhD
Department of Otolaryngology-Head and Neck Surgery, Institut Gustave Roussy, Villejuif, France

HEINRICH IRO, MD
Professor, Chair, and Director, Department of Otolaryngology-Head and Neck Surgery, University of Erlangen, Erlangen, Germany

PHILIPPE KATZ, MD
Head, Salivary Glands Functional Explorations Institut, Paris, France

MICHAEL KOCH, MD
Senior Physician, Department of Otorhinolaryngology-Head and Neck Surgery, University of Erlangen, Erlangen, Germany

MARK McGURK, MD, FRCS, FDSRCS, DLO
Professor of Oral and Maxillofacial Surgery, Department of Maxillofacial Surgery, King's College London, Dental Institute of Guy's, King's College, St Thomas' Hospitals, Guy's Hospital, London, United Kingdom

KRISTINE M. MOSIER, DMD, PhD
Chief, Head & Neck Imaging; Associate Professor of Radiology, Section of Neuroradiology, Department of Radiology, Indiana University School of Medicine, Indianapolis, Indiana

ODED NAHLIELI, DMD
Professor and Chairman, Department of Oral and Maxillofacial Surgery, Barzilai Medical Center, Ashkelon; Faculty of Medicine, Ben Gurion University of the Negev, Beer Sheva, Israel

LORENZO PIGNATARO, MD
Professor of Otolaryngology and Director of Otolaryngology Unit, Department of Specialist Surgical Sciences, Fondazione I.R.C.C.S. Ospedale Maggiore Policlinico, Mangiagalli e Regina Elena, University of Milan, Milano, Italy

SARA TORRETTA, MD
Resident, Department of Specialist Surgical Sciences, Fondazione I.R.C.C.S. Ospedale Maggiore Policlinico, Mangiagalli e Regina Elena, University of Milan, Milano, Italy

JOHANNES ZENK, MD
Professor and Vice Chair, Department of Otorhinolaryngology-Head and Neck Surgery, University of Erlangen, Erlangen, Germany

Contents

Preface **xiii**
Michael H. Fritsch

Sialendoscopy and Lithotripsy: Literature Review **915**
Michael H. Fritsch

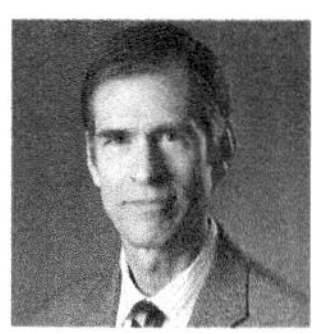

This article presents a brief literature review of sialendoscopy and lithotripsy highlights from journal articles and presentations spanning from 1953 to 2009. Seventy-seven sources were reviewed for this article.

Causes, Natural History, and Incidence of Salivary Stones and Obstructions **927**
John D. Harrison

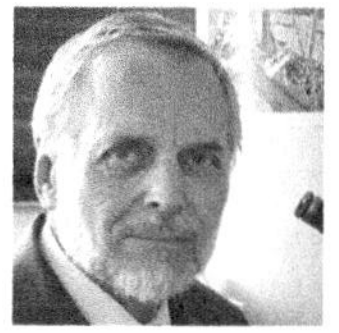

Uncertainty about the causes and natural history of salivary stones (sialoliths) and other obstructions is being dispelled by clinical and experimental research. Sialoliths are now shown to be secondary to chronic obstructive sialadenitis. Microscopic stones (sialomicroliths) accumulate during secretory inactivity in normal salivary glands and produce atrophic foci by obstruction. Microbes ascend the main salivary duct during secretory inactivity and proliferate in atrophic foci and cause spreading inflammation, leading to inflammatory swelling and fibrosis that can compress large ducts. This leads to stagnation of secretory material rich in calcium that precipitates onto degenerating cellular membranes to form a sialolith.

Diagnostic Radiographic Imaging for Salivary Endoscopy 949
Kristine M. Mosier

The advent of sialoendoscopy techniques presents new challenges in the diagnostic imaging of the salivary glands. This article reviews the different diagnostic imaging approaches for work-up of patients before sialoendoscopy. The relative advantages and disadvantages of each technique and guidelines for application of the different techniques are discussed.

Clinical Ultrasound of the Salivary Glands 973
Philippe Katz, Dana M. Hartl, and Agnès Guerre

Ultrasound investigation of the major salivary glands has been routinely used for the past 25 years. Ultrasound provides an immediate diagnosis in acute or chronic inflammatory salivary diseases and can visualize sialolithiasis as small as 0.4 mm. Ultrasound is also an important imaging modality for salivary gland tumors, guiding fine needle aspiration (FNA) for cytological diagnosis. It is particularly sensitive in detecting suspicious lymph nodes in the neck and helps to guide FNA. Ultrasound is a first-line tool for diagnosis of salivary pathology. It is simple to use, noninvasive, and well tolerated, even in children.

Technology of Sialendoscopy 1001
Urban W. Geisthoff

Technical developments have taken place since the first endoscopes suitable for sialendoscopy appeared. Now, a variety of endoscopes are available. Ranging from rigid to flexible, each type has its own properties. Light sources, imaging, recording instrumentation, and other equipment used with the endoscopes facilitate or extend the range of their use. Experiences using different endoscopes in more than 300 endoscopies are discussed.

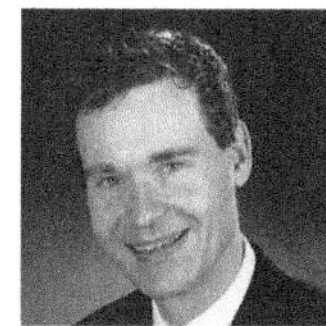

When basic surgical principles are followed diagnostic salivary endoscopy is a relatively safe operative procedure. Therapeutic sialendoscopy uses such instrumentation as lasers, forceps, baskets, and balloons for endoductal fragmentation, retrieval, and dilatation. Based on experience acquired from more than 300 salivary endoscopy procedures and a review of the current literature, the most relevant operative techniques are presented.

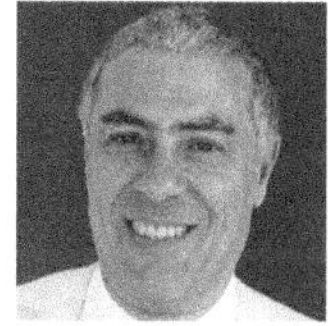

This article presents and discusses advanced minimally invasive sialoendoscopy and combined methods: endoscopy, endoscopic-assisted techniques, and external-lithotripsy combined procedures. It also presents rare situations and complications encountered during sialoendoscopic procedures. Sialoendoscopy is a relatively novel technique, which adds significant new dimensions to the surgeon's armamentarium for management of inflammatory salivary gland diseases. Because of the rapid development in minimally invasive surgical techniques, surgeons are capable of more facilely treating complicated inflammatory and obstructive conditions of the salivary glands.

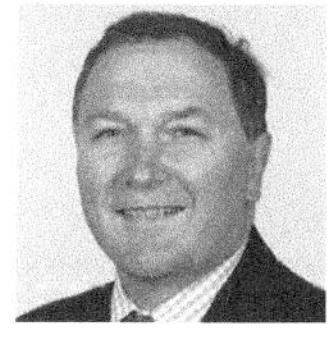

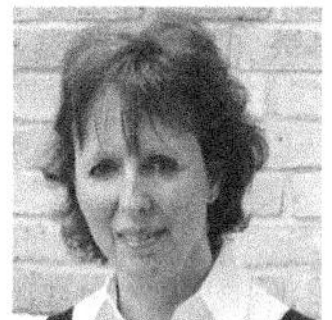

Minimally invasive alternatives for treatment of salivary duct obstruction are discussed. Radiologically- and endoscopically-guided interventions using wire baskets and dilating balloons, including cutting balloons, are covered as are combined endoscopic and open approaches.

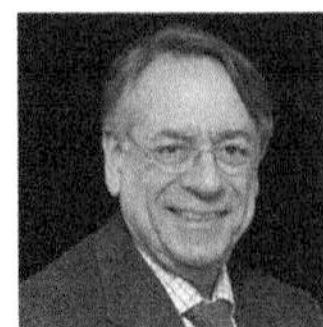
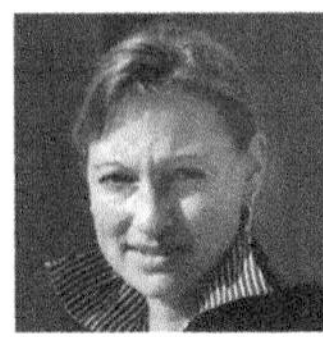
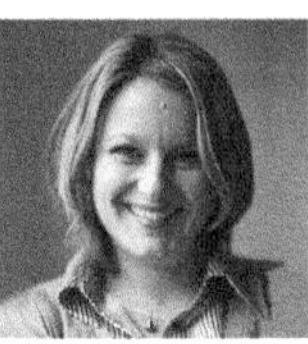

Juvenile recurrent parotitis (JRP) can be a debilitating illness in children. Knowing how to recognize and diagnose it for early treatment avoids recurrences that could lead to significant destruction of the glandular parenchyma. This article discusses the various therapeutic modalities proposed in the literature (medical treatment or sialendoscopy) and describes the authors' treatment of choice of combining antibiotics and iodinated oil sialography.

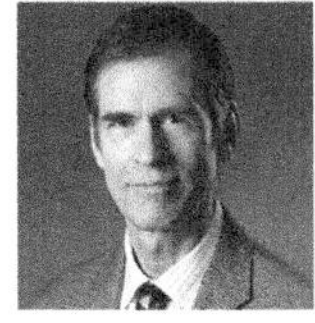

Salivary gland preservation during treatment for obstructive duct and gland problems is a goal worth pursuing. Difficult cases may seem to be candidates for sialadenectomy. However, progress in endoscopic and open-surgical procedures can help the physician to find solutions that overcome difficult problems without removing the gland. Broader application of these sialendoscopic and open preservation procedures may be especially useful for physicians without access to extracorporeal lithotriptors.

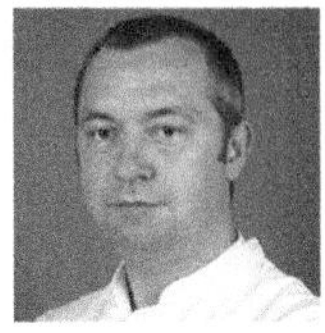
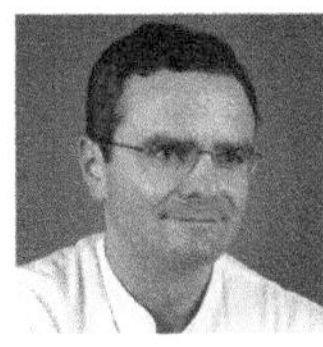
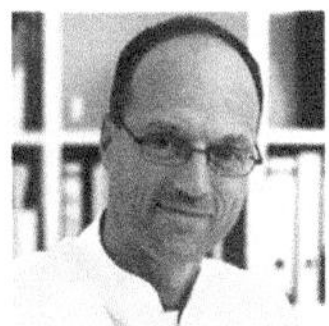

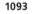

The traditional treatment for sialolithiasis was extirpation of the affected gland. It is now known, however, that salivary gland function can recover completely after stone extraction alone. Since the mid-1980s, much thought has been given to treating sialolithiasis with extracorporeal or intracorporeal shock waves in a manner similar to that used for urinary tract or biliary tract stones, and this has been implemented successfully. This article provides an overview of the various methods of extracorporeal and intracorporeal lithotripsy that have been used or proposed for salivary calculi to date, considering the advantages and disadvantages of each of the techniques.

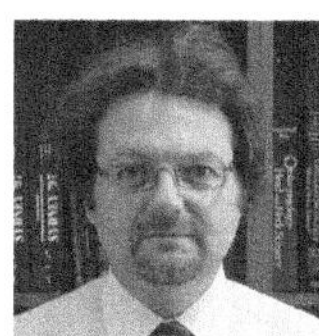 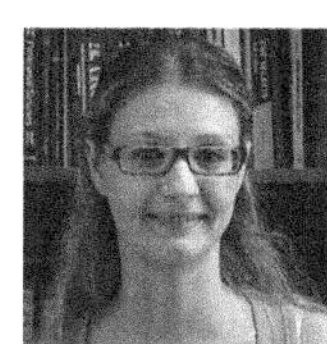 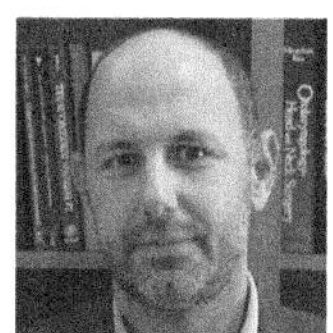

Over the past 20 years, development of minimally invasive therapies has led to the use of extracorporeal shock wave lithotripsy (ESWL) to treat salivary stones. The two main energy sources are piezoelectric and electromagnetic extracorporeal lithotripsy. Both have the aim of fragmenting the stones. ESWL is considered the treatment of choice for all parotid calculi and submandibular perihilar or intraparenchymal stones of less than 7 mm. Continuous ultrasonographic monitoring during the procedure reduces the number of untoward effects. The main limitations are the need for multiple sessions and residual stone fragments inside the duct system.

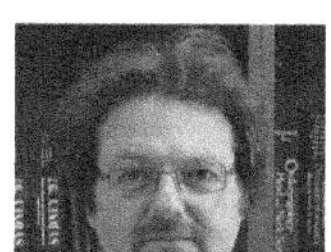 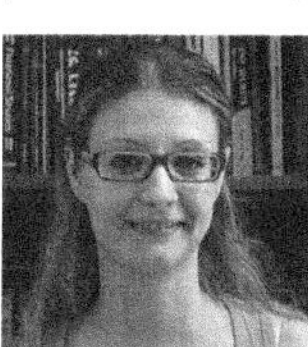 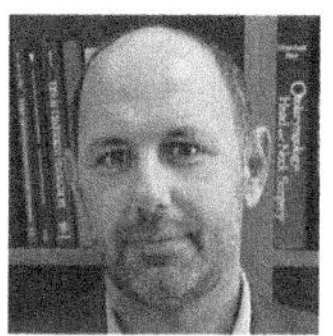

Salivary gland ductal obstructions are common, being the most frequent nonneoplastic salivary disorders in adults. Salivary calculi are the main cause of obstruction. Traditional and invasive transcervical sialadenectomy is still the most widely used treatment for perihilar and intraparenchymal obstructive salivary diseases worldwide despite the well-known morbidity related to its functional, neurologic, and aesthetic sequelae. However, improved radiologic imaging, better optical systems and endoscopic devices, and the introduction of minimally invasive therapeutic options have allowed the development of conservative gland-preserving techniques for managing salivary gland obstructions, including extracorporeal shock wave lithotripsy, operative sialoendoscopy, video-assisted transoral and transcervical stone removal, and ductal rehabilitation through interventional radiology and sialoendoscopy. Through adopting a minimally invasive and multimodal policy, a significant number (74%–100%, technique dependent) of salivary calculi can be safely and successfully retrieved while leaving an intact and functional salivary gland system. Only 2% to 5% of patients require gland excision. However, long-term follow-up evaluations of obstructive symptom recurrence are needed before the ultimate benefits of a gland-preserving conservative approach and the residual role of adenectomy can be assessed.

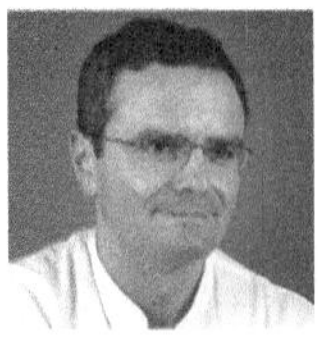
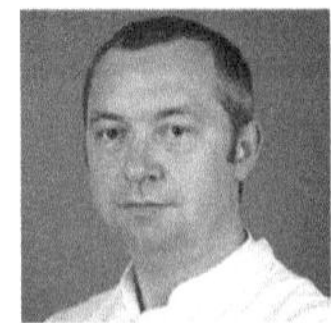
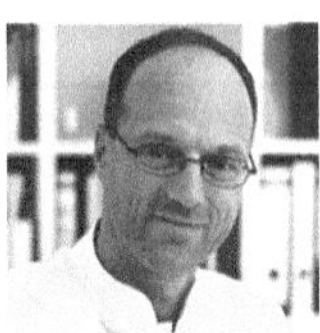

Treatment of obstructive diseases of the major salivary glands has undergone a dramatic change in the last 10 to 15 years. New minimally invasive techniques have been developed, covering all different entities that are included in the complex of salivary gland obstruction, and can help the physician to find the right diagnosis and an adequate treatment plan and to perform a gland-preserving form of therapy. Sialolithiasis or stenosis is the cause of about 90% of all obstructive salivary gland diseases. The development of radiologically or fluoroscopically controlled methods, but especially the introduction of sialendoscopy, has led to changes in the treatment protocol. Knowledge from the authors' experience and from a thorough investigation of the literature has been combined to elaborate algorithms for the treatment of the different obstructive diseases of the salivary glands. Sialoliths and stenoses can be successfully treated by radiologically or fluoroscopically controlled or sialendoscopically based methods in approximately 80% of cases. Extracorporeal shock-wave lithotripsy (ESWL) is successful in up to 50% of cases. Transoral duct slitting is an important method for extraparenchymal submandibular stones, with a success rate of 90%. Operative duct procedures and the combined endoscopic-transcutaneous approach complete the spectrum of treatment modalities of the parotid gland. Sialendoscopy plays a central role in the treatment of obstructive salivary gland diseases, but maximum success can only be attained by the reasonable combination of all these new minimally invasive techniques. Altogether, in well over 95% of cases, resection of the gland can be prevented, thus reducing morbidity and the surgical risks for patients.

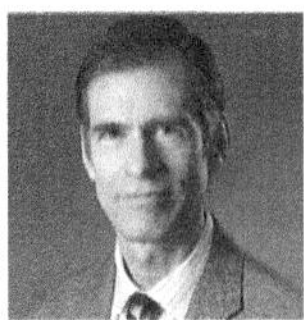

Algorithms for treatment of salivary stones for physicians without access to an extracorporeal lithotriptor are proposed. Strategies for stones of different sizes and for salivary duct stenoses and strictures are discussed.

BONUS Article – Facial Plastic Surgery

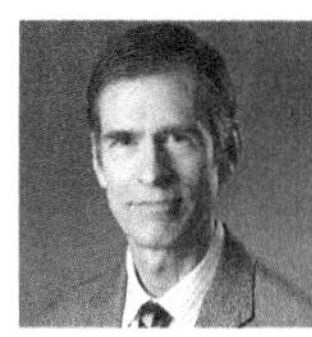

Incisionless Otoplasty surgery for lop (protuberant) ears has evolved through three major steps in technique since its inception in 1992. Improvement was seen with each progressive technical advance. The previously published 2.0 version of 2004 has undergone evolution to streamline placement of the percutaneous retention sutures. The new 3.0 version technique greatly reduces the number of operative steps required. In this article, technical instructions for the 3.0 version are explained, and multiple applications of the 3.0 procedure and the 2.0 are illustrated.

BONUS Article – Otology – Neurotology Surgery

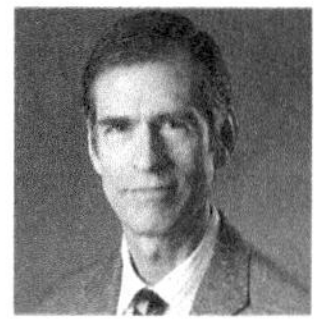

Endoscopic surgery of the inner ear may be a useful, minimally invasive approach to remove pathologic lesions and yet retain inner ear function. Several different endoscopic inner ear surgical entry sites and strategies that may help to preserve otologic function are described. These endoscopic surgical method alternatives are based on temporal bone studies, prior literature, and clinical patient experiences. Endoscopic inner ear surgery is a challenging, but potentially very useful method to address inner ear problems.

FORTHCOMING ISSUES

Cough: An Interdisciplinary Problem
Kenneth W. Altman, MD, PhD, and Richard S. Irwin, MD, *Guest Editors*

Thyroid and Parathyroid Surgery
Ralph Tufano, MD, and Sara Pai, MD, *Guest Editors*

Head and Neck Ultrasound
Joseph Sniezek, MD, and Robert Sofferman, MD, *Guest Editors*

Rhinology: Evolution of Science and Surgery
Rodney Schlosser, MD, and Richard Harvey, MD, *Guest Editors*

Meniere's Disease: Current Diagnostic and Treatment Methods
Jeffrey Harris, MD, and Quyen Nguyen, MD, *Guest Editors*

RECENT ISSUES

October 2009
Technologic Innovations in Rhinology
Raj Sidwani, MD, *Guest Editor*

August 2009
Radiosurgery and Radiotherapy for Benign Skull Base Tumors
Robert A. Battista, MD, *Guest Editor*

June 2009
Surgical Management of Nasal Obstruction: Facial Plastic Surgery Perspective
Daniel G. Becker, MD, *Guest Editor*

Preface: Salivary Endoscopy and Lithotripsy

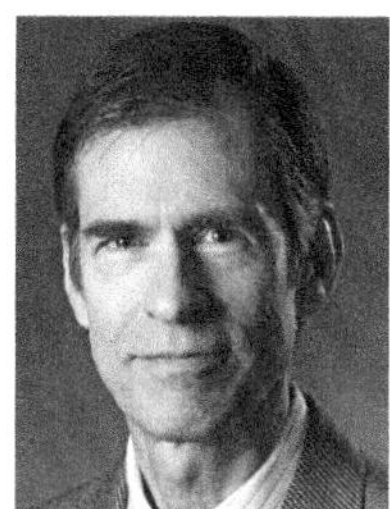

Michael H. Fritsch, MD, FACS
Guest Editor

The contributors to this issue are dedicated to a better understanding of salivary gland disease and the advancement of minimally-invasive means of diagnosis and treatment. They are at the forefront of knowledge and experience in the field of sialendoscopy and lithotripsy. By sharing their experiences in this book-sized collection of articles, a review of the present-day breadth of these fields can be gained from one source. From queries into the initiation of pathologic salivary processes to improved patient treatment techniques, knowledge that previously would have taken much time to garner is assembled in this issue for the readers.

Challenging salivary problems encountered by clinicians may lead to patient treatment using conventional gland resection surgery when other solutions may not be immediately obvious. The consequences of losing a gland, however, can be important to patients who may seem "not to need the gland." By removing even one major gland, an immediate large percentage decrease in salivary function is imposed for the rest of a patient's lifetime. If a functional gland is saved, it can have major advantages for a patient. Therefore, treating physicians should adopt and press forward with all the advances that salivary gland science can offer. Progress includes new ways of repairing and preserving salivary glands and ducts. By conscientiously using endoscopic and lithotripsy approaches, more functioning glands can be preserved. The immediate advantages are no incision, avoidance of open-surgical complications, immediate return to normal activities, and preservation of full oral function. Long term, consider that during the course of a lifetime, a healthy person's salivary gland function may become impaired for a variety of reasons, such as autoimmune disease, Iodine-131 treatments, certain medications, or age-related decline of function. Many middle-aged and elderly persons suffer from dry mouth symptoms. Therefore, a 20-year-old patient may not realize the full benefits and be thankful for a physician's vigorous efforts to conserve the major salivary glands for a further 40 to 50 years. Salivary gland preservation surgery for challenging problems is desirable at all levels.

Otolaryngol Clin N Am 42 (2009) xiii–xiv
doi:10.1016/j.otc.2009.08.017
oto.theclinics.com
0030-6665/09/$ – see front matter

As guest editor for this issue, I would like to personally thank all of the contributing authors for their diligent and enlightening work. Their collective expertise will be the foundation for a solid first step into sialendoscopy and lithotripsy for many North American physicians. Even for experienced physicians, the nuances found in these pages will help enhance their base of knowledge in sialendoscopy and lithotripsy.

Michael H. Fritsch, MD, FACS
Professor, Department of Otolaryngology-Head and Neck Surgery
Indiana University Medical Center
Indianapolis, IN, USA

E-mail address:
mfritsch@iupui.edu (M.H. Fritsch)

Sialendoscopy and Lithotripsy: Literature Review

Michael H. Fritsch, MD, FACS

KEYWORDS

• Sialendoscopy • Lithotripsy • Salivary • Parotid
• Submandibular • Review article

The last 15 years have seen rapid development of nonsurgical and minimally invasive techniques for diagnosing and treating salivary gland duct obstructions. The conventional treatment has shifted from open surgical or gland resection procedures to endoscopic and gland preservation techniques. The goal of treatment now is to leave a physiologically intact gland for the patient. Extracorporeal shock wave lithotriptors, endoscopes, mini-instruments, and corresponding surgical techniques and approaches all have become focused on and tailored to salivary duct and gland pathologies. Originally developed to treat salivary duct stones, progress in equipment designs and surgical techniques has allowed for precise diagnosis and treatment of previously unrecognized nuances of duct pathology. Worldwide, researchers' and physicians' understanding, experience, and skills have accumulated rapidly. Multiple medical specialties have contributed to the present clinical algorithms. These algorithms, which have brought marked improvements in patient care, include nonsurgical, minimally invasive, and conventional open surgical procedures to produce the best diagnostic and treatment possibilities. To obtain better insight into the current state of diagnosis and treatment of salivary obstructive pathologies, a brief review of the literature can give perspective.

LITERATURE REVIEW

In 1965, Mandel and Baurmash[1] studied 14 different radio-opaque contrast solutions, including Sinografin and Ethiodol, for use in sialography. Viscosity, opacity, granuloma formation, irritant effects on mucous membranes, and duration of opacity were analyzed.

Yamamoto and colleagues[2] in 1984 reported on salivary stone chemical and structural composition with scanning electron microscopy and radiograph diffraction analyses of 18 submandibular stones. Lamellar patterned cross-sections revealed

Department of Otolaryngology–Head and Neck Surgery, Indiana University School of Medicine, Indiana University Medical Center, 702 Barnhill Drive, Suite 0860, Indianapolis, IN 46202, USA
E-mail address: mfritsch@iupui.edu

Otolaryngol Clin N Am 42 (2009) 915–926
doi:10.1016/j.otc.2009.09.001 **oto.theclinics.com**

numerous shapes of mineral deposits within the lamella and led to possible explanations of sialolith formation. The main stone components were noted to be apatite and whitlock; calcium and phosphorous were the main constituent elements present, with magnesium and sulfur also occurring frequently.

Riesco and colleagues[3] in 1989 reported on the electron microscopic structure of a minor salivary gland stone. It appeared to be only a crystal without bacterial content, undergoing early external coating toward becoming a stone.

Galili and Marmary[4] in 1986 described the beneficial clinical effects on juvenile recurrent parotitis after sialography. They used Pantopaque and felt that the clinical improvements were caused by the dilation and flushing effects and because of the antiseptic properties of iodine. For salivary stones, Marmary[5] in 1986 proposed electrohydraulic Dornier shock waves as a noninvasive technique based on his in vitro experiences.

Brouns[6] reported in 1989 on his in vitro experience with the destructive effects of an electrohydraulic extracorporeal renal lithotriptor on a salivary stone and a molar tooth and the possible patient safety issues involved with using a renal lithotriptor.

In 1989, Iro and colleagues[7] reported the first successful clinical case of shock wave extracorporeal lithotripsy; they proposed piezoelectric shock waves as a safer source. They cautioned against electrohydraulic Dornier shock waves due to tissue damage based on several animal studies. In 1990, Iro's group reported on clinical experiences with extracorporeal piezoelectric shock wave treatment of stones in 14 patients.[8] A 50% success rate at 3 months without complications was reported.

Briffa and Callum[9] in 1989 described use of an interventional radiology embolectomy catheter for removal of a submandibular duct stone.

Sterenborg and colleagues[10] in 1990 described in vitro laser lithotripsy comparing the pulse dye laser (Candela LFDL/3, Candela Corp, Wayland, Massachusetts, USA) and the Ho-YSGG laser (Laser 1-2-3, Schwartz Electro-optics, Orlando, Florida). The lasers were deemed inefficient at power levels safe for tissues. Eleven stones were analyzed and mainly composed of hydroxyapatite mixed with other minerals.

Grundlach and colleagues[11] reported a 12-patient and in vitro experience using endoscopic intracorporeal lithotripsy in 1990. Eighteen stones were analyzed for stone photo-reflective and absorptive characteristics to help ascertain which laser might be most useful; maximal absorption was at 300 to 400 nm, while maximum reflection was at 500 to 600 nm. The XeCl excimer laser system (308 to 351nm) was judged most efficacious for stone fragmentation, with the CO_2 and ND:YAG laser less applicable. Currently used urologic and salivary holmium lasers operate at 2100 nm.

In 1990 and 1993, Konigsberger and colleagues[12,13] published a case report and series, respectively, using intracorporeal endoscopic-guided laser lithotripsy and intracorporeal electrohydraulic shock wave lithotripsy. The excimer laser was successful in the clinical case report; in the series, 19 of 23 patients had complete stone fragmentation. The shock wave probe tip was placed 1.0 mm in front of the stone, and had a pulse energy of 150 mJ at 10 Hz. Two patients had mucoproteid stones deemed too soft for lithotripsy, and six patients were excluded because of ductal stenosis barring endoscopic passage.

In 1990 and 1991, Katz[14,15] wrote about flexible endoscopy of the salivary ducts. He used a 0.8 mm miniendoscope that was passively flexible, starting in 1988. Stone pathology was visualized, as well as intraductal anatomy such as the first genu of Stensens duct as it crossed the anterior border of the masseter muscle, a valve at the parotid hilum, and the genu of Wharton's duct at the mylohyoid.

Kater and colleagues[16,17] described their experiences using a shock wave device in 1990 with a 3-year update in 1993.

In 1992, Buckenham and colleagues[18] reported on strictures treated with balloon dilation by interventional radiology.

Katz[19] in 1993 reported on use of the Dormia basket and dye laser lithotripsy on yellow-colored stones.

Nahlieli and colleagues[20–25] reported multiple times on endoscopic experiences starting in 1994. The evolution of endoscopic intervention starting with a 2.7 mm rigid arthroscope is chronicled. Initially, stones were removed by suction vacuum. Larger stones were crushed with a forceps before vacuum extraction. The CO_2 laser was used to incise the submandibular duct for anterior stones. Unusual etiologies for stones were noted, such as hair and plant fiber niduses. In 1997, Nahlieli and colleagues provided a treatment algorithm, wherein stones were removed endoscopically by forceps, suction, or basket. Larger stones were crushed with a forceps or laser fragmented (Calcutrip, K. Storz, Tuttlingen, Germany). Sialadenectomy was reserved for large stones or those proximal to a stenosis. Intraparenchymal stones, severe duct angles, and strictures also caused endoscopic failures. Bupivacaine 0.5% totaling 2 mL intraductally allowed 30- to 60-minute operative durations. Postoperative antibiotics were used for 7 days. In 1999, Nahlieli and colleagues forwarded two endoscope designs: a 1.1 mm diameter diagnostic type and a 2.3 mm treatment type. Acute sialadenitis and stones larger than 10 mm were contraindications. The overall success rate was 82%. A 2 mm wide polyethylene tubing stent was placed for 2 weeks. Specific recommendations for treatment of strictures and duct kinks were given in 2001.

In 1994, Arzoz and colleagues[26] reported on a lithiasis case using a #7fr urethroscope (K. Storz) with a 1 mm working channel and using an Alexandrite laser at 60 mJ and 2000 pulses to fragment the stone. In 1996, Arzoz and colleagues[27] described a 19-patient series with sialolithiasis. A Pneumoblastic energy source was deemed most effective compared with laser or electromagnetic Dornier sources. Two patients were treated using a renal lithotriptor. Duct dilation problems were noted to be obstacles to endoscopic progress. Stones were analyzed and noted to be composed of calcium carbonate and octacalcium.

Iro and colleagues[28] in 1995 described use of the Rhodamine 6-G Flashlamp pumped dye laser (Technomed International, France) for lithiasis. An energy of 120 mJ with 1500 pulses delivered was used; the unit featured an automatic feedback cut-out to prevent duct injury by laser mistargeting. In vitro success of 75% translated to 65% total or partial fragmentation in vivo. The authors cautioned against using electrohydraulic and eximer laser lithotripsy because of duct damage. Their in vitro studies showed poor stone fragmentation with the Nd:YAG and Alexandrite (Lithognost, Telemit Co, Munich, Germany) lasers.

Ottaviani and colleagues[29] in 1996 reported on using the Minilith SL-1 lithotriptor (K. Storz). Fifty-two patients with prior salivary duct dissection or obstacles to endoscopic access were treated. Acute sialadenitis patients first were treated using antibiotics until quiescent. Overall, 46% were free of stones; 31% had sand of less than 2.0 mm, and 23% had fragments larger than 2.0 mm after treatment. Seven percent needed sialadenectomy because of stones larger than 2.0 mm.

Harrison and colleagues[30] in 1997 reported on the etiologies and mechanisms of submandibular sialolithiasis formation and the histopathology, having also published on ultrastructure of microliths in 1993 with Triantalyllou.[31]

Zenk and colleagues[32] in 1998 reported on duct diameters. The mean diameters of normal ducts were 0.5 to 1.4 mm for Stensen ducts and 0.5 to 1.5 mm for Wharton's ducts. The minimum width of the ducts was at the ostium. The upper limit for instrument design was recommended to be 1.2 mm.

In 2001, Marchal and colleagues[33] found that among 48 consecutive submandibular adenectomy patients with proven stones, 10 had normal histology; 18 had intermediate alterations, and 20 glands had extensive atrophy and fibrous. The implications were that most glands are near normal except for the ductal calculus, and therefore, gland-preserving techniques should be attempted when removing the stones. Also in 2001, Marchal and colleagues expanded on Nahlieli's findings of foreign bodies as a nidus for stone formation.[21,34]

Guerrissi and Taborda[35] in 2001 reported on the first endoscopic intraoral resection of the submandibular gland on two patients. Both patients had sialolithiasis as the underlying problem. The main technical difficulty was with "the vascular pole...posterior third of gland" and the narrow confines between jaw and tongue.

Terris and colleagues[36,37] used a laparoscopic endoscope to achieve total excision of the submandibular gland in a porcine model in 2001 and on a cadaver lower neck entry in 2004. The cadaver procedure duration ranged from 50 to 150 minutes depending on experience. Balloon dissection was used to allow for a field of view through three incisions in the lower neck to accommodate the endoscope and two instruments.

In 2002, Drage and colleagues[38] investigated if the submandibular duct genu was related to sialolithiasis or adenitis. No correlation was found from 102 sialograms; there was a wide variation in the angle in unaffected normals ranging from 24° to 178°, with a mean of 103°, 108° in those with duct calculi, and 91° in those with adenitis.

Lewkowicz and colleagues[39] in 2002 reported on experiences with parotid gland and duct traumatic injuries. They formulated a decision tree. Primary closure was indicated if no leakage was seen coming from the traumatic gland and facial wound after retrograde infusion of saline into the duct. End-to-end anastomosis with an intraductal stent for 14 days was recommended if leakage occurred and both duct ends were found. If leakage occurred and only the proximal end was found, or if the laceration was extensive, then end-to-end anastomosis was recommended with an intraductal stent for 14 days; if only the proximal end was found, or if the laceration was extensive, then clamping of the remaining proximal portion was indicated with suturing. Traumatic sialocele treatment also was discussed. Although not mentioned, facial nerve considerations would need simultaneous attention.

The combined approach was reported in 2002 on 12 patients by Nahlieli and colleagues.[40] Some parotid stones may present as impossible to treat endoscopically; yet they can be seen intraductally with the endoscope. The endoscope was used intraductally as a skin transilluminator to locate the stone and was combined with a 1 cm vertical cheek skin incision over the stone. After stone removal by incising the duct, endoscopy was performed to explore the remaining duct for secondary stones. The duct was closed with 4-0 Vicryl and allowed to heal over a stent (1.7 mm polyethylene tube) for 2 weeks. Perioperative antibiotics were given, and a 48-hour compression bandage was placed over the site.

In 2002, Morimoto and colleagues[41] reported on their new magnetic resonance imaging (MRI) protocol allowing for virtual endoscopy of the salivary duct, modeled on similar virtual endoscopy protocols for the bronchial tree, colon, vascular structures, and urinary tract. An update was offered in 2004.[42] Su and colleagues[43] in 2006 compared their virtual endoscopy protocol with actual endoscopy and found clear, detailed views.

In 2003, Marchal and Dulguerov[44] forwarded their treatment algorithm. They combined submandibular and parotid gland endoscopic treatments into one decision tree. If a small stone (less than 4 mm/submandibular and 3.0 mm/parotid) was found, then wire basket extraction was recommended. If the stones were greater than 4.0 mm and 3.0 mm for the submandibular and parotid glands, respectively, then either extracorporeal shock wave lithotripsy or laser intracorporeal lithotripsy (2100 nm holmium laser) would be followed by wire basket extraction. Stenoses were corrected with metallic dilators or soft balloon catheters.

In 2004, Zenk and colleagues[45] reported a 10-year experience with extracorporeal shock wave lithotripsy for submandibular stones. Over 10 years, 191 patients were treated with the Piezolith 2500 (R. Wolf Company, Knittlingen, Germany). Stones were treated at 80 Megapascals, 3000 shock waves, and monitored by a B-mode 7.5 MHz ultrasound scanner. The shock wave treatment was followed by massage, duct bougienage, and Dormia basket extraction. Results showed that of the originally treated group, 71% had some residual asymptomatic stone material in the ducts, of which half had long-term symptoms requiring further therapy such as transoral removal of stones or adenectomy. There was an upper size limit of 12 mm for shock wave treatment. The sole prognostic criterion for certain shock wave success was being free of stones after treatment.

Katz[46] reported in 2004 on 1773 cases of sialendoscopy and extracorporeal lithotripsy. Overall, 96% of patients had elimination of stones endoscopically. In 63% of lithotriptor cases, the stones were completely destroyed, with 35% resulting in fragmentation with spontaneous or endoscopically assisted expulsion. One case required parotidectomy because of a basket wire snare that became lodged in the duct around a large stone fragment. Ultimately, 4% of endoscopic cases and 2% of lithotriptor cases required gland removal.

In 2004, McGurk and colleagues[47] reported conservative open surgical procedures of the parotid and submandibular glands. For the parotid gland, a combination endoscopic intraductal and open surgical approach was used. The intraductally situated endoscope transilluminated the cheek soft tissues at the stone site, while a preauricular incision parotid flap allowed access to the parenchyma overlying the stone. Incising directly through the Superficial Musculoaponeurotic System (SMAS) and gland overlaying the stone down to the duct, the stone could be removed. The duct with a stent in place and gland were oversewn. A pressure dressing was applied for 48 hours, and perioperative antibiotics were used. The authors also discussed selected parotid tumor removal by capsule dissection. The submandibular gland stones were removed through the floor of the mouth, in a transoral approach similar to that reported by Van den Akker and colleagues,[48] who also evaluated postoperative function in 1983.

Makdissi and colleagues[49] in 2004 evaluated submandibular gland function after intraoral calculus removal in 43 patients. Technetium pertechnetate 0.5 milliseverts was given preoperatively, and the abnormal gland was compared with its paired normal gland; 3 months postoperatively, scintigraphic examination also was performed. Stones were removed in 97% of cases. In 52% of stone removal cases, gland function was improved; 14% remained unchanged, and 34% deteriorated. Gland recovery was related inversely to size of the stone. Recently, Su[50] reported on 15 patients with technetium scintigraphy before and after stone removal by endoscopy. Compared with the preoperative status, after stone removal treatment, both the 13 submandibular and 4 affected parotid glands showed no statistically significant side-to-side difference. Nishi,[51] in 1987, and Yoshimura in 1989 also evaluated submandibular salivary gland function after sialolithectomy.[52] Also in 2004, Jongerius and colleagues[53] studied salivary flow rates. They found that salivary flow rates varied considerably between individuals, but were relatively constant within a given individual.

Nahlieli and colleagues[54] in 2004 reviewed management of chronic recurrent parotitis. Although complete adenectomy was the only cure for persistent-symptom patients, some patients had treatable findings. Of endoscopic interest were sausage-like ducts amenable to balloon dilation, strictures helped by expansion with the miniforceps, and mucous plugs removed by flushing. The balloon technique was either through the endoscope working lumen or next to the endoscope. Among the etiologies reviewed, nanobacteria were cited from another journal, although there has been no further substantiation of these. Chronic enlargement of the salivary glands also was noted to be caused by Mikulicz disease, Sjögren syndrome, recurrent childhood parotitis, and lymphoepithelial lesion of Godwin.

Nahlieli and colleagues[55] in 2004 also reviewed their treatment modality for juvenile recurrent parotitis and again in 2009 by Sracham[56] with a total of 70 children. Endoscopic findings included white appearance of the ducts without typical blood vessels. Strictures and kinks were seen in the most severe cases. Treatment consisted of preoperative sialography (Ultravist, Schering, Berlin) followed by sialendoscopy with vigorous 60 mL saline lavages. Any strictures were treated with a balloon or microdrill (0.3 mm). Finishing the case, hydrocortisone 100 mg was injected through the endoscope. Postoperative antibiotics were used. Only five patients (7.1%) needed a repeat endoscopy; nine (12.9%) had another mild episode after treatment. Also reporting on juvenile recurrent parotitis were Quenin and colleagues[57] in 2008 with a similar protocol to Nahlieli and with 10 patients. One patient (10%) needed a repeat sialendoscopy; two patients (20%) had a contralateral episode.

Qi and colleagues[58] in 2005 microscopically analyzed sialendoscopic irrigation fluid in obstructed parotid glands. Fiber-like substances, which were connected to the duct wall and floating and blocking the lumen were seen to be composed of desquamative epithelial and inflammatory cells.

Zenk and colleagues[59] in 2005 reviewed their series of intraoral submandibular stone extractions. In the 683 patients, no distinct area for stone location was noted. The stone was approached by incising from the punctum in a posterior direction. The lingual nerve was identified, and the incision continued until the stone was found. When the stone was located further into the parenchyma of the gland, a submandibulotomy external incision approach was used to assist removal. There were 98.3% symptom-free patients, although 6.9% had stone rests; 1.7% required adenectomy for symptom relief.

Capaccio and colleagues[60] in 2005 reported on 11 patients using conservative transoral stone removal for submandibular glands. The stones, ranging from 8 to 25 mm, were removed successfully. Closure of the hilum area was by a net of fibrillar surgicel (Tabotamp, Johnson & Johnson, Skipton, United Kingdom) to achieve hemostasis and antimicrobial properties and avoid risk of stricture and stenosis.

Chossegros and colleagues[61] in 2006 described entering a tight duct by first placing a guidewire, followed by threading the endoscope over the guidewire and into the duct, as a variation of standard interventional radiology procedure described as a novel technique in 1953 by Seldinger.[62]

In 2006 and earlier, Fritsch reported on his experiences with the endoscopic open approach as an extension of McGurk's work but without access to extracorporeal lithotripsy.[47,63] Further developments included Segmental gland resection of the irreversibly diseased gland drainage basin proximal to the stone; leaving postresection normally draining gland tissue for cosmesis; retrograde saline duct irrigations to locate any cross-cut duct openings in the parenchyma, allowing for oversewing to prevent sialocele; use of the NIMS facial nerve monitor; Staged techniques; and microvascular technique for duct or vein anastomoses. These were later partially reported on by Marchal.[64]

Geisthoff and colleagues[65] in 2006 reported on their using ultrasonographic visualization of the duct in sialolithiasis cases. Sialendoscopic instrumentation with the 0.8 mm endoscopic microforceps may not be effective for stone fragmentation because of the fragile nature of the forceps. In their new technique, using an ear surgery alligator forceps, the relatively robust nature of the forceps was able to efficiently crush the stones and also retrieve the fragments all under real-time ultrasonographic observation without any need of an endoscope.

The issue of I-131 parotiditis continues to be a problem for patients. In 2007, Kim and colleagues[66] outlined their treatment for I-131 sialadenitis in 21 patients and reviewed the pertinent literature. The parotid gland was involved 90% of the time. Symptoms began about 5 months after administration of I-131 and appeared to be dose-related. For 70% of cases, conservative therapy using a regime of aggressive massage, sialogogues, steroids, antibiotics, nonsteroidal anti-inflammatory drugs, vitamin B12, zinc, and pilocarpine was successful. For the remainder, a 50% success rate was achieved by sialendoscopy. The major problem encountered was stenosis, and it was treated by dilation with various diameter endoscopes or with balloons. Unsuccessful cases ended in resection of the involved gland. Another protocol, forwarded by Silberstein[67] in 2008, is conservative but is started before the I-131 administration. Despite the article title, pilocarpine resulted in no additional protection compared with his routine and effective regime incorporating dexamethasone, dolsetron, 2400 mL nondairy fluids, and sialogogues starting before I-131. There were 60 patients in his study with reference to 109 prior cases using the same treatment. His overall strategy was to quickly remove any I-131 accumulated in the gland by expectoration so that it did not linger. The regime continued for both daytime and nights. Remarkable results were achieved in this series, with sialadenitis present in only 3% to 7% of patients. Lastly, amifostine has been used successfully, although unremitting nausea in people is a frequent reason for noncompliance. There is also concern regarding suppression of radiation effects in the target tissue.[68]

In 2007, Nakayama and colleagues[69] described their experiences with an intracorporeal electrohydraulic lithotripsy system through an endoscope (Salivascope T PD-ZS-2002, 1.35 mm O.D. Polydiagnost, Pfaffenhofen, Germany). Acrinol (ethacrine lactate) was instilled into the duct as an antimicrobial at the end of the procedure, with no dosage given. Previously, Iro in 1989 and Konigsberger in 1993 had experiences with electrohydraulic extracorporeal and intracorporeal lithotripsy, respectively.[7,13]

Nahlieli and colleagues[70] in 2007 reported on the ductal stretching technique. The endoscope is introduced first to locate the stone, followed by a lacrimal probe. The duct is dissected and isolated; the gland and stone are pushed from below to herniate the stone forward. Incision of the duct follows with lithectomy, then reattachment of the anterior duct to the mouth floor, having excised the anterior 5 mm of duct. The stretching appears to mean straightening of the duct to allow the stone to slip past the obstacle of the lingual nerve before incision and extraction from a more anterior location.

In 2008, Walvekar and colleagues[71] reported on their initial 56-case experience and complications. Major complications occurred in one case with avulsion of the duct, and minor complications occurred in 13 patients. The minor complications were mainly attributable to stenotic duct segments, duct bends, and a narrow papilla opening that gave rise to retained stones, duct tears, mucosal necrosis, and failure of the procedure. Salvage of the problems was by applying standard salivary surgery. An observation was that despite its apparent simplicity, sialendoscopy is technically challenging and requires sequential learning. Overall, sialendoscopy was judged to be a safe and effective diagnostic and treatment modality.

Nahlieli and colleagues[72] in 2008 reviewed their experiences with Stensen's duct injuries caused by facial rejuvenation cosmetic procedures. Fourteen patients were treated by sialendoscopy. Four groups of injuries with four corresponding specific treatment types were given. Type 1 was comprised of compression of the duct caused by SMAS tightening. In type 2 injuries, a laceration to the gland caused swelling that resulted in duct compression. Both types 1 and 2 were treated conservatively. Type 3 had both a compression of the duct by SMAS fascia tightening over the masseter and edema associated with gland laceration. Type 3 was treated by sialendoscopic drainage of the duct sialocele with a facial compression garment applied until facial swelling resolved. Type 4 was a complete cut of the Stensen's duct. It was treated by sialendoscopy to find the proximal duct end through the sialocele and also the distal duct end, followed by high-pressure balloon dilation of the distal duct, an endoscopic anastomosis by a sialodrain stent inserted for 4 weeks into the entire duct to allow healing. Any sialocele was aspirated and a compression garment placed. No external ancillary incisions were used, only the stent to connect the two duct ends. In Type 4 injury repair, two of five patients had no function after 6 weeks. One of five patients for type 3 had no function; the rest had function.

Luers and colleagues[73] in 2008 reported on a methylene blue dye swab technique of the papilla to find a nonapparent punctum. If not immediately visible, pressure on the gland could release a microdrop of saliva through the blue dye and mark the spot of the punctum.

In 2008, Fritsch reported on reported on decibel levels generated during extracorporeal shock wave lithotripsy with an 80 dB peak found. Because of the acoustic stress of shock waves administered by the thousands, hearing protection was thought advisable.[74] Also in 2008, he reported on using a sponge and flesh-colored plastic tubing model as a reliable dry laboratory approach to teaching sialendoscopy; other wet laboratory animal and human cadaver models were deemed expensive and time-consuming to use.[75]

Woo and colleagues[76] in 2009 described their experiences with long-term intraoral submandibular stone removal in 14 children versus 40 adults. Although sialolithiasis is uncommon in children, a similar technique was used as in adults, with both groups having an 83% symptom-free long-term result.

Iro and colleagues[77] in 2009 reported on a comprehensive five-group multi-institutional experience of 4691 patients regarding all diagnostic and therapeutic aspects of salivary calculi over a 14-year period. It is the most extensive clinical review to date. Submandibular stones outnumbered parotid stones by a three to one ratio. Acute sialadenitis was treated with antibiotics. Extensive algorithms were shown. Extracorporeal shock wave lithotripsy was curative in 51% of patients, partially successful in 25%, and needed repeat extracorporeal shock wave lithotripsy treatment in 23%. Further follow-up treatments included endoscopy, intraoral surgery, and gland removal. For endoscopic basket microforceps retrieval, a 92% success rate was reported. Intraoral submandibular surgery was curative in 93% of cases.

SUMMARY

Much can be learned by reviewing the earlier salivary research and clinical experiences from the last 25 years. These research efforts have advanced diagnostic and treatment possibilities and allowed for ever more physiologic and gland conservation approaches and results. This brief outline of the literature cannot fully discuss all of the contributions to salivary endoscopy and salivary lithotripsy made by many hardworking and talented individuals. By reading the cited author's journal articles, a bud of knowledge is provided that can blossom by reading the article references. The clinical problems that one encounters on a daily basis are made more understandable, and the patients seen every day will benefit from the practitioner's familiarity with the prior sialendoscopy and lithotripsy literature.

ACKNOWLEDGMENTS

The author wishes to thank Ms. Rebecca Colson, administrative assistant, for her help in preparing this manuscript.

REFERENCES

1. Mandel L, Baurmash H. Radiopaque contrast solutions for sialography. J Oral Ther Pharmacol 1965;2:73–80.
2. Yamamoto H, Sakae T, Takagi M, et al. Scanning electron microscopic and x-ray microdiffractometeric studies on sialolith crystals in human submandibular glands. Acta Pathol Jpn 1984;34:47–53.
3. Riesco JM, Juanes JA, Diaz-Gonzalez MP, et al. Crystalloid architecture of a sialolith in a minor salivary gland. J Oral Pathol Med 1999;28:451–5.
4. Galili D, Marmary Y. Juvenile recurrent parotitis: clinicoradiological follow-up study and the beneficial effect of sialography. Oral Surg Oral Med Oral Pathol 1986;61:550–6.
5. Marmary Y. A novel and non-invasive method for the removal of salivary gland stones. Int J Oral Maxillofac Surg 1986;15:585–7.
6. Brouns JJ, Hendrikx AJ, Bierkens AF. Removal of salivary stones with the aid of a lithotripter. J Craniomaxillofac Surg 1989;17:329–30.
7. Iro H, Nitsche N, Schneider HT, et al. Extracorporeal shockwave lithotripsy of salivary gland stones. Lancet 1989;2:115.
8. Iro H, Schneider T, Nitsche N, et al. Extrakorpale piezoelectrische Lithotripsie von Speichelsteinen: erste klinische erfahrungen. HNO 1990;38:251–5 [in German].
9. Briffa NP, Callum KG. Use of an embolectomy catheter to remove a submandibular duct stone. Br J Surg 1989;76:814.
10. Sterenborg H, Van den Akker H, Van der Meulen C, et al. Laserlithotripsy of salivary stones: a comparison between the pulsed dye laser and HO-YSGG laser. J Med Sci 1990;5:357–62.
11. Grundlach P, Scherer H, Hopf J, et al. Die endoscopisch kontrollierte Laserlithotripsie von Speichelsteinen. HNO 1990;38:247–50 [in German].
12. Konigsberger R, Feyh J, Goetz A, et al. Die endosscopisch kontrollierte Laserlithotripsie zur Behandlung der Sialolithiasis. Laryngorhinootologie 1990;69: 322–3 [in German].
13. Konigsberger R, Feyh J, Goetz A, et al. Endoscopically controlled electrohydraulic intracorporeal shock wave lithotripsy (EISL) of salivary stones. J Otolaryngol 1993;22:12–3.
14. Katz PH. Un nouveau mode d' exploration des glandes salivaries: la fibroscopie. Inf Dent 1990;8:785–6 [in French].
15. Katz PH. Endoscopie des glands salivaries. Ann Radiol (Paris) 1991;34:110–3 [in French].
16. Kater W, Meyer WW, Rachel U, et al. Lithotripsy of salivary calculi as a non-invasive treatment alternative to surgical removal of calculi. Biomed Tech (Berl) 1990; 35:239–40.
17. Kater W. Die fortentwicklung des extrakorporalen stosswellen Lithotripsie von Speichelsteinen mit dem Minilith. Presented at 65 jahresversammlung desdeutschen Gesellschaff fur orl heilkunde Kopf and Halschirugie. Chemnitz (Germany), May, 1994 [in German].

18. Buckenham TM, Page JE, Jeddy T. Technical report: interventional sialography balloon dilation of a stenosis duct stricture using digital subfraction sialography. Clin Radiol 1991;45:34.
19. Katz PH. Traitement endoscopique des lithiasis salivares. J Otorhinolaryngol 1993;42:33–6 [in French].
20. Nahlieli O, Neder A, Baruchin AM. Salivary gland endoscopy: a new technique for diagnosis and treatment of sialolithiasis. J Oral Maxillofac Surg 1994;52:1240–2.
21. Nahlieli O, Baruchin AM. Sialoendoscopy: three years experience as a diagnostic and treatment modality. J Oral Maxillofac Surg 1997;55:912–8.
22. Nahlieli O, Baruchin AM. Endoscopic technique for the diagnosis and treatment of obstructive salivary gland diseases. J Oral Maxillofac Surg 1999;57:1394–401.
23. Nahlieli O, Eliav E, Hasson O, et al. Pediatric sialolithiasis. Oral Surg Oral Med Oral Pathol Oral Radiol Endod 2000;90:709–12.
24. Nahlieli O, Baruchin AM. Long-term experience with endoscopic diagnosis and treatment of salivary gland inflammatory diseases. Laryngoscope 2000;110:988–93.
25. Nahlieli O, Shacham R, Yoffe B, et al. Diagnosis and treatment of strictures and kinks in salivary gland ducts. J Oral Maxillofac Surg 2001;59:484–90.
26. Arzoz E, Santiago A, Garatea J, et al. Removal of a stone in Stensen's duct with endoscopic laser lithotripsy: report of a case. J Oral Maxillofac Surg 1994;52:1329–30.
27. Arzoz E, Santiago A, Esnal F, et al. Endoscopic intracorporeal lithotripsy for sialolithiasis. J Oral Maxillofac Surg 1996;54:847–50.
28. Iro H, Zenk J, Benzel W. Laser lithotripsy of salivary duct stones. Adv Otorhinolaryngol 1995;49:148–52.
29. Ottaviani F, Capaccio P, Campi M, et al. Extracorporeal electromagnetic shockwave lithotripsy for salivary gland stones. Laryngoscope 1996;106:761–4.
30. Harrison JD, Epivatianos A, Bhatia SN. Role of microliths in the aetiology of chronic submandibular sialadenitis: a clinicopathological investigation of 154 cases. Histopathology 1997;31:237–51.
31. Triantalyllon A, Harrison JD, Garrett JR. Analytical ultrastructure investigation of microliths in salivary glands of cat. Hist Jahrb 1993;25:183–90.
32. Zenk J, Zikarsky B, Hosemann WG, et al. The diameter of the Stensen's and Wharton ducts. Significance for diagnosis and therapy. HNO 1998;46:980–5.
33. Marchal F, Kurt A, Dulgerov P, et al. Histopathology of submandibular glands removed for sialolithiasis. Ann Otol Rhinol Laryngol 2001;110:464–9.
34. Marchal F, Kurta AM, Dulgerov P, et al. Retrograde theory in sialolithiasis formation. Arch Otolaryngol Head Neck Surg 2001;127:66–8.
35. Guerrissi JO, Taborda G. Endoscopic excision of the submandibular gland by an intraoral approach. J Craniofac Surg 2001;12:299–303.
36. Terris DJ, MonFared A, Thomas A, et al. Endoscopic resection of the submandibular gland in a porcine model. Laryngoscope 2001;112:1089–93.
37. Terris DJ, Haus BM, Gourin CG. Endoscopic neck surgery: resection of the submanidbular gland in a cadaver model. Laryngoscope 2004;114:407–10.
38. Drage NA, Wilson RF, McGurk M. The genu of the submandibular duct—is the angle significant in salivary gland disease? Dentomaxillofac Radiol 2002;31:15–8.
39. Lewkowicz AA, Hasson O, Nahlieli O. Traumatic injuries to the parotid gland and duct. J Oral Maxillofac Surg 2002;60:676–80.
40. Nahlieli O, London D, Zagury A, et al. Combined approach to impacted parotid stones. J Oral Maxillofac Surg 2002;60:1418–23.
41. Morimoto Y, Tanaka T, Yoshioka I, et al. Virtual endoscopic view of salivary gland duct using magnetic resonance sialography data from three-dimension fast

asymmetric spin echo (3D-FASE) sequences: a preliminary study. Oral Dis 2002; 8:268–72.
42. Morimoto Y, Tanaka T, Tominaga K, et al. Clinical application of magnetic resonance sialogtraphic 3-dimensional reconstruction imaging and magnetic resonance virtual endoscopy for salivary gland duct analysis. J Oral Maxillofac Surg 2004;62:1237–45.
43. Su YX, Liao GQ, Kang Z, et al. Application of magnetic resonance virtual endoscopy as a presurgical procedure before sialendoscopy. Laryngoscope 2006;116:1899–906.
44. Marchal D, Dulgerov P. Sialolithiasis management. Arch Otolaryngol Head Neck Surg 2003;129:951–6.
45. Zenk J, Bozzato A, Winter M, et al. Extracorporeal shockwave lithotripsy of submandibular stones: evaluation after 10 years. Ann Otol Rhinol Laryngol 2004;113:378–83.
46. Katz P. New techniques for the treatment of salivary lithiasis: sialendoscopy and extracorporeal lithotripsy: 1773 cases. Ann Otolaryngol Chir Cervicofac 2004; 121:123–32.
47. McGurk M, MacBean A, Ian KF, et al. Conservative management of salivary stones and benign parotid tumours: a description of the surgical techniques involved. Ann R Australas Coll Dent Surg 2004;17:14–44.
48. van den Akker HP, Busemann-Sokole E. Submandibular gland function following transoral sialolithectomy. Oral Surg Oral Med Oral Pathol 1983;56:351–6.
49. Makdissi J, Escudier MP, Brown JE, et al. Glandular function after intraoval removal of salivary calculi from the hilum of the submandibular gland. Br J Oral Maxillofac Surg 2004;42:538–41.
50. Su YX, Xu JH, Liao GQ, et al. Salivary gland functional recovery after sialendoscopy. Laryngoscope 2009;119:646–52.
51. Nishi M, Mimura T, Marutani K, et al. Evaluation of submandibular gland function by sialo-scintigraphy following sialolithectomy. J Oral Maxillofac Surg 1987;45:567–71.
52. Yoshimura Y, Morishita T, Sugihara T. Salivary gland function after sialolithiasis: scintigraphic examination of submandibular glands with 99m Tc-pertechnetate. J Oral Maxillofac Surg 1989;47:704–10.
53. Jongerius PH, Limbeek JV, Rotleveel JJ. Assessment of salivary flow rate: biologic variation and measure error. Laryngoscope 2004;114:1801–4.
54. Nahlieli O, Bar T, Shacham R, et al. Management of chronic recurrent parotitis: current therapy. J Oral Maxillofac Surg 2004;62:1150–5.
55. Nahlieli O, Shachem R, Shlesinger M, et al. Juvenile recurrent parotitis: a new method of diagnosis and treatment. Pediatrics 2004;114:9–12.
56. Shacham R, Droma EB, London D, et al. Long-term experience with endoscopic diagnosis and treatment of juvenile recurrent parotitis. J Oral Maxillofac Surg 2009;67:162–7.
57. Quenin S, Plou-Gaudon I, Marchal P, et al. Juvenile recurrent parotitis: sialendoscopic approach. Arch Otolaryngol Head Neck Surg 2008;134:715–9.
58. Qi S, Liu X, Wang S. Sialoendsocopic and irrigation findings in chronic obstructive parotitis. Laryngoscope 2005;115:541–5.
59. Zenk J, Gottwald F, Bozzato A, et al. Submandibular sialoliths. Stone removal with organ preservation. HNO 2005;53:243–9.
60. Capaccio P, Bottero A, Pompilio M, et al. Conservative transoral removal of hilar submandibular salivary calculi. Laryngoscope 2005;115:750–2.
61. Chossegros C, Guyot L, Richard O, et al. A technical improvement in sialendoscopy to enter the salivary ducts. Laryngoscope 2006;116:842–4.

62. Seldinger SI. Catheter replacement of the needle in percutaneous arteriography; a new technique. Acta Radiol 1953;39:368–76.
63. Fritsch MH. Sialo-endoscopic intervention for salivary duct obstructions: additional strategies for difficult and staged cases. Presented at the AAO-HNS National meeting 2004–2008 courses; Triological Society, COSM, Chicago, Ill, April 2006; 1st North American Meeting on Sialendoscopy and Lithotripsy. Indianapolis, June, 2006.
64. Marchal P. A combined endoscopic and external approach for extraction of large stones with preservation of parotid and submandibular glands. Laryngoscope 2007;117:373–7.
65. Geisthoff UW, Lehnert BK, Verse T. Ultrasound-guided mechanical intraductal stone fragmentation and removal for sialolithiasis: a new technique. Surg Endosc 2006;20:690–4.
66. Kim JW, Han GS, Lee SH, et al. Sialendoscopic treatment for radioiodine induced sialadenitis. Laryngoscope 2007;117:133–6.
67. Silberstein EB. Reducing the incidence of I-131 induced sialadenitis: the role of pilocarpine. J Nucl Med 2008;49:546–9.
68. Bohuslavizki KH, Klutmann S, Brenner W, et al. Salivary gland protection by amifostine in high-dose radioiodine treatment: results of a double-blind placebo-controlled study. J Clin Oncol 1998;16:3542–9.
69. Nakayama E, Okamura K, Mitsuyasu T, et al. A newly developed interventional sialendoscope for a completely nonsurgical sialolithectomy using intracorporeal electrohydraulic lithotripsy. J Oral Maxillofac Surg 2007;65:1402–5.
70. Nahlieli O, Shacham R, Zagury A, et al. The ductal stretching technique: an endoscopic-assisted technique for removal of submandibular stones. Laryngoscope 2007;117:1031–5.
71. Walvekar RR, Razfar A, Carrau RL, et al. Sialendoscopy and associated complications: a preliminary experience. Laryngoscope 2008;118:776–9.
72. Nahlieli O, Abramson A, Shacham R, et al. Endoscopic treatment of salivary gland injuries due to facial rejuvenation procedures. Laryngoscope 2008;118:763–7.
73. Luers JC, Vent J, Beutner D. Methylene blue for easy and safe detection of salivary duct papilla in sialendoscopy. Otolaryngol Head Neck Surg 2008;139:466–7.
74. Fritsch MH. Decibel levels during extracorporeal lithotripsy for salivary stones. J Laryngol Otol 2008;10:1–4.
75. Fritsch MH. A new sialendoscopy teaching model of the duct and gland. J Oral Maxillofac Surg 2008;66:2409–11.
76. Woo SH, Jang JY, Park GY, et al. Long-term outcomes of intraoral submandibular stone removal in children as compared with adults. Laryngoscope 2008;119:116–20.
77. Iro H, Zenk J, Escudier MP, et al. Outcome of minimally invasive management of salivary calculi in 4691 patients. Laryngoscope 2009;119:263–8.

Causes, Natural History, and Incidence of Salivary Stones and Obstructions

John D. Harrison, PhD, FDSRCSEng, FRCPath[a,*]

KEYWORDS

- Salivary gland disease • Sialolithiasis • Calculi
- Sialadenitis • Küttner's tumor • Calcification

HISTORICAL REVIEW

A brief historical review, which begins with Küttner in the late nineteenth century and finishes with research in progress, is necessary to appreciate current understanding. A detailed historical review has been presented elsewhere.[1]

Clinical Investigations

Küttner[2] in 1896 published the results of his microscopic examinations of two patients' chronically swollen submandibular glands that attracted a clinical diagnosis of malignancy. He realized that the swelling was caused by chronic inflammation that, together with fibrosis, led to a clinical appearance of malignancy. He found a sialolith the size of a cherrystone associated with the gland in one of the patients, who had complained of a submandibular swelling for 10 years. He considered the sialolith secondary to the inflammation because the sialolith was far too small for a concretion of 10 years' accumulation and because of the absence of a sialolith in the other case, in which the duration was only 1.5 months. Küttner was of the opinion that chronic sialadenitis is primary and arises by inflammation that ascends Wharton's duct from the mouth. He considered three ways in which a sialolith could form: inflammation may roughen the lining of ducts and precipation occurs on this; inflammation may compress the intraglandular collecting ducts of lobules and precipitation occurs in the obstructed lobules; and precipitation may occur in bacterial deposits.

Küttner's seminal publication in 1896 established chronic obstructive sialadenitis as an entity, which became known in continental Europe as Küttner's tumor. Küttner's subsequent practice and research confirmed his opinion that sialoliths are secondary to sialadenitis (see his *Handbuch der Praktischen Chirurgie*, 1926)[3,4]

[a] Department of Oral Pathology, King's College London Dental Institute at Guy's, King's College and St Thomas' Hospitals, London, SE1 9RT, UK
* Department of Oral Pathology, Floor 28, Guy's Tower, Guy's Hospital, London, SE1 9RT, UK
E-mail address: john.harrison@kcl.ac.uk

Otolaryngol Clin N Am 42 (2009) 927–947
doi:10.1016/j.otc.2009.08.012 oto.theclinics.com
0030-6665/09/$ – see front matter

(**Fig. 1**). Rauch, in his monograph, *Die Speicheldrüsen des Menschen*, in 1959, considered Küttner's tumor a mycosis and did not mention Küttner's opinion about sialoliths. Instead, he described various other theories to explain the production of sialoliths.[5,6]

Küttner's work, however, was developed by Seifert and Donath in their 1977 clinicopathologic investigation of chronic submandibular sialadenitis.[7] They divided it into progressive stages that ranged from focal sialadenitis to severe chronic sialadenitis with fibrosis. The first stage occurs when sialomicroliths cause obstruction of small intraglandular ducts, followed by an inflammatory reaction. In the subsequent stages, there is increasing atrophy, fibrosis, and inflammation. The decreased secretory activity of glandular atrophy facilitates ascending invasion by microbes that sustain the inflammation, thus creating a vicious circle.

A major problem of the classification into histologic stages is that the overall microscopic appearance is graded, although there can be great variation between the different features that make up this appearance, even within different parts of the same gland. Harrison and colleagues analyzed this problem by investigating 154 cases of chronic submandibular sialadenitis and statistically reviewing 18 different clinical and histologic features.[8]

This investigation found that sialoliths, atrophy, fibrosis, and other histologic features are all related to inflammation. Inflammation is of the greatest importance in the progression of sialadenitis and the development of sialoliths. Inflammation, atrophy, fibrosis, and sialoliths are all related to the duration of symptoms, which supports Seifert and Donath's concept of a chronologic progression through increasingly severe histologic stages with secondary production of sialoliths.

Previous investigations of chronic submandibular sialadenitis, however, did not reveal the etiologic factors that could transform a normal gland into a diseased gland.

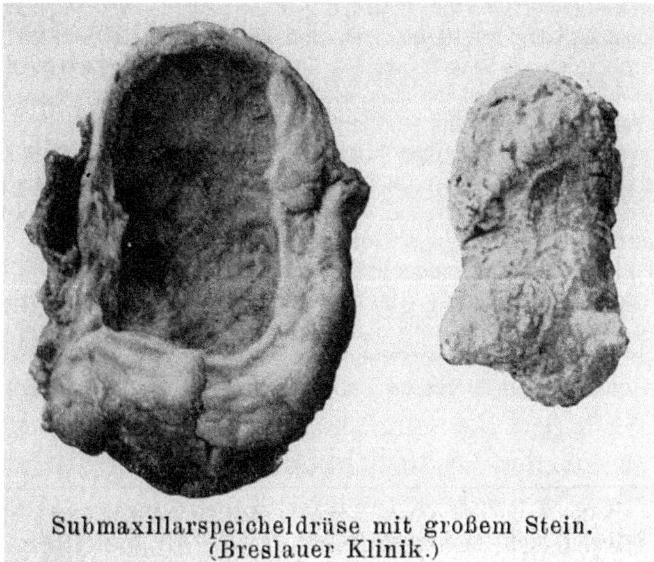

Submaxillarspeicheldrüse mit großem Stein.
(Breslauer Klinik.)

Fig. 1. Submandibular gland with a large sialolith to the right that fits into the cavity in the gland. (*From* Küttner H. Speichelsteine. In: Garrè C, Küttner H, Lexer E, editors. Handbuch der Praktischen Chirurgie. Vol. 1. Chirurgie des Kopfes. 6th edition. Stuttgart: Ferdinand Enke; 1926:929–35 [Fig. 357])

The 1970s, observations by Scott[9,10] that sialomicroliths and foci of obstructive sialadenitis occur in normal submandibular glands were what eventually led Harrison and colleagues to find this missing link. A postmortem investigation found sialomicroliths in all normal submandibular glands and in a minority of normal parotids[11] (**Fig. 2**). These findings correspond to a higher concentration of calcium in the submandibular gland.[12] Calcium is sequestered in secretory granules, where it is present as a cationic shield that allows the condensation of acidic secretory glycoprotein[13] (**Fig. 3**). The level of calcium can be far higher than in the serum and corresponds to the acidity of the glycoprotein in the secretory granules, which is greater in the submandibular gland.

Harrison and colleagues investigated the hypothesis that sialomicroliths impact in ducts and accrete to form sialoliths. A search for sialomicroliths in cases of chronic submandibular sialadenitis was successful[14] (**Figs 4** and **5**). Although this success supported the hypothesis, Harrison and colleagues were unable to find any relation between sialomicroliths and sialoliths or between sialomicroliths and duration of symptoms in chronic submandibular sialadenitis.[8] This was a surprise and did not support the hypothesis that sialomicroliths are inchoate sialoliths.

The mystery was solved only after experimental investigations.

Experimental Investigations

Animal experiments led to major breakthroughs in understanding the origins and pathogenesis of sialadenitis and sialolithiasis and much of this work relates to sialomicrolith formation.

The earliest model for the investigation of the origins and pathogenesis of sialadenitis and sialolithiasis was the salivary glands of rat. Sialomicroliths and obstructive sialadenitis were produced in the submandibular and parotid glands of rats made hypercalcemic and given repeated high doses of isoprenaline.[15] Isoprenaline given

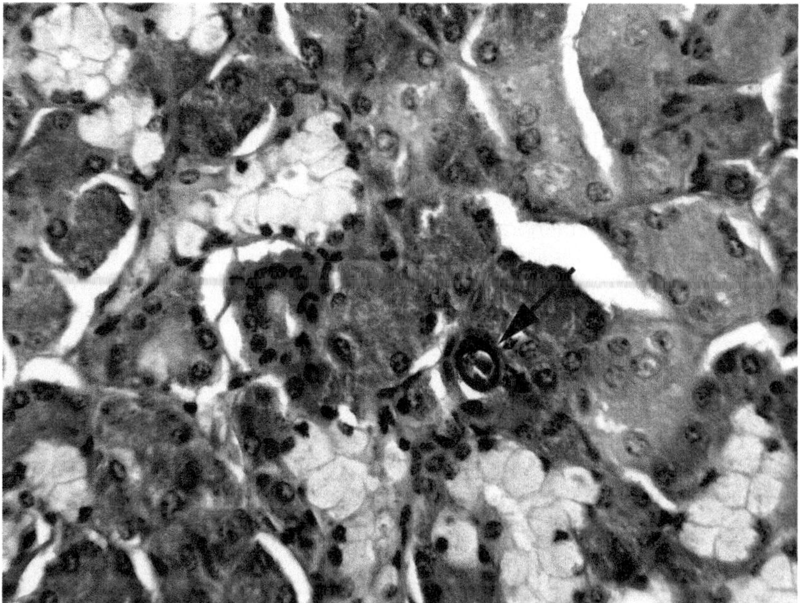

Fig. 2. Arrow points to a sialomicrolith in a serious acinus. Normal submandibular gland (section stained with hematoxylin-eosin, magnification ×390).

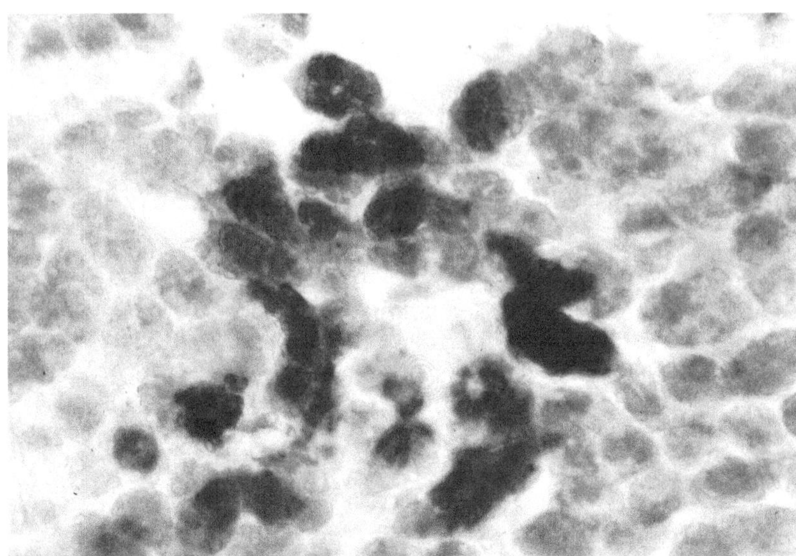

Fig. 3. The orange stain indicates the ionized and ionizable calcium present in secretory granules. The strongly stained structures are mucous acinar cells and the moderately stained structures are serous acinar cells. Normal submandibular gland (section stained by Schäfer's modification of the histochemical technique using glyoxal bis[2-hydroxyanil] for the demonstration of ionized and ionizable calcium as described by Harrison and colleagues,[12] magnification ×304).

in repeated high doses soon produces a great increase in the size and weight of the submandibular and parotid glands of rats as a result of hyperplasia and hypertrophy of the acinar cells. The acinar enlargement is sufficient to result in compression of the intraglandular ducts. Every dose of isoprenaline is followed by an explosive release of secretory material from the acinar cells, which is unable to flow freely through the lumina of the compressed ducts, and the resultant increase of luminal pressure damages acinar cells. The partial obstruction thus results in a mixture of stagnant secretory material, which is particularly rich in calcium because of the hypercalcemia, and cellular debris. An important component of the cellular debris appertaining to calcification is damaged membranes. Cellular membranes contain phospholipid that becomes exposed when they are damaged. This exposed phospholipid is the potent nucleator of calcification.[16–19] The combination of stagnant calcium-rich secretory material together with phospholipid allows the calcium to precipitate on the phospholipid to form sialomicroliths. This occurs in the small intraglandular ducts and gives rise to obstructive sialadenitis (**Fig. 6**).

Harrison and colleagues found the salivary glands of cat to be a better experimental model than those of rat for the investigation of the origins and pathogenesis of sialadenitis and sialolithiasis, and investigations included ductal ligation, stimulation of the parasympathetic and sympathetic nerves, parasympathectomy, and sympathectomy.[20–28] Sialomicroliths were detected in 1 out of 75 normal parotids, 9 out of 93 normal submandibular glands, and 17 out of 63 normal sublingual glands (**Fig. 7**). A greatly increased occurrence of sialomicroliths in submandibular glands that had been parasympathectomized, in which sialomicroliths were found in 31 out of 41 glands, led to the pivotal realization that the lack of parasympathetic secretory stimulation had caused the pathologic accumulation of sialomicroliths[21,26] (**Fig. 8**).

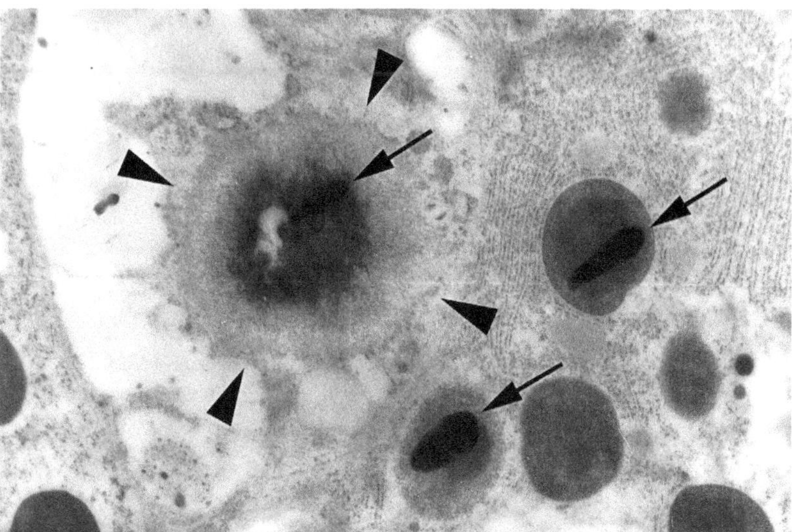

Fig. 4. Transmission electron micrograph shows a sialomicrolith in an autophagosome (*arrowheads*) in a serous acinar cell. The sialomicrolith consists of fine needle-shaped crystals that are concentrated centrally and are finely dispersed in surrounding granular material. The three arrows point to three burn marks caused by energy-dispersive x-ray microanalysis (**Fig. 5**) of the sialomicrolith and two adjacent secretory granules. Chronic submandibular sialadenitis without sialolithiasis; tissue retrieved from routine formaldehyde fixative, immersion-fixed in glutaraldehyde and formaldehyde and subsequently in osmium tetroxide (section stained with uranyl acetate and lead citrate, magnification ×19,700).

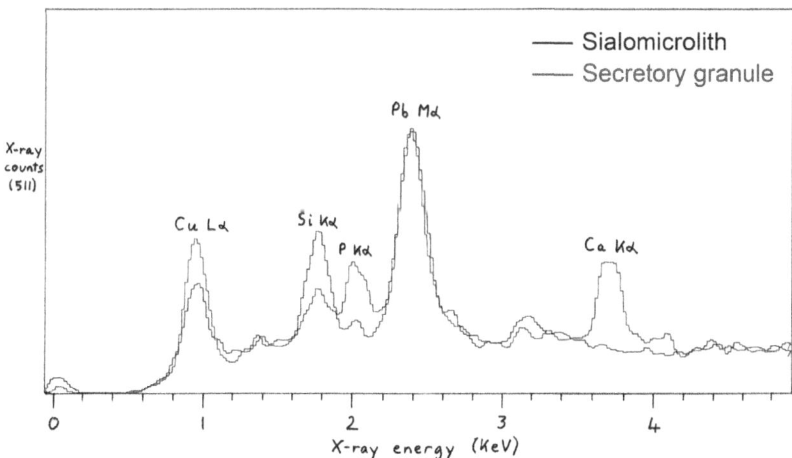

Fig. 5. Electron-microscopic microanalysis of the sialomicrolith and one of the secretory granules of **Fig. 4**. Comparison of the energy-dispersive x-ray spectra shows that there are peaks for calcium and phosphorus in the sialomicrolith. These elements are present in the needle-shaped crystals, which are hydroxyapatite. The peaks for copper, silicon, and lead in both spectra are artifacts introduced by the system and the stain.

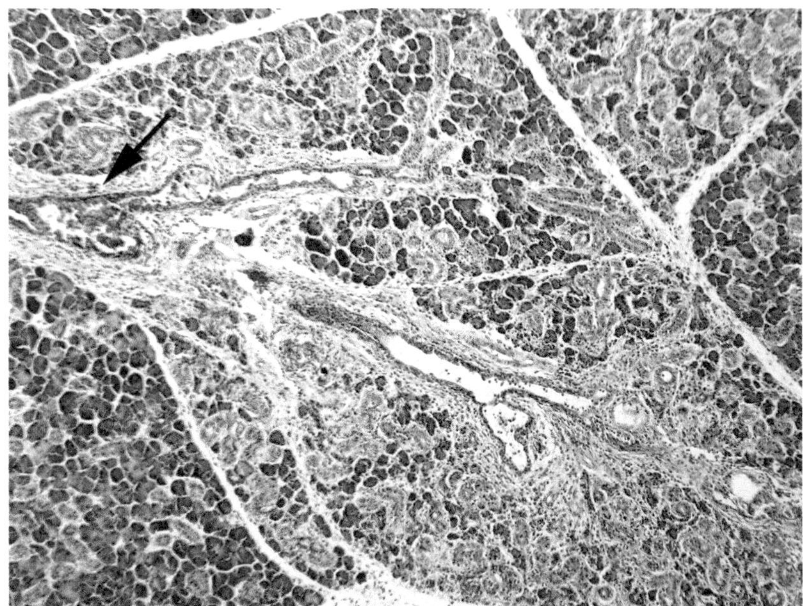

Fig. 6. Arrow points to a sialomicrolith impacted in a collecting duct causing obstructive atrophy and inflammation of the lower right lobule. Sialomicroliths are also present in the lumina of other ducts. The lower left lobule is unaffected and is of normal appearance. Submandibular gland of a rat given isoprenaline and calcium gluconate as described by Harrison and Epivatianos[15] (section stained with hematoxylin-eosin, magnification ×62).

The acinar secretory granules of the submandibular gland of cat contain a high level of sequestered calcium associated with acidic glycoprotein.[27] The sequestered calcium is released in an ionized form during the normal release of glycoprotein from secretory granules or during the degradation of secretory granules in autophagosomes when there is secretory inactivity, such as that caused by parasympathectomy. The phospholipid of degraded cellular membranes becomes exposed and the ionized calcium precipitates on the phospholipid to form calcified sialomicroliths (see **Fig. 7**). The cell thereby is saved from toxic death owing to an overwhelming release of ionized calcium. Sialomicroliths may be expelled from the cells and pass into the lumina. There they may also be formed in stagnant secretory material (see **Fig. 8**). Luminal sialomicroliths may be flushed away in the saliva, although if they impact in a small intraglandular duct, a focus of obstructive atrophy may be produced. This is more likely when a pathologic accumulation of sialomicroliths occurs, such as when there is secretory inactivity. Sialomicroliths are also removed by macrophages, which helps prevent an accumulation under normal conditions.

The contrast between the accumulation of sialomicroliths in the parasympathectomized submandibular glands and the lack of accumulation in the parotids relates to the impossibility of making an adequate parasympathectomy in the parotid and to the low level of sequestered calcium in the secretory granules of this gland. Although the secretory granules of the sublingual gland contain a high level of sequestered calcium, this gland secretes spontaneously in the absence of nervous stimulation, and this spontaneous secretion is sufficient to prevent an accumulation of sialomicroliths after parasympathectomy.

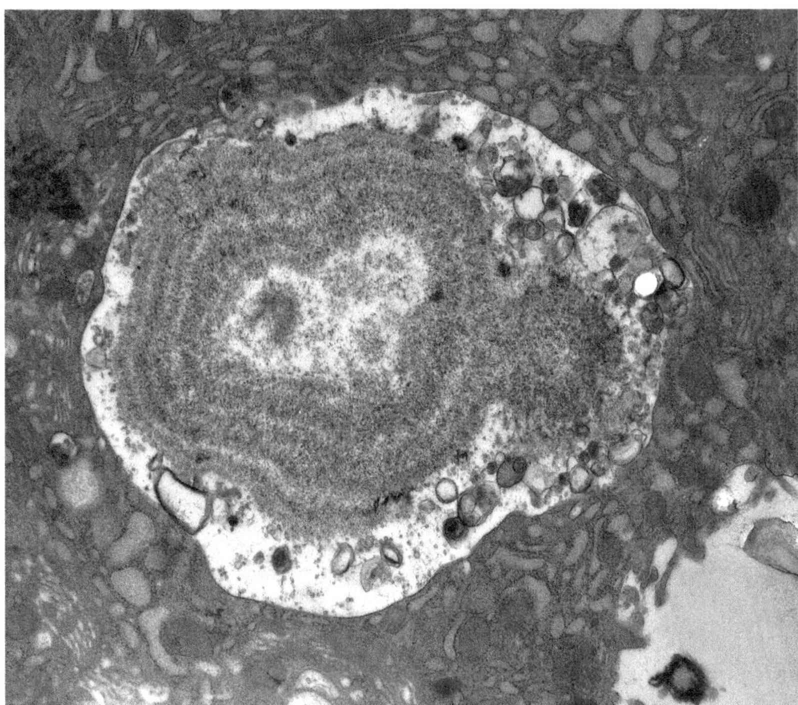

Fig. 7. Transmission electron micrograph in which an autophagosome in an acinar cell contains a lamellar sialomicrolith consisting of fine needle-shaped crystals and granular material surrounded by membraneous debris. The autophagosome is close to the lumen, part of which is present in the lower right corner. Sublingual gland of cat; tissue immersion fixed in glutaraldehyde and formaldehyde and subsequently in osmium tetroxide (section stained with uranyl acetate and lead citrate, magnification ×11,890).

Another model, established by Triantafyllou and colleagues,[29–32] is the parotid of ferret, which frequently contains sialomicroliths and in which the association between secretory inactivity and sialomicrolithiasis has been confirmed. Secretory inactivity and stagnation and autophagy of calcium-rich secretory material were found to lead to the production of sialomicroliths, which were seen obstructing small intraglandular ducts.

Experimental investigations have also yielded information on obstructive atrophy and recovery. Investigations of ductal ligation have shown that: the parotid is the most susceptible to obstruction, with progressive atrophy; the submandibular gland is more resistant, with variable atrophy; the sublingual gland is the most resistant, with not only variable atrophy but also extravasation of mucus that sometimes forms an extravasation mucocele; the parenchyma of obstructed glands can adapt and survive; and obstructed glands are capable of recovery, which depends on the duration and degree of obstruction.[33–40] Complete obstruction, however, does not lead to an accumulation of sialomicroliths or produce sialoliths.[25]

CAUSES AND NATURAL HISTORY OF CHRONIC OBSTRUCTIVE SIALADENITIS AND SIALOLITHIASIS

Obstruction Primarily Caused by Inflammation

Secretory inactivity in a normal gland leads to an accumulation of sialomicroliths and ascent of the main duct by microbes. Impaction of a sialomicrolith in a small

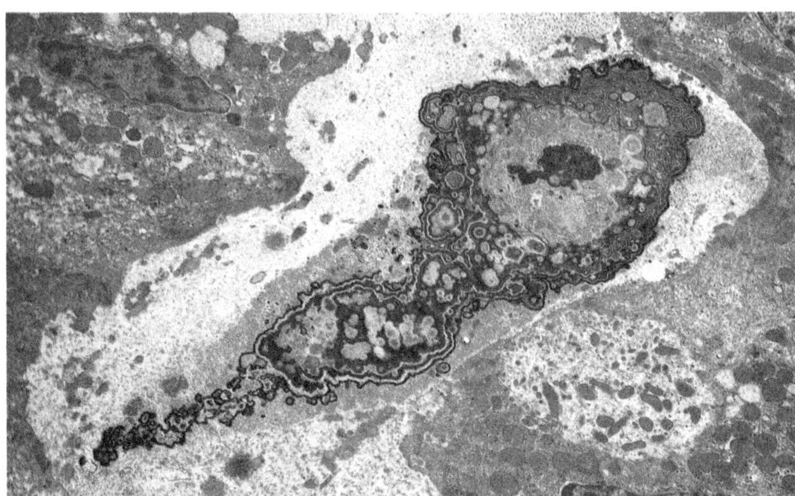

Fig. 8. Transmission electron micrograph in which a sialomicrolith is present in the lumen of a duct and consists of numerous lamellae and cores that indicate growth by accretion. Stagnant secretory material and some membraneous debris are also present in the lumen. Submandibular gland of a cat 14 days after parasympathectomy, as described by Triantafyllou and colleagues[26]; tissue immersion-fixed in glutaraldehyde and formaldehyde and subsequently in osmium tetroxide (section stained with lead citrate, magnification ×4640). (*Courtesy of* A. Triantafyllou, PhD, FRCPath, Liverpool, England.)

intraglandular duct causes focal obstructive atrophy (**Fig. 9**). Microbes proliferate in atrophic parenchyma, where they are protected from the flushing and microbicidal activity of saliva and from systemic immunity by the surrounding fibrosis. The diffusion of their waste products and local invasion cause inflammation, the fluid and cellular exudate of which compresses surrounding parenchyma and causes further atrophy (**Fig. 10**). The process eventually spreads to involve more of the lobules until the inflammatory swelling and fibrosis compress large intraglandular ducts. This causes partial obstruction that leads to ductal dilatation and stagnation of the calcium-rich secretory material. This can precipitate on the phospholipid exposed in degenerating cellular membranes to form a sialolith (**Figs 11–13**). As the process progresses, the gland becomes increasingly inflamed, atrophic, and fibrosed (**Fig. 14**). The process may sometimes eventually end as a symptomless sialolith in a very fibrosed duct together with completely obstructed, uninflamed, atrophic remnants of the gland.

Stenosis of the main duct is sometimes found in chronic sialadenitis and is likely secondary to chronic inflammation. The partial obstruction caused by the stenosis is an important factor in the persistence of sialadenitis and formation of sialoliths.[41–48] Also, the lining of Stensen's duct in juvenile recurrent parotitis has been seen endoscopically as white and avascular and the duct as stenotic, likely representing fibrosis of chronic inflammation, and could itself cause partial obstruction.[49,50]

Plugs described as mucous, fibrinous, or fiber-like have been seen endoscopically. They have been found associated with inflammatory stenoses.[48] Microscopic examination shows that they contain desquamated parenchymal cells and inflammatory cells.[46] They also include the albuminous coagulum found when plasma proteins leak into the lumina of inflamed glands.[51] The plugs are secondary to inflammation and are obstructive.

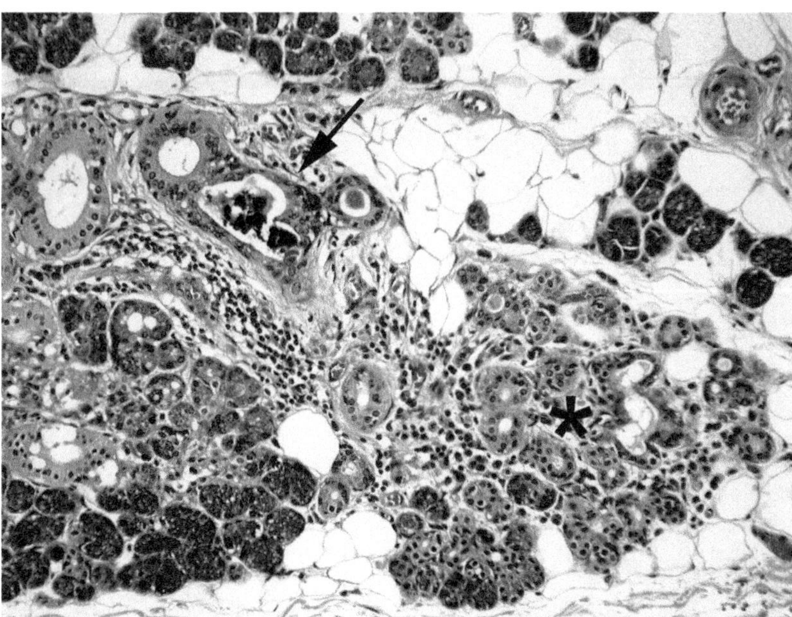

Fig. 9. Sialomicroliths (*arrow*) are impacted in a striated duct causing focal obstructive atrophy of the parenchyma (*asterisk*). Normal submandibular gland (section stained with hematoxylin-eosin, magnification ×156).

A sphincter has been seen endoscopically in Stensen's and Wharton's ducts, and a layer of smooth muscle has been found histologically in the wall of both ducts.[41,52–55] Skeletal muscle fibers from the buccinator muscle are inserted into the terminal part of Stensen's duct, other fibers from the buccinator muscle run parallel to the duct, and a valve-like structure is present in the terminal part.[55] These muscles are likely of importance in the flow of saliva and to function as sphincters. Malfunction could allow ascent by microbes or cause partial obstruction, and microbes have been found histologically in normal Stensen's ducts.[53]

Foreign bodies that migrate from the orifice of the main duct or penetrate the main duct have occasionally been found and cause inflammation leading to partial obstruction and the consequent formation of a sialolith.[1] Malfunction of ductal muscle is a likely factor in the introduction of foreign bodies via the orifice.

Many cases of chronic sialadenitis are of normal appearance on diagnostic imaging or endoscopy.[45,47] These cases correspond to the 12% to 21% of cases of a normal histologic appearance.[8,56]

Irrigation, even by saline alone, is effective in many cases of chronic submandibular and parotid sialadenitis because the irrigation: dilutes and flushes microbes out of atrophic foci into regions where the microbicidal capacity of the saliva is effective; flushes out obstructing plugs; dilates ducts, thus allowing small sialoliths to be passed; and dislodges sialoliths adherent to the walls of ducts.[57]

The concentration of sequestered calcium in the secretory granules is lower in the parotid than in the submandibular gland because the secretory glycoprotein is not acidic, which accounts for the lower incidence of sialomicroliths and sialoliths in the parotid. The parotid, however, is much less resistant to noxious stimuli than the submandibular gland, and diminished or absent secretory activity facilitates ascending infection.[33]

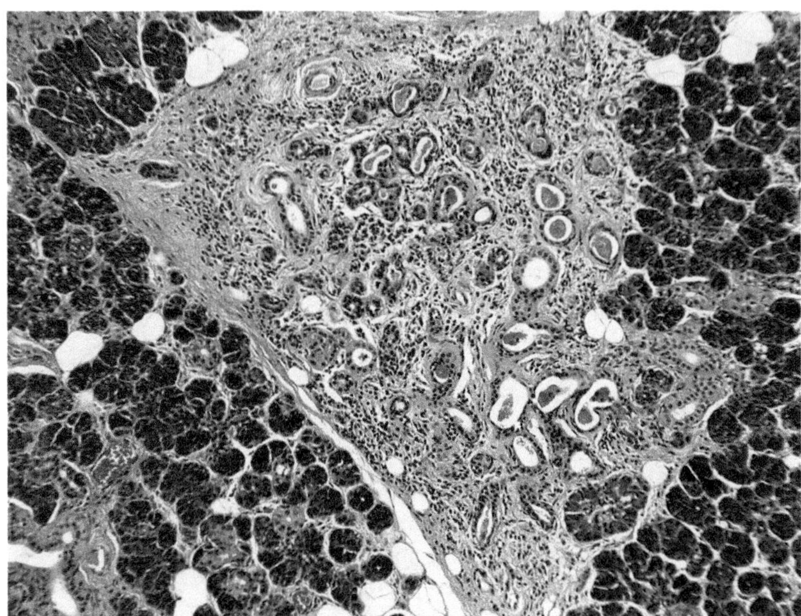

Fig. 10. A large focus of very atrophic parenchyma that is inflamed and fibrotic occupies much of a lobule and contrasts with adjacent acini. Chronic submandibular sialadenitis without sialolithiasis (section stained with hematoxylin-eosin, magnification ×98).

Sialoliths are found in the minor salivary glands, although rarely and somewhat later than in the submandibular and parotid glands.[58] This relates to the ongoing spontaneous secretion of the minor glands, and also the sublingual gland, that occurs in the absence of nervous stimulation. This is in contrast to the submandibular and parotid glands, in which secretion is dependent on nervous stimulation, in the absence of which there is secretory inactivity.[59,60] Thus, the spontaneous secretion safeguards the minor and sublingual salivary glands, which are histologically and functionally identical, until eventually age-related degenerative changes occur, including acinar atrophy, reduced discharge of secretory granules, organic sialomicroliths in ductal lumina, and an increase of inflammatory cells.[61,62] This degeneration may lead to stagnation of the calcium-rich secretory material, and ultimately to the formation of sialoliths.[12]

Obstruction not Primarily Caused by Inflammation

Noninflammatory factors of obstructive etiologic importance are kinks of Wharton's duct, ductal polyps, ductal invaginations, and pelvis-like abnormalities of the duct at the submandibular hilum.[41,43]

An obstructive etiologic factor in juvenile recurrent parotitis arising from occlusal disharmony that leads to increased tone of the masseter muscle, which then obstructs Stensen's duct, was cured by orthodontic therapy.[63] Support for the notion that ductal obstruction can be caused by adjacent skeletal muscle is given by the findings that fibers of the buccinator muscle are inserted into the anterior part of Stensen's duct, fibers also run parallel to the duct, and atrophy in von Ebner's glands is related to adjacent skeletal muscle.[55,64]

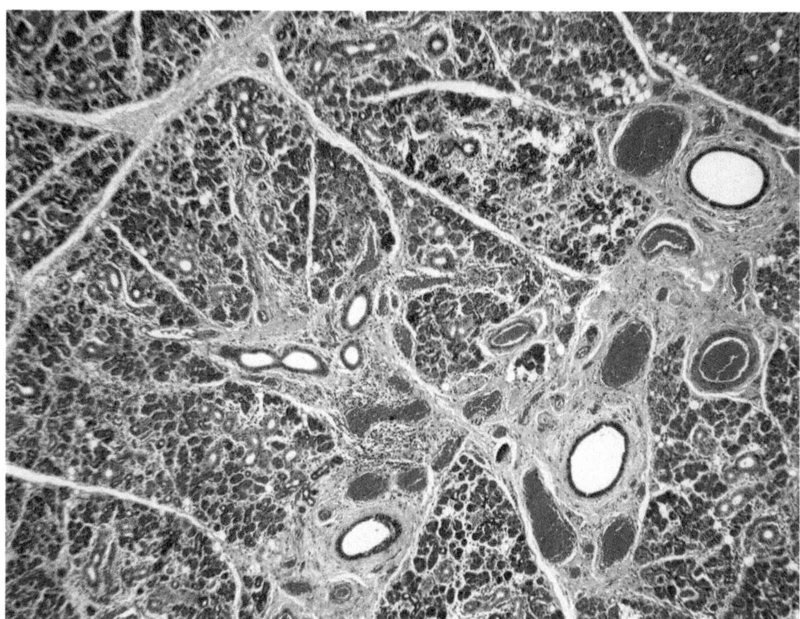

Fig. 11. A submandibular gland is moderately inflamed, atrophic, and fibrosed with dilated ducts. Chronic submandibular sialadenitis without sialolithiasis (section stained with hematoxylin-eosin, magnification ×40).

Autoimmunity

The term *Küttner's tumor* only became familiar to the English-speaking medical profession after 1991, when it was included in the second edition of the WHO *Histologic Typing of Salivary Gland Tumours*.[65] This led to a crop of case reports purporting to be of a rare, exotic condition, namely Küttner's tumor, without the realization that it was the mundane chronic obstructive sialadenitis without sialolithiasis. Then, recently, a rare, IgG4-related, autoimmune form of chronic sialadenitis, was named Küttner's tumor, or Mikulicz's disease when the lacrimal glands are involved.[66–68] Unfortunately, the use of these eponyms is fraught with confusion. Küttner had no doubt that the disease that he described was chronic obstructive sialadenitis that may or may not lead to sialolithiasis.[3,4] Furthermore, examination of the original detailed illustration of the histology in Mikulicz's 1892 article revealed that the disease he described is MALT lymphoma.[69] This confusion indicates that these eponyms should no longer be used.

Nevertheless, it is established that the rare, autoimmune disease, best named *IgG4-related sclerosing disease*, can involve many organs, especially the pancreas, bile duct, retroperitoneum, and salivary glands. Although the term *IgG4-related sialadenitis* is cumbersome compared with *Küttner's tumor*, it is accurate and should not lead to confusion and possible mismanagement.

Relation to Other Diseases

Patients with sialolithiasis suffer from nephrolithiasis more often than the general population.[70] Patients with hyperparathyroidism exhibit an increased incidence of sialolithiasis, and those with hyperparathyroidism and sialolithiasis exhibit a greater incidence of nephrolithiasis than those without sialolithiasis.[71] This indicates that

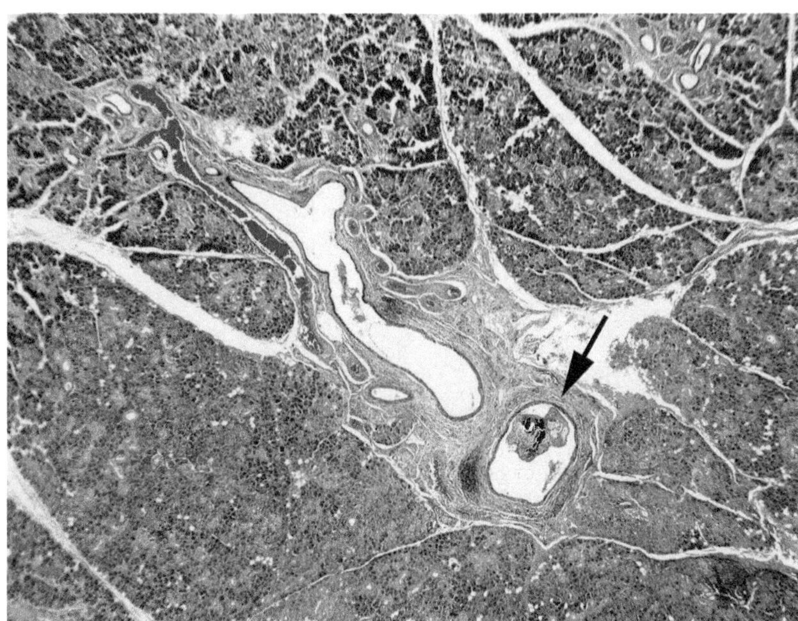

Fig. 12. A submandibular gland is moderately inflamed, atrophic, and fibrosed with dilated ducts. A dilated duct (*arrow*) is seen in which there is an inchoate sialolith that consists of foci of calcification mixed with mucopus. Mucopus consists of secretory material, inflammatory cells and degenerate parenchymal cells. Chronic submandibular sialadenitis with sialolithiasis (section stained with hematoxylin-eosin, magnification ×16).

hypercalcemia can be a factor in the development of sialolithiasis, as demonstrated in animal experiments.[15]

Survival and Recovery of Glands

Salivary glands affected by chronic obstructive sialadenitis adapt to the altered environment by cell death through apoptosis and necrosis and by autophagy in which redundant secretory granules and organelles associated with synthesis of secretory material are digested by lysosomal enzymes.[72–74] Ihrler and colleagues[73,74] found immunohistochemical evidence of a profound inducible capacity for regeneration in the salivary glands, which is the biologic basis for the good functional results from conservative therapies that improve the internal environment of the glands.

The function of submandibular glands affected by sialolithiasis has been investigated scintigraphically after surgical removal of the sialoliths, and improvement was inversely related to age.[75–77] This is similar to the finding that a favorable clinical outcome after extracorporeal lithotripsy of the submandibular gland and parotid is inversely related to age.[78] There is a decreased resistance and potential for recovery of the glands with increasing age, which is also shown by the greater proportion of cases of chronic submandibular sialadenitis with widespread atrophy in older patients.[8,56] Additionally, a good functional recovery or favorable clinical outcome that was inversely related to the size of the sialolith probably relates to a more complete obstruction by a larger sialolith that results in greater atrophy of the

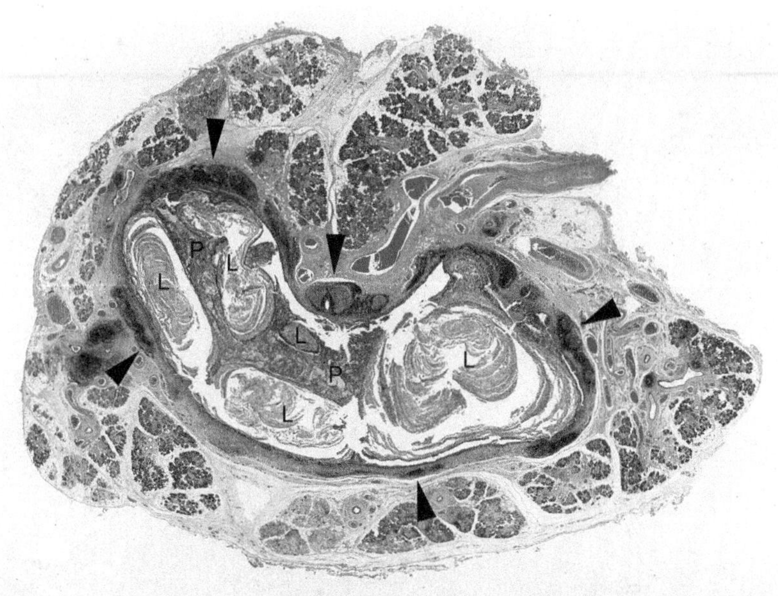

Fig. 13. A submandibular gland is moderately inflamed, atrophic, and fibrosed with a collection of lamellar sialoliths (L) mixed with mucopus (P) in a dilated duct. Dense periductal inflammatory infiltrate (*arrowheads*) is lymphocytic and contains germinal centers. Chronic submandibular sialadenitis with sialolithiasis; tissue decalcified in formic acid (section stained with hematoxylin-eosin, magnification ×4).

gland.[76,78] Support for this explanation is given by scintigraphy in which the preoperative glandular function was poor in the two cases that failed to recover.[77]

Structure and Composition of Sialomicroliths and Sialoliths

Investigations on the structure and composition of sialomicroliths and sialoliths have yielded information about the causes and natural history of chronic obstructive sialadenitis and sialolithiasis; they are reviewed elsewhere[1] and summarized as follows:

A sialomicrolith is defined as a concretion in a salivary gland that can only be seen microscopically and is most often calcified.[23]

Sialomicroliths range from consisting of hydroxyapatite crystals to condensed degenerate secretory material (see **Figs. 4, 5, 7** and **8**).[11,14,20,23,30,32,79] Sialomicroliths grow and fuse by accretion, and the presence or absence of crystals relates to the local concentration of calcium when a particular part is forming.

A sialolith is defined as a concretion in a salivary gland or main duct that can be seen with the naked eye and is most often calcified.

Sialoliths share many features with sialomicroliths, including great variation in structure and in the content of mineral and organic matrix. The organic matrix contains glycoprotein and lipids derived from secretory material and cellular membranes, which indicates a mechanism of formation similar to that of sialomicroliths.

Sialoliths contain cores, which are single or multiple, vary from purely organic to heavily calcified, and have surrounding calcified lamellae that alternate with less calcified or purely organic lamellae. The core is considered the initial sialolith, yet it sometimes

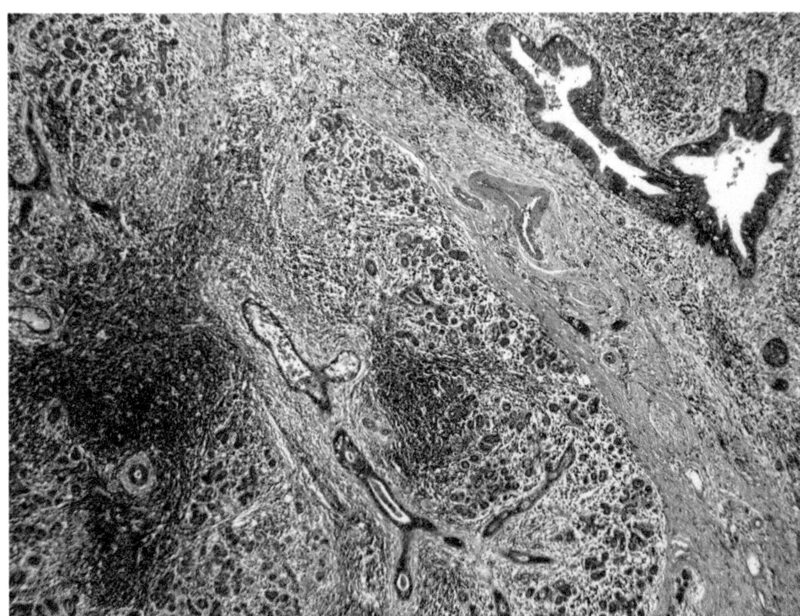

Fig. 14. A submandibular gland is very inflamed, atrophic, and fibrosed with dilated ducts. Chronic submandibular sialadenitis with sialolithiasis (section stained with hematoxylin-eosin, magnification ×40).

exhibits a substructure, which indicates a formation by accretion and fusion of smaller sialoliths, and this process possibly also includes sialomicroliths.

The absence of bacteria in sialomicroliths shows that bacteria are unnecessary for calcification, and they are absent from the cores of sialoliths. The partial obstruction caused by a sialolith enables bacteria to ascend more easily from the mouth to reach and colonize the surface of the sialolith and to become incorporated.

Hydroxyapatite is the most widespread mineral in sialoliths, but other minerals are variably present, such as whitlockite and octacalcium phosphate. The microenvironment and its variations with time determine the type of mineral formed and the degree of calcification. Thus, the saliva of patients with calcified sialoliths was found to contain more calcium and less phytate than that of a healthy group and of patients with purely organic sialoliths.[80] Phytate is obtained in the diet from the seeds of plants and particularly cereals and is a potent inhibitor of hydroxyapatite crystallization.

Causes and natural history of chronic obstructive sialadenitis and sialolithiasis are outlined in **Fig. 15**.

INCIDENCE OF CHRONIC OBSTRUCTIVE SIALADENITIS AND SIALOLITHIASIS

The universally quoted figure for the prevalence of sialolithiasis is 1.2%, found in Rauch's monograph: "*De Temino* u. a. (1949) geben 1,15% ihrer Autopsien an," which is translated as "De Temino and colleagues (1949) state 1.15% of their autopsies."[6] However, reference to this article, in Excerpta Medica reveals that de Temiño and Villar y Pérez de los Ríos reported 23 clinical cases of sialolithiasis.[81] This article is an excerpt of their original article, in which they state that the 23 cases were found among 20,000 patients during 18 years in the stomatologic service of their

Involvement of sialomicrolithiasis

Secretory inactivity in normal gland

↓

Accumulation of sialomicroliths causes foci of obstructive atrophy

↓

Microbes ascend main duct and proliferate in foci of obstructive atrophy

↓

Inflammation with fluid and cellular exudate

Compression of surrounding parenchyma with further atrophy

Further ascent by and proliferation of microbes

↓

Further inflammation with fluid and cellular exudate and fibrosis

Compression of large duct with partial obstruction

Involvement of other factors

Kink in Wharton's duct causes partial obstruction.

Malfunction of ductal muscle causes partial obstruction.

Malfunction of ductal muscle allows ascent by microbes or introduction of foreign body, which lead to inflammation and resultant partial obstruction.

Adjacent skeletal muscle causes partial obstruction.

Ductal polyp, ductal invagination and pelvislike abnormality of submandibular hilum cause partial obstruction.

Inflammation causes formation of plugs, which cause partial obstruction.

Inflammation of the main duct from any of the above causes leads to stenosis, which causes partial obstruction.

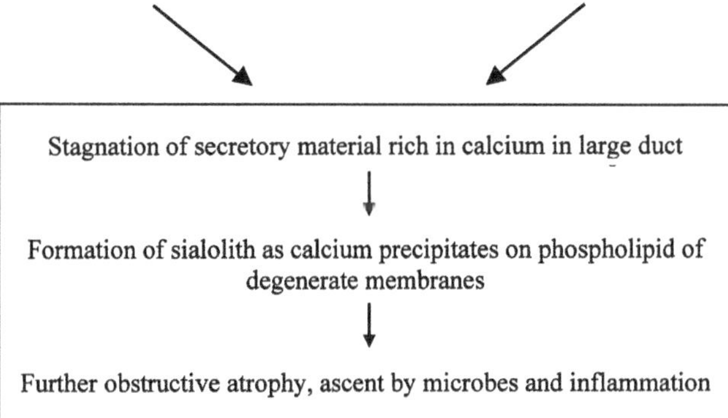

Fig. 15. Causes and natural history of chronic obstructive sialadenitis and sialolithiasis.

institution.[82] Thus, this was neither a postmortem investigation nor a statement of prevalence but a statement that the incidence of sialolithiasis in their stomatologic service was 0.115%.

Rauch presented a table of the incidence of sialolithiasis in the major glands that was obtained from the published work of several investigators.[6] A corrected summary of this table is that out of 1251 cases of sialolithiasis, 80% involved the submandibular gland, 13% the parotid, and 7% the sublingual gland. The stated incidence for the sublingual gland is far higher than the real figure, because the part of the submandibular gland superior to the mylohyoid muscle usually merges with the posterior part of the sublingual gland and is indistinguishable from it except histologically.[83] Therefore, sialoliths in this part of the submandibular gland or associated Wharton's duct could easily be incorrectly classified as sublingual sialoliths. That this occurred in the past is shown by Zenk and colleagues[84] recent series of 635 patients with sialolithiasis of the major glands in which 79 % involved the submandibular gland, 21% the parotid, and none the sublingual gland.

Sialolithiasis of the minor salivary glands is rare compared with that of the submandibular and parotid glands. In a series of 245 patients with sialolithiasis, Lustmann and colleagues reported that a minor salivary gland was involved in only 2 cases.[70] The most common site of sialolithiasis of the minor salivary glands was the upper lip, closely followed by the inner aspect of the cheeks, and the least common sites were the lower lip, vestibule, tongue, and palate.[58]

An attempt to estimate the prevalence of sialolithiasis in the general population was made by Escudier and McGurk.[85] They calculated that the incidence of symptomatic sialolithiasis in England is at least 27.5 cases per million population per annum and possibly as much as 59 cases per million population per annum. The latter figure expressed as 0.0059% per annum multiplied by the figure for average life expectancy of 76 years produces an estimated prevalence for symptomatic sialolithiasis of 0.45%, which is higher than the incidence of 0.115% found by de Temiño and Villar y Pérez de los Ríos[82,86] in their stomatologic service and, therefore, may be an overestimate.

The average age of patients with sialolithiasis was 40.5 years for the submandibular gland, 47.8 years for the parotid, and 50 years for the minor salivary glands.[58,84] The higher age for the parotid may relate to the lower level of calcium in this gland, which makes it less favorable for the formation of sialoliths.[12] The highest age for the minor salivary glands relates to the spontaneous secretion that protects the glands until degenerative age changes become established.

There has been little attempt to separate series of cases of sialadenitis without sialolithiasis from those with sialolithiasis and the data usually are given together. Thus, the mean age at submandibular sialadenectomy in our series was 42 years.[8] This is similar to the finding of Seifert and Donath of the peak incidence in the fifth decade.[7] Data were given separately, however, by Escudier and McGurk,[85] Drage and colleagues,[87] and Preuss and colleagues.[88] These investigations reported that the peak incidence of sialadenitis with sialolithiasis preceded that for sialadenitis without sialolithiasis. Ngu and colleagues,[47] however, showed a peak incidence from 40 to 69 years for sialadenitis with stricture and without sialolithiasis for the submandibular and parotid glands, which is older than the peak incidence of sialadenitis without sialolithiasis from 30 to 64 years for the submandibular and parotid glands shown by Escudier and McGurk[85] but younger than 50 to 69 years for the submandibular gland shown by Preuss and colleagues.[88] Furthermore, our database of chronic submandibular sialadenitis reveals an increase in the proportion of cases with sialolithiasis with increasing age (**Table 1**).

Table 1
Chronic submandibular sialadenitis stratified by age

	Age in Years							
	0–19	20–29	30–39	40–49	50–59	60–69	70 and Over	Total
Without sialolithiasis	3	10	7	7	7	6	1	41
With sialolithiasis	3	24	18	13	16	11	5	90
Ratio of proportion of cases with sialolithiasis to proportion of cases without sialolithiasis	0.5	1.1	1.2	0.8	1.0	0.8	2.3	

Data from database used in Harrison JD, Epivatianos A, Bhatia SN. Role of microliths in the aetiology of chronic submandibular sialadenitis: a clinicopathological investigation of 154 cases. Histopathology 1997;31:237–51.

SUMMARY

It is more than a century since Küttner's seminal work based on his intelligent observation of two cases. Today's greater understanding of the causes, natural history, and incidence of sialadenitis and sialolithiasis reflects the advances made in science since 1896. Every patient's chronic salivary problem is unique. A better understanding of the underlying pathology will help arriving at a better diagnosis and treatment plan for every patient.

REFERENCES

1. Harrison JD. Natural history of chronic sialadenitis and sialolithiasis. In: Nahlieli O, Iro H, McGurk M, editors. Modern management preserving the salivary glands. Herzeliya: Isradon; 2007. p. 93–135.
2. Küttner H. Ueber entzündliche Tumoren Der Submaxillar-Speicheldrüse [On the inflammatory tumors of the submandibular salivary gland]. Beiträge zur klinischen Chirurgie 1896;15:815–28.
3. Küttner H. Speichelsteine [Salivary stones]. In: Garrè C, Küttner H, Lexer L, editors. Handbuch der Praktischen Chirurgie. 6th edition. Chirurgie des Kopfes, Vol. 1. Stuttgart: Ferdinand Enke; 1926. p. 929–35.
4. Küttner H. Chronische Entzündungen [Chronic inflammations]. Entzündliche Tumoren. In: Garrè C, Küttner H, Lexer E, editors. Handbuch der Praktischen Chirurgie. 6th edition. Chirurgie des Kopfes, vol. 1. Stuttgart: Ferdinand Enke; 1926. p. 948–51.
5. Rauch S. Mykose, Pollinose und Parasiten der Speicheldrüsen [Mycosis, pollinosis and parasites of the salivary glands]. Die Speicheldrüsen des Menschen. Anatomie, Physiologie und Klinische Pathologie. Stuttgart: Georg Thieme; 1959. p. 218–23.
6. Rauch S. Speichelsteine (sialolithiasis) [Salivary stones (sialolithiasis)]. Die Speicheldrüsen des Menschen. Anatomie, Physiologie und Klinische Pathologie. Stuttgart: Georg Thieme; 1959. p. 434–50.

7. Seifert G, Donath K. Zur Pathogenese des Küttner-Tumors der Submandibularis. Analyse von 349 Fällen mit Chronischer Sialadenitis der Submandibularis [On the pathogenesis of the Küttner tumor of the submandibular gland. Analysis of 349 cases with chronic sialadenitis of the submandibular gland]. HNO 1977;25:81–92.
8. Harrison JD, Epivatianos A, Bhatia SN. Role of microliths in the aetiology of chronic submandibular sialadenitis: a clinicopathological investigation of 154 cases. Histopathology 1997;31:237–51.
9. Scott J. The incidence of focal chronic inflammatory changes in human submandibular salivary glands. J Oral Pathol 1976;5:334–46.
10. Scott J. The prevalence of consolidated salivary deposits in the small ducts of human submandibular glands. J Oral Pathol 1978;7:28–37.
11. Epivatianos A, Harrison JD. The presence of microcalculi in normal human submandibular and parotid salivary glands. Arch Oral Biol 1989;34(4):261–5.
12. Harrison JD, Triantafyllou A, Baldwin D, et al. Histochemical and biochemical determination of calcium in salivary glands with particular reference to chronic submandibular sialadenitis. Virchows Archiv A Pathol Anat Histopathol 1993; 423:29–32.
13. Verdugo P, Deyrup-Olsen I, Aitken M, et al. Molecular mechanism of mucin secretion: I. The role of intragranular charge shielding. J Dent Res 1987;66(2):506–8.
14. Epivatianos A, Harrison JD, Dimitriou T. Ultrastructural and histochemical observations on microcalculi in chronic submandibular sialadenitis. J Oral Pathol 1987; 16:514–7.
15. Harrison JD, Epivatianos A. Production of microliths and sialadenitis in rats by a short combined course of isoprenaline and calcium gluconate. Oral Surg Oral Med Oral Pathol 1992;73(5):585–90.
16. Boskey AL, Boyan-Salyers BD, Burstein LS, et al. Lipids associated with mineralization of human submandibular gland sialoliths. Arch Oral Biol 1981;26:779–85.
17. Slomiany BL, Murty VLN, Aono M, et al. Lipid composition of the matrix of human submandibular salivary gland stones. Arch Oral Biol 1982;27:673–7.
18. Boskey AL, Burstein LS, Mandel ID. Phospholipids associated with human parotid gland sialoliths. Arch Oral Biol 1983;28(7):655–7.
19. Slomiany BL, Murty VLN, Aono M, et al. Lipid composition of human parotid salivary gland stones. J Dent Res 1983;62(8):866–9.
20. Epivatianos A, Harrison JD, Garrett JR, et al. Ultrastructural and histochemical observations on intracellular and luminal microcalculi in the feline sublingual salivary gland. J Oral Pathol 1986;15:513–7.
21. Triantafyllou A, Harrison JD, Garrett JR, et al. Increase of microliths in inactive salivary glands of cat. Arch Oral Biol 1992;37(8):663–6.
22. Triantafyllou A, Harrison JD, Garrett JR. Microliths in normal salivary glands of cat investigated by light and electron microscopy. Cell Tissue Res 1993;272:321–7.
23. Triantafyllou A, Harrison JD, Garrett JR. Analytical ultrastructural investigation of microliths in salivary glands of cat. Histochem J 1993;25:183–90.
24. Harrison JD, Triantafyllou A, Garrett JR. The effect of sympathectomy on the occurrence of microliths in salivary glands of cat as studied by light and electron microscopy. Arch Oral Biol 1993;38(1):79–84.
25. Harrison JD, Triantafyllou A, Garrett JR. The effects of obstruction and secretory stimulation on microlithiasis in salivary glands of cat: light and electron microscopy. Virchows Archiv B Cell Pathol 1993;64:29–35.
26. Triantafyllou A, Harrison JD, Garrett JR. Production of salivary microlithiasis in cats by parasympathectomy: light and electron microscopy. Int J Exp Pathol 1993;74:103–12.

27. Harrison JD, Triantafyllou A, Baldwin D, et al. Histochemical and biochemical determination of calcium in salivary glands of cat. Histochemistry 1993;100: 155–9.
28. Harrison JD, Triantafyllou A, Garrett JR. Ultrastructural localization of microliths in salivary glands of cat. J Oral Pathol Med 1993;22:358–62.
29. Triantafyllou A, Fletcher D, Scott J. Organic secretory products, adaptive responses and innervation in the parotid gland of ferret: a histochemical study. Arch Oral Biol 2005;50:769–77.
30. Triantafyllou A, Fletcher D, Scott J. Histological and histochemical observations on salivary microliths in ferret. Arch Oral Biol 2006;51:198–205.
31. Triantafyllou A, Harrison JD, Garrett JR. Microenvironmental adaptations in the parotid of ferret investigated by electron microscopy. Arch Oral Biol 2007;52(8): 768–77.
32. Triantafyllou A, Harrison JD, Garrett JR. Microliths in the parotid of ferret investigated by electon microscopy and microanalysis. Int J Exp Pathol 2009;90(4): 439–47.
33. Harrison JD, Garrett JR. Histological effects of ductal ligation of salivary glands of the cat. J Pathol 1976;118:245–54.
34. Shimizu M, Yoshiura K, Kanda S. Radiological and histological analysis of the structural changes in the rat parotid gland following release of Stensen's duct obstruction. Dentomaxillofac Radiol 1994;23:197–205.
35. Takahashi S, Schoch E, Walker NI. Origin of acinar cell regeneration after atrophy of the rat parotid induced by duct obstruction. Int J Exp Pathol 1998;79:293–301.
36. Scott J, Liu P, Smith PM. Morphologial and functional characteristics of acinar atrophy and recovery in the duct-ligated parotid gland of the rat. J Dent Res 1999;78(11):1711–9.
37. Harrison JD, Fouad HMA, Garrett JR. The effects of ductal obstruction on the acinar cells of the parotid of cat. Arch Oral Biol 2000;45:945–9.
38. Harrison JD, Fouad HMA, Garrett JR. Variation in the response to ductal obstruction of feline submandibular and sublingual salivary glands and the importance of the innervation. J Oral Pathol Med 2001;30:29–34.
39. Takahashi S, Shinzato K, Nakamura S, et al. Cell death and cell proliferation in the regeneration of atrophied rat submandibular glands after duct ligation. J Oral Pathol Med 2004;33:23–9.
40. Osailan SM, Proctor GB, Carpenter GH, et al. Recovery of rat submandibular salivary gland function following removal of obstruction: a sialometrical and sialochemical study. Int J Exp Pathol 2006;87:411–23.
41. Nahlieli O, Baruchin AM. Long-term experience with endoscopic diagnosis and treatment of salivary gland inflammatory diseases. Laryngoscope 2000;110: 988–93.
42. Marchal F, Dulguerov P, Becker M, et al. Specificity of parotid sialendoscopy. Laryngoscope 2001;111:264–71.
43. Nahlieli O, Shacham R, Yoffe B, et al. Diagnosis and treatment of strictures and kinks in salivary gland ducts. J Oral Maxillofac Surg 2001;59:484–90.
44. Marchal F, Dulguerov P, Becker M, et al. Submandibular diagnostic and interventional sialendoscopy: new procedure for ductal disorders. Ann Otol Rhinol Laryngol 2002;111:27–35.
45. Koch M, Zenk J, Bozzato A, et al. Sialoscopy in cases of unclear swelling of the major salivary glands. Otolaryngol Head Neck Surg 2005;133(6):863–8.
46. Qi S, Liu X, Wang S. Sialoendoscopic and irrigation findings in chronic obstructive parotitis. Laryngoscope 2005;115:541–5.

47. Ngu RK, Brown JE, Whaites EJ, et al. Salivary duct strictures: nature and incidence in benign salivary obstruction. Dentomaxillofac Radiol 2007;36:63–7.
48. Koch M, Iro H, Zenk J. Role of sialoscopy in the treatment of Stensen's duct strictures. Ann Otol Rhinol Laryngol 2008;117(4):271–8.
49. Nahlieli O, Shacham R, Shlesinger M, et al. Juvenile recurrent parotitis: a new method of diagnosis and treatment. Pediatrics 2004;114:9–12.
50. Quenin S, Plouin-Gaudon I, Marchal F, et al. Juvenile recurrent parotitis. Sialendoscopic approach. Arch Otolaryngol Head Neck Surg 2008;134(7):715–9.
51. Baurmash HD. Chronic recurrent parotitis: a closer look at its origin, diagnosis, and management. J Oral Maxillofac Surg 2004;62:1010–8.
52. Marchal F, Kurt A-M, Dulguerov P, et al. Retrograde theory in sialolithiasis formation. Arch Otolaryngol Head Neck Surg 2001;127:66–8.
53. Takeda Y. Histoarchitecture of the human parotid duct. Light-microscopic study. Acta Anat (Basel) 1987;128(4):291–4.
54. Teymoortash A, Ramaswamy A, Werner JA. Is there evidence of a sphincter system in Wharton's duct? Etiological factors related to sialolith formation. J Oral Sci 2003;45(4):233–5.
55. Kang H-C, Kwak H-H, Hu K-S, et al. An anatomical study of the buccinator muscle fibres that extend to the terminal portion of the parotid duct, and their functional roles in salivary secretion. J Anat 2006;208:601–7.
56. Marchal F, Kurt A-M, Dulguerov P, et al. Histopathology of submandibular glands removed for sialolithiasis. Ann Otol Rhinol Laryngol 2001;110:464–9.
57. Antoniades D, Harrison JD, Epivatianos A, et al. Treatment of chronic sialadenitis by intraductal penicillin or saline. J Oral Maxillofac Surg 2004;62:431–4.
58. Ben Lagha N, Alantar A, Samson J, et al. Lithiasis of minor salivary glands: current data. Oral Surg Oral Med Oral Pathol Oral Radiol Endod 2005;100(3):345–8.
59. Harrison JD. Salivary mucoceles. Oral Surg Oral Med Oral Pathol 1975;39(2): 268–78.
60. McGurk M, Eyeson J, Thomas B, et al. Conservative treatment of oral ranula by excision with minimal excision of the sublingual gland: histologic support for a traumatic etiology. J Oral Maxillofac Surg 2008;66(10):2050–7.
61. Scott J. Qualitative and quantitative observations on the histology of human labial salivary glands obtained post mortem. J Biol Buccale 1980;8:187–200.
62. Vered M, Buchner A, Bolden P, et al. Age-related histomorphometric changes in labial salivary glands with special reference to the acinar component. Exp Gerontol 2000;35:1075–84.
63. Bernkopf E, Colleselli P, Broia V, et al. Is recurrent parotitis in childhod still an enigma? A pilot experience. Acta Paediatr 2008;97:478–82.
64. Triantafyllou A, Fletcher D, Scott J. Histochemical phenotypes of von Ebner's gland of ferret and their functional implications. Histochem J 2001;33:173–81.
65. Seifert G. Chronic sclerosing sialadenitis of submandibular gland [Küttner tumour]. In: Seifert G, editor. Histological typing of salivary gland tumours. 2nd edition. Berlin: Springer; 1991. p. 37.
66. Kitagawa S, Zen Y, Harada K, et al. Abundant IgG4-positive plasma cell infiltration characterizes chronic sclerosing sialadenitis (Küttner's tumor). Am J Surg Pathol 2005;29(6):783–91.
67. Kamisawa T, Okamoto A. Autoimmune pancreatitis: proposal of IgG4-related sclerosing disease. J Gastroenterol 2006;41:613–25.
68. Yamamoto M, Takahashi H, Ohara M, et al. A new conceptualization for Mikulicz's disease as an IgG4-related plasmacytic disease. Mod Rheumatol 2006;16: 335–40.

69. Ihrler S, Harrison JD. Mikulicz's disease and Mikulicz's syndrome: analysis of the original case report of 1892 in the light of current knowledge identifies a MALT lymphoma. Oral Surg Oral Med Oral Pathol Oral Radiol Endod 2005;100(3):334–9.
70. Lustmann J, Regev E, Melamed Y. Sialolithiasis. A survey of 245 patients and a review of the literature. Int J Oral Maxillofac Surg 1990;19:135–8.
71. Stack BC Jr, Norman JG. Sialolithiasis and primary hyperparathyroidism. ORL J Otorhinolaryngol Relat Spec 2008;70(5):331–4.
72. Harrison JD, Badir MS. Chronic submandibular sialadenitis: ultrastructure and phosphatase histochemistry. Ultrastruct Pathol 1998;22:431–7.
73. Ihrler S, Zietz C, Sendelhofert A, et al. A morphogenetic concept of salivary duct regeneration and metaplasia. Virchows Arch 2002;440:519–26.
74. Ihrler S, Blasenbreu-Vogt S, Sendelhofert A, et al. Regeneration in chronic sialadenitis: an analysis of proliferation and apoptosis based on double immunohistochemical labelling. Virchows Arch 2004;444:356–61.
75. van den Akker HP, Busemann-Sokole E. Submandibular gland function following transoral sialolithectomy. Oral Surg Oral Med Oral Pathol 1983;56(4):351–6.
76. Nishi M, Mimura T, Marutani K, et al. Evaluation of submandibular gland function by sialo-scintigraphy following sialolithectomy. J Oral Maxillofac Surg 1987;45(7):567–71.
77. Yoshimura Y, Morishita T, Sugihara T. Salivary gland function after sialolithiasis: scintigraphic examination of submandibular glands with ^{99m}Tc-pertechnetate. J Oral Maxillofac Surg 1989;47:704–10.
78. Capaccio P, Ottaviani F, Manzo R, et al. Extracorporeal lithotripsy for salivary calculi: a long-term clinical experience. Laryngoscope 2004;114:1069–73.
79. Triantafyllou A, Harrison JD, Donath K. Microlithiasis in parotid sialadenosis and chronic submandibular sialadenitis is related to the microenvironment: an ultra-strutural and microanalytical investigation. Histopathology 1998;32:530–5.
80. Grases F, Santiago C, Simonet BM, et al. Sialolithiasis: mechanism of calculi formation and etiologic factors. Clin Chim Acta 2003;334:131–6.
81. de Temiño PR, Villar y Pérez de los Ríos F. Càlculos salivales *salivary calculi* anales españoles de odontoestomatologia. Madrid 1948, 7/8 (661–673) Illus. 15. Excerpta Medica, Section 11, 1949;2:349.
82. de Temiño PR, Villar y Pérez de los Ríos F. Cálculos salivales [Salivary calculi]. An Esp Odontoestomatol 1948;7(8):661–73.
83. Leppi TJ. Gross anatomical relationships between primate submandibular and sublingual salivary glands. J Dent Res 1967;46(2):359–65.
84. Zenk J, Constantinidis J, Kydles S, et al. Klinische und diagnostische Befunde bei der Sialolithiasis [Clinical and diagnostic findings in sialolithiasis]. HNO 1999;47:963–9.
85. Escudier MP, McGurk M. Symptomatic sialoadenitis and sialolithiasis in the English population, an estimate of the cost of hospital treatment. Br Dent J 1999;186(9):463–6.
86. Escudier M. Epidemiology and aetiology of salivary calculi. In: McGurk M, Renehan A, editors. Controversies in the management of salivary gland disease. Oxford and New York: Oxford University Press; 2001. p. 249–55.
87. Drage NA, Wilson RF, McGurk M. The genu of the submandibular duct—is the angle significant in salivary gland disease? Dentomaxillofac Radiol 2002;31:15–8.
88. Preuss SF, Klussmann JP, Wittekindt C, et al. Submandibular gland excision: 15 years of experience. J Oral Maxillofac Surg 2007;65:953–7.

Diagnostic Radiographic Imaging for Salivary Endoscopy

Kristine M. Mosier, DMD, PhD

KEYWORDS

• Salivary glands • Sialography • CT • MRI • Endoscopy

Diagnostic imaging of the salivary glands has undergone significant evolution with advances in cross-sectional imaging techniques. Prior to the advent of CT and MRI, sialography performed with x-ray techniques or under fluoroscopic guidance was the mainstay of evaluation of the salivary glands. The emergence of sialoendoscopy as a diagnostic and therapeutic technique for salivary disorders creates unique challenges in imaging. Each pathologic condition of the gland and duct is treated differently by sialoendoscopic technique; thus, radiographic identification of the various pathologies and their potential endoscopic complications is imperative. This article discusses the different diagnostic imaging approaches to evaluation of the salivary ductal system and the advantages of each technique in the diagnostic work-up for sialoendoscopy.

CONVENTIONAL SIALOGRAPHY

Conventional or x-ray sialography was first described by Carpy in 1904[1] and, although x-ray sources, contrast agents, and techniques have evolved, the essential technique remains the same. The examination begins with identification of the papilla of Stensen's duct or Whartons' duct (**Fig. 1**). An important next step in the diagnostic evaluation before sialoendoscopy is the dilatation of the ductal orifice. Although sialographic techniques can be performed without dilatation, dilatation of the ductal orifice determines whether or not a sialoendoscope can be inserted without surgical papillotomy and whether or not there is significant stenosis at the orifice. Dilatation of the duct is achieved using incremental sizes of lacrimal probes. The lacrimal probes range in tip dimension from 0000 to 4 (**Fig. 2**). The probe is inserted into the papilla (**Fig. 3**) and gently advanced until resistance is met and the duct dilated using a circular motion of the probe. The next incremental size probe is introduced until the duct is dilated to the largest achievable size.

Section of Neuroradiology, Head & Neck Imaging, Department of Radiology, Indiana University School of Medicine, 950 West Walnut Street, RII E124, Indianapolis, IN 46202, USA
E-mail address: kmosier@iupui.edu

Otolaryngol Clin N Am 42 (2009) 949–972
doi:10.1016/j.otc.2009.08.010

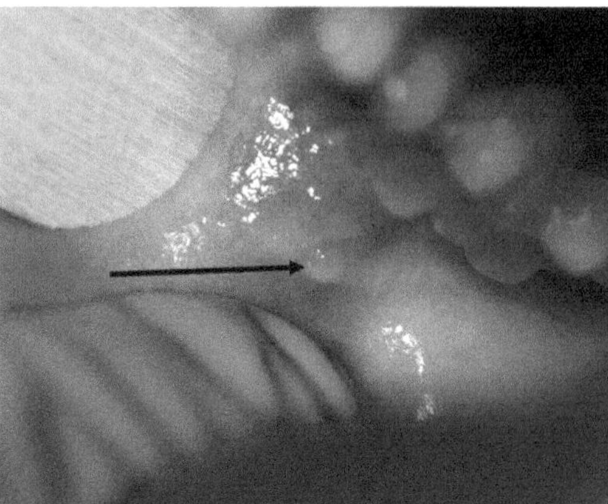

Fig. 1. Intraoral photographic view of the papilla of Stensen's duct (*black arrow*) in the buccal mucosa. The papilla is typically located adjacent to the second maxillary molar. Mild digital pressure typically expresses a droplet of saliva in patients with normal salivary flow.

Once maximum ductal dilatation is obtained, the sialographic catheter is introduced. There are a variety of sialographic catheters available of different dimensions and end-hole or side-hole configuration. The Yune-Klatte catheter (Cook Medical, Bloomington, Indiana) was developed by Drs Heun Y. Yune and Eugene Klatte of Indiana University and is an end-hole teflon catheter (**Fig. 4**) available in two sizes: 19 and 39. Generally, this catheter is more suitable for most Stensen's ducts; however, the orifice of Wharton's duct is not infrequently too small, even when dilated, to easily accommodate this catheter. Ranfac Corporation (Avon, Massachusetts) manufactures sialographic catheters in three sizes: 27, 30, and 31; the latter two sizes are likewise used for galatography. These are stainless steel end-hole catheters useful for Wharton's duct and stenotic Stensen's ducts (**Fig. 5**). An alternative to commercially available sialographic catheters is to use the semirigid plastic sheath of a #24 angiocatheter (BD Angiocath peripheral venous catheter, Hamilton Medical Products,

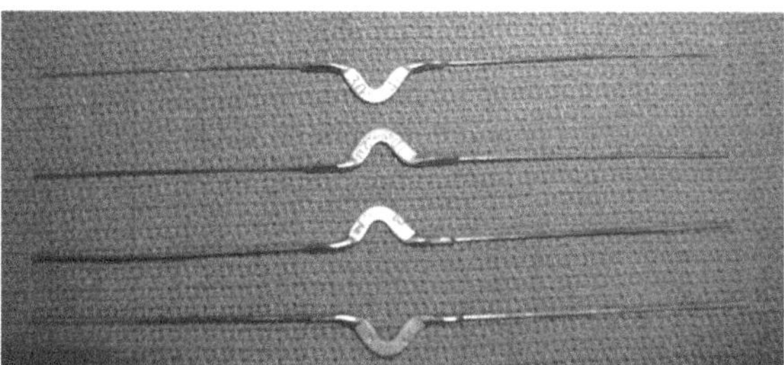

Fig. 2. Standard set of lacrimal probes used to dilate the salivary ducts. Sizes are incremental across the two blunt ends of each probe. Pictured are Bowman dilators ranging from 0000/000 (*top*), to 00/0 (*second from top*), to 1 to 2 (*third from top*), and to 3 to 4 (*bottom*). Wilder or Castroviejo lacrimal dilators may likewise be used; however, these are limited to 1–3 tip dimensions and three different tapers (Wilder). Generally, the submandibular ducts or stenotic Stensen's duct accommodates the smallest probes whereas a normal Stensen's duct accommodates sizes 00 to 4. Dilation to a size 1 or beyond is sufficient to accommodate a sialoendoscope without further dilation or papillotomy.

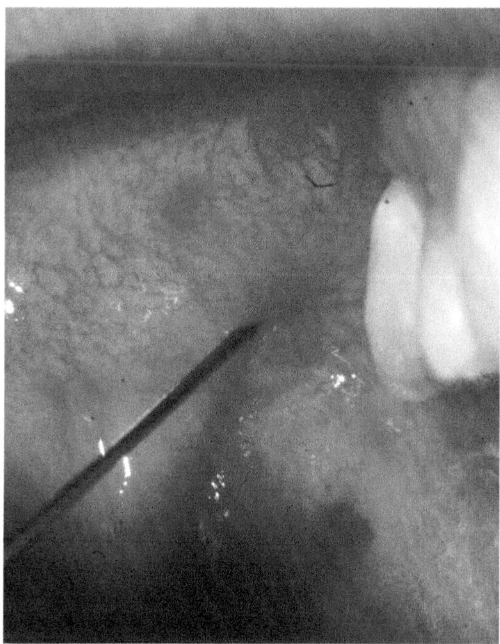

Fig. 3. Intraoral photograph of a Bowman size 2 lacrimal probe in Stensen's duct.

Mill Valley, California) (**Fig. 6**), which is intermediate in tip dimension between the Yune-Klatte catheters and the Ranfac catheters.

There are two iodinated contrast agents primarily used in conventional sialography: the oil-based agent, Ethiodol (Savage Laboratories, Melville, New York), or a water-soluble agent, Sinografin (Bracco Diagnostics, Princeton, New Jersey). Ethiodol contains 37% iodine in a poppy seed oil base. Due to its significantly reduced viscosity (0.5 to 1.0 poise at 15°C) and the fatty acid composition, which limit significant trans-ductal permeability, Ethiodol provides better contrast of ductal walls, permitting improved identification of wall irregularities, including polyps, mucous/fibrin plugs,

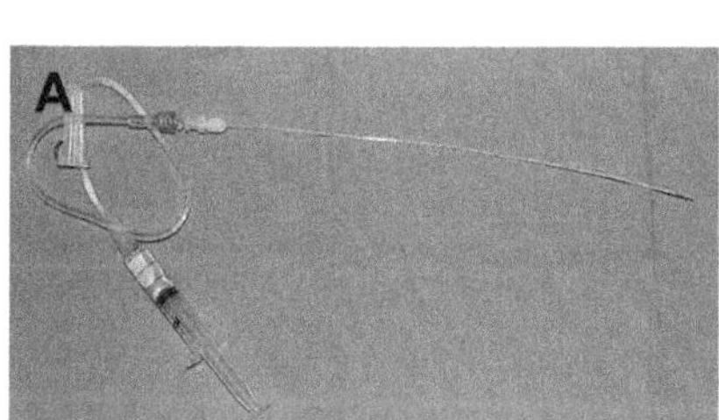

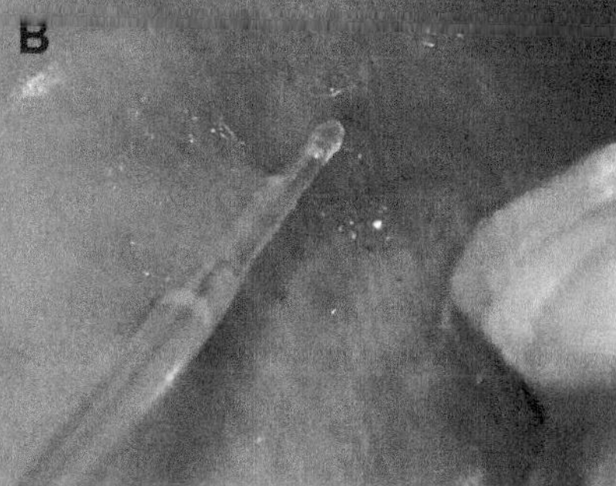

Fig. 4. (*A*) Photograph of a Yune-Klatte size 39 catheter. Care must be taken to extrude any air bubbles before insertion (*B*) Intraoral photograph of the end-hole configuration and taper of the semirigid Yune-Klatte 39 catheter.

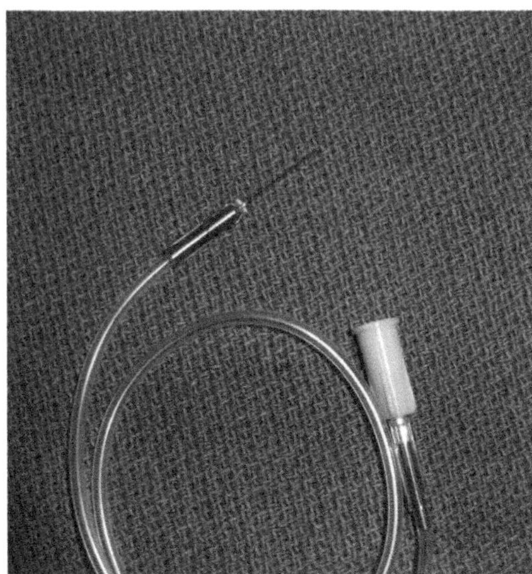

Fig. 5. Photograph of a Ranfac size 27 catheter. The stainless steel, rigid, end-hole design of this catheter is particularly useful for stenoses or kinks near the orifice which on initial filling tend to produce back presssure that expulses or leaks around a semirigid catheter.

or granulomatous areas (**Fig. 7**). It is advisable, however, to substitute Ethiodol with a water-soluble agent if sialoendoscopy is to be performed within 24 to 48 hours, as retained intraductal Ethiodol creates oil droplets or bubbles that may interfere with visualization at the endoscope tip.

Prior to infusion of the sialographic contrast agent, a radiograph (or when performing the examination under fluoroscopy, a spot film) of the relevant area is obtained to verify the presence or absence of calcified sialoliths. Filling is accomplished using moderate constant hand pressure on the syringe plunger. Fluoroscopic filming should begin with the start of filling to identify obstruction or stenosis of the orifice or buccal (Stensen's) or distal (Wharton's) segment and should be performed in the

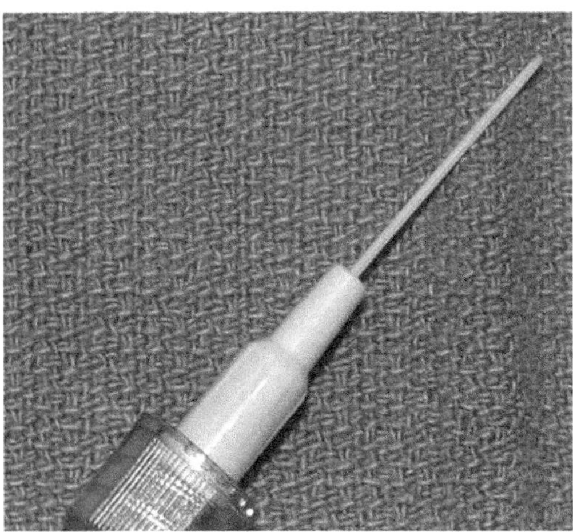

Fig. 6. Photograph of the size 24 angiocatheter guide sheath.

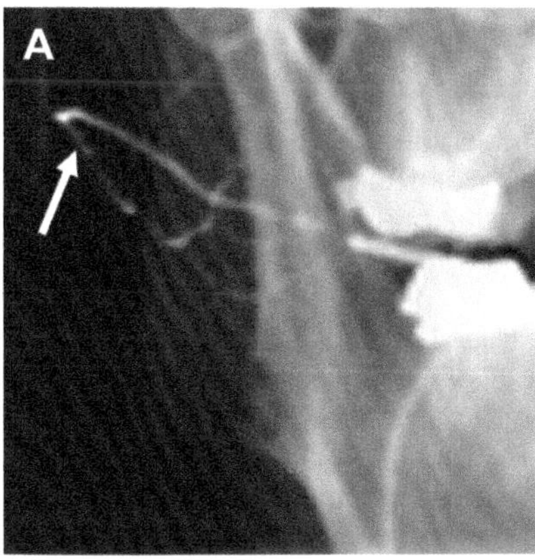

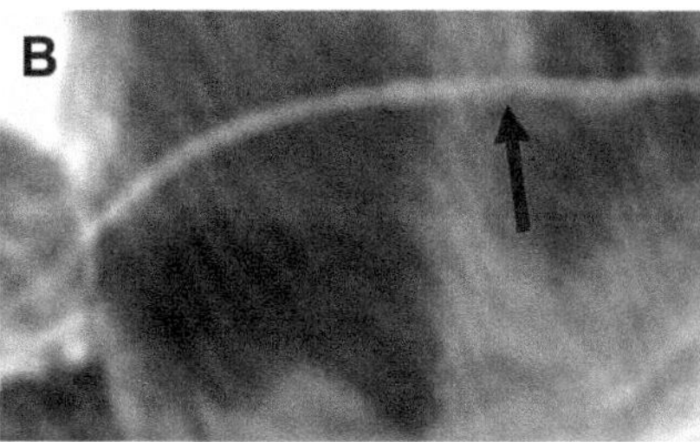

Fig. 7. (*A*) AP sialographic view of right Stensen's duct opacified with Ethiodol. The superior contrast of the ductal walls permits identification of small (1–3mm)–sized radiolucent fibrin plugs (*white arrow*) seen in the masseteric and proximal intraparenchymal segments. (*B*) Lateral sialographic view of Stensen's duct opacified with Ethiodol in a different patient shows a lenticular-shaped radiolucent defect (*black arrow*) extending from the sidewall. This is the typical appearance of granulomatous accumulations along the sidewall.

anteroposterior (AP) plane (**Fig. 8**). Moderate constant hand pressure on the syringe is important to ensure that ductal walls weakened by prior episodes of sialodochitis are not ruptured by the contrast bolus. Moreover, the relative amount of hand pressure required to infuse the contrast provides additional qualitative tactile information about the degree of stenosis and the need for balloon dilatation. On initial filling of the duct to

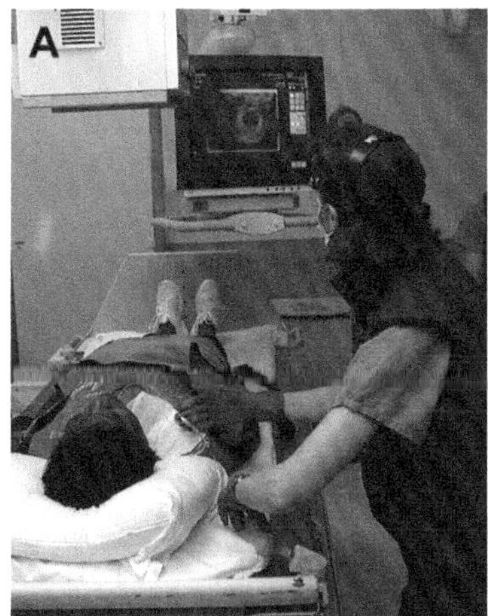

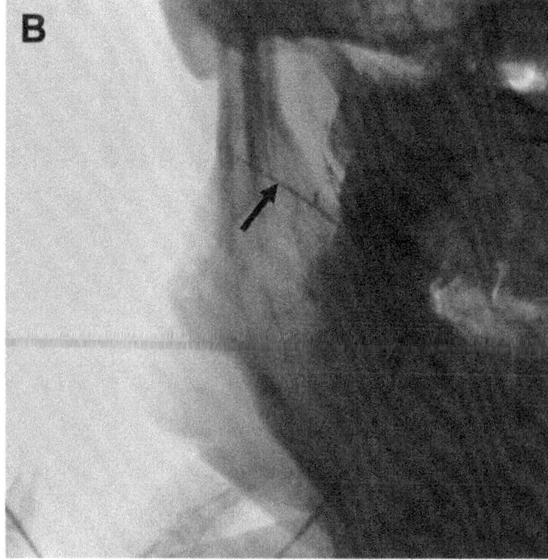

Fig. 8. (*A*) Photograph of the set up for fluoroscopically guided conventional sialography. The examination begins with a single exposure in the AP plane (shown as the image on the monitor) to identify the presence of opacified salioliths (not present in this patient). Filling begins in the AP plane, and once contrast reaches the hilum, the patient's head is repositioned for lateral views. The sialographer must be aware of digital sensations of decreased ductal compliance or stenoses to avoid excess injection pressure that could result in contrast extravasations. (*B*) AP sialographic view of the initial filling of the buccal segment of right Stensen's duct (*black arrow*) using Ethiodol contrast.

the hilum, patients are turned to the lateral position and the remainder of the examination filmed with lateral views.

There are two major phases of contrast filling in conventional sialography: ductal and acinar (**Fig. 9**). The ductal phase constitutes the majority of filling and consists of filling the major duct, hilum, and secondary and tertiary ducts. Acinar filling is achieved with contrast "blush" of the parenchyma and, before the advent of cross-sectional imaging techniques, was the preferred method for evaluation of salivary gland parenchyma. In diagnostic sialography performed for sialoendoscopic purposes, the acinar phase is not performed; filling is completed with contrast opacification of the tertiary ducts or as much as ductal pathology permits. Typically, parotid ducts can be sufficiently opacified with 1 to 2 mL of contrast, whereas the submandibular ducts may require as much as 3 to 5 mL of contrast. At completion of filling, the catheter is removed; patients are administered a sialogogue (typically approximately 1 to 2 ounces/approximately 30 mL undiluted lemon juice) that is expectorated. Post-evacuation AP and lateral views are obtained to evaluate the presence or absence of

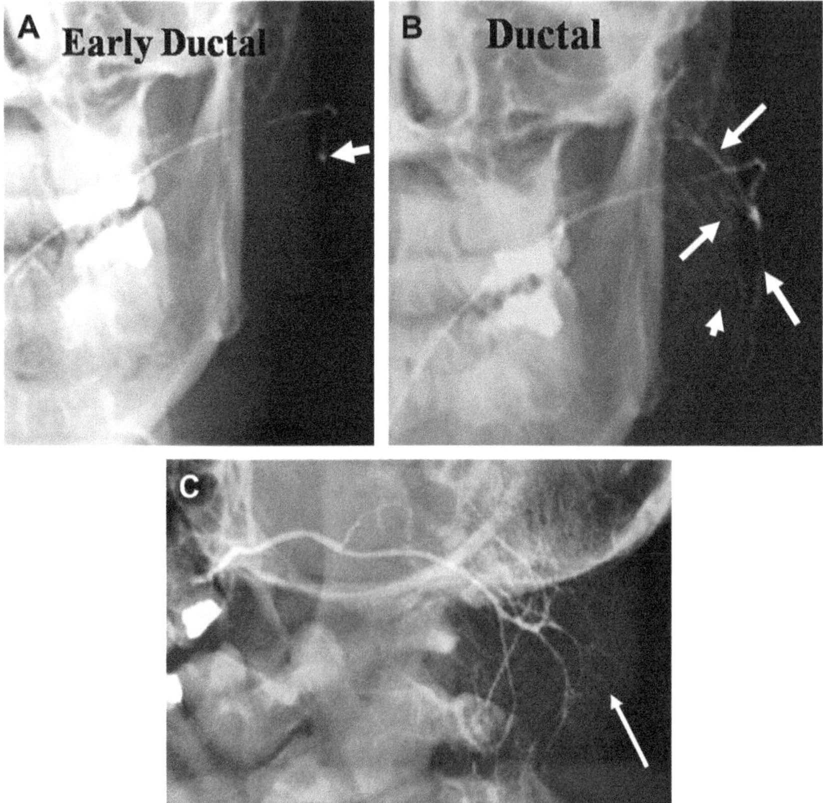

Fig. 9. (*A*) AP sialographic view of early ductal filling of the buccal, masseteric and intraparenchymal segments of left Stensen's duct to the hilum of the parotid gland (*white arrow*). (*B*) AP sialographic view of ductal filling of the secondary ducts (*white arrows*) and teritary ducts (*white arrowhead*). (*C*) Lateral sialographic view of acinar filling obtained by filling beyond the secondary and teritary ducts to achieve a contrast "blush" of the acini (*white arrow*).

contrast retention. Retention of contrast in the main duct or secondary/tertiary ducts in the absence of obstruction or significant stenosis is indicative of sialoparesis that may benefit from sialoendoscopic lavage.

Traditional conventional sialographic techniques use digital subtraction techniques to mask out the underlying osseous structures that limit visualization of the ductal and acinar phases.[2–4] Conventional sialography performed for sialoendoscopy at the author's institution does not use digital subtraction techniques. Although the author's interpretation provides a quantitative roadmap from the orifice of obstruction, stenosis, or kinks, it is nevertheless useful to retain anatomic landmarks on the sialographic image for co-localizing the endoscope tip intraoperatively.

There are several sialographic findings relevant to sialoendoscopy, including calcified sialolithiasis; noncalcified obstructive lesions, including fibrin or mucous plugs; granulomatous collections on ductal walls; stenosis; stricture; and significant kinks in the duct. Calcified sialoliths are found more commonly in Wharton's duct due to increased alkalinity of submandibular saliva, increased calcium and phosphate concentration, and increased mucin content.[5] Calcified sialoliths are most commonly found at the mylohyoid turn of the duct at the unicate (deep lobe) of the submandibular gland (**Fig. 10**) due predominately to the relative stasis at this approximately 90° turn. Calcified sialoliths are likewise commonly encountered at the orifice to Wharton's duct. The size of the calcified sialolith is most accurately measured on conventional sialography or CT and provides an indication as to whether or not basket retrieval or laser lithotripsy is a more suitable approach (**Fig. 11**). Noncalcified obstructions due to fibrin or mucous plugs are more commonly encountered in Stensen's duct and secondary ducts of the parotid, although they are also found with Wharton's duct and the submandibular secondary ducts. On conventional sialography, these appear as radiolucent filling defects within the lumen or extending from the sidewall (**Fig. 12**). Granulomatous deposits on the sidewall are seen as irregular linear- or lenticular-shaped areas of radiolucency along the ductal wall (**Fig. 13**). Significant

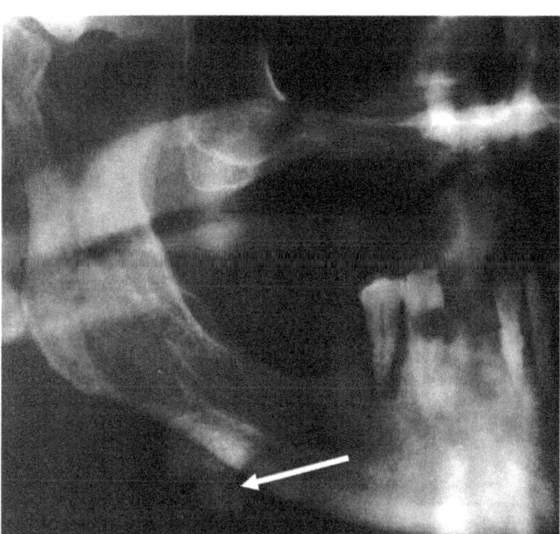

Fig. 10. Plain film radiograph demonstrating a large calcified sialolith (*white arrow*) involving the mylohyoid turn of Wharton's duct and the uncinate (deep) lobe of the submandibular gland. A stone of this size at the turn would require likely require laser fragmentation with forceps or basket retrieval, extacorpreal shockwave lithotripsy, or an open intraoral approach.

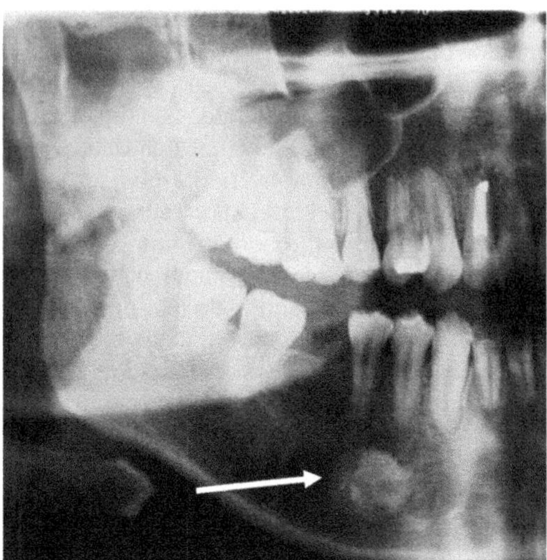

Fig. 11. Plain film radiograph of a large stone in right Wharton's duct. The magnification of this panoramic radiograph overestimates the size of the stone and the superimposition of structures necessitates differentiation from intra-alveolar pathology. Nevertheless, this stone measured greater than 1 cm in dimension, which would likely require shock wave fragmentation or an open intraoral approach.

stenosis at the orifice (**Fig. 14**) precludes sialoendoscopy without papillotomy. Stenosis may occur anywhere from the orifice to the hilum. The location, relative degree of stenosis, and segmental length of the stenosis dictate the choice of balloon for balloon dilatation (**Fig. 15**). Kinks are severe serpentine bends in the duct, which potentially impair advancement of the endoscope (**Fig. 16**).[6] These occur as a result of chronic sialodochitis and significant kinks are often associated with proximal or distal stenosis, stricture, and dilatation. The degree and location of the kink assists in determining whether or not ductoplasty or balloon recontouring is indicated. Severe segmental kinks may limit sialoendoscopy to diagnostic localization only (**Fig. 17**).

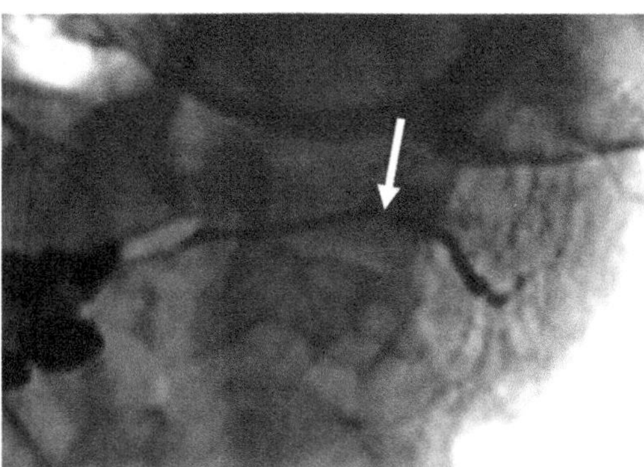

Fig. 12. Lateral sialographic view of left Stensen's duct showing an intraluminal filling defect (*white arrow*) which was not calcified on spot films. Note the well-delineated margins of the defect and the surrounding beaded appearance of the remaining proximal segments of the duct. This is an appearance typical of mucous/fibrin plugs.

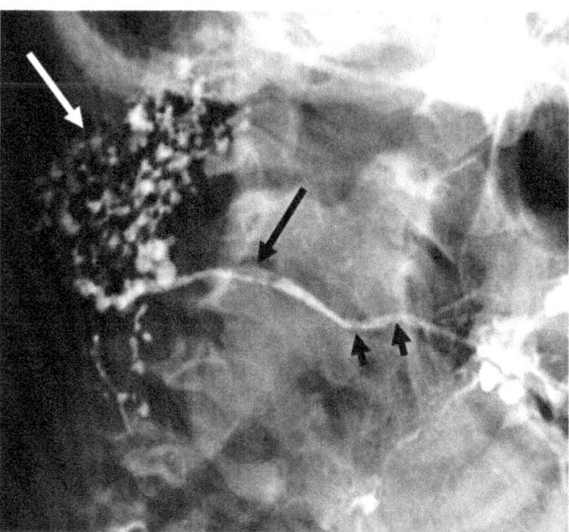

Fig. 13. Lateral sialographic view of a patient with a large lenticular-shaped filling defect extending from the sidewall of the masseteric segment (*black arrow*), representing significant granulomatous deposits in this patient with sarcoid. Note the mucous plugs/fibrin plugs in the buccal segment (*short black arrow*) and the extensive acinar atrophy with cavitary sialoectasia (*white arrow*).

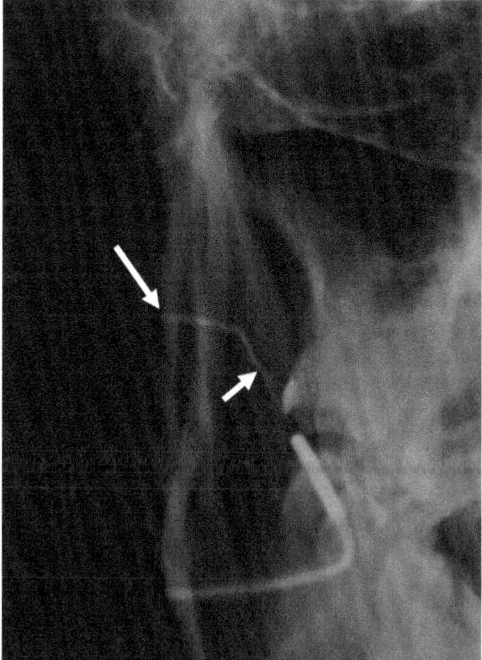

Fig. 14. AP sialographic view of a patient with significant stenosis of right Stensen's duct. The catheter is a 27 Ranfac; this patient was maximally dilated to a size 00 lacrimal probe. The orifice dimension is approximately 1 mm (*short arrow*) and although the buccal segment marginally widens, there is complete stenosis at the buccal turn (*long arrow*). This patient would require aggressive dilation under sedation or general anesthesia or papillotomy to insert the sialoendoscope. The complete stenosis would likely require balloon dilation or possibly ductoplasty and stenting.

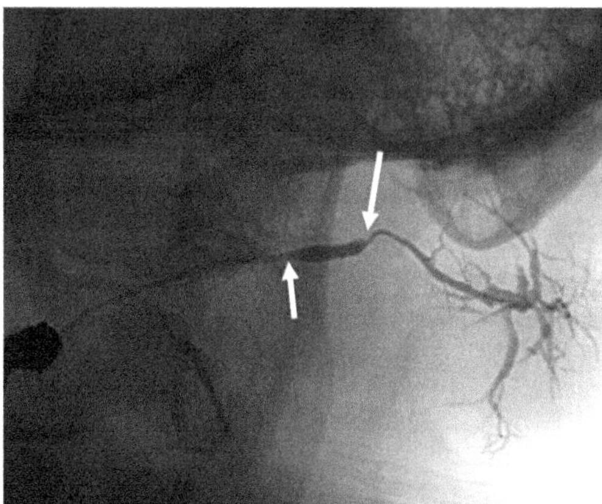

Fig. 15. Lateral sialographic view of a patient with stricture (*white arrows*) on either side of a moderate segment of dilation in the masseteric segment of Stensen's duct and a mild kink at the proximal intraparenchymal segment. These findings suggest stenoses that could be successfully addressed with soft balloon dilation.

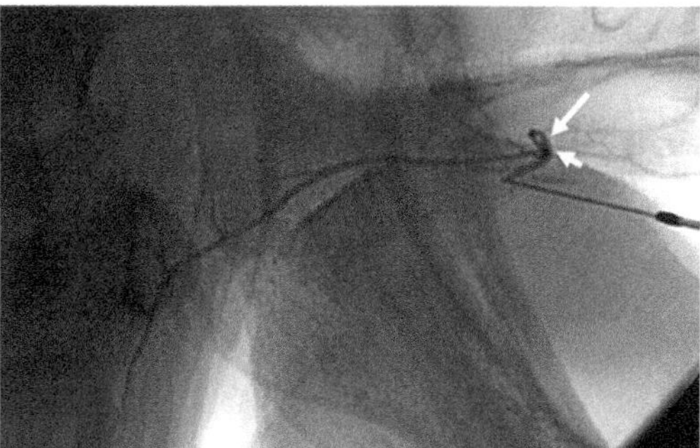

Fig. 16. Lateral sialographic view of right Stensen's duct with a severe kink in the buccal segment (*short arrow*) such that it folds back on itself (*long arrow*). Severe kinks, such as this, may be most amenable to advancement dochoplasty.

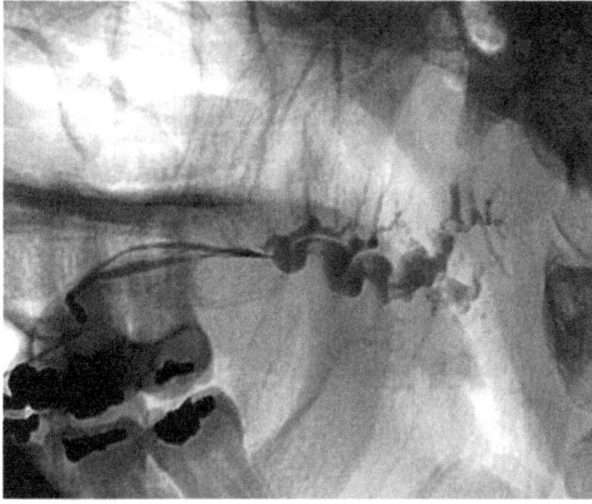

Fig. 17. Lateral sialographic view of left Stensen's duct with severe sialodochitis and multiple severe kinks involving the entire masseteric and intraparenchymal segments. The number and severity of kinks in this patient would likely preclude sialoendoscopy.

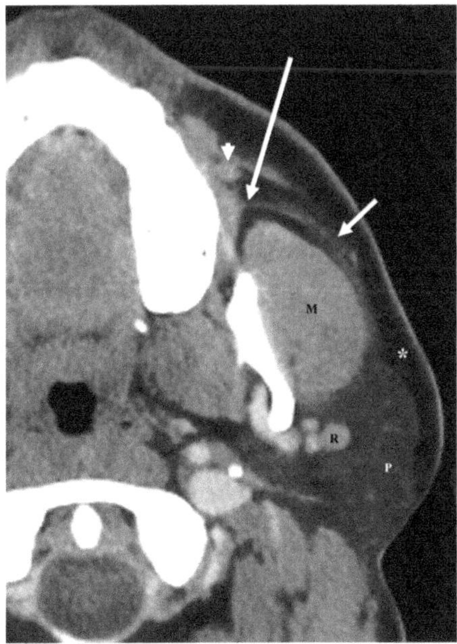

Fig. 18. Axial contrast-enhanced CT view of a normal left Stensen's duct and parotid. Stensen's duct emerges through the buccinator muscle (*long arrow*) immediately posterior to the anterior facial vein (*arrowhead*). Note that the masseteric segment of the duct is surrounded by accessory parotid gland (*short arrow*). On contrast-enhanced CT, the parotid parenchyma (P) is hypodense relative to muscle (M, masseter muscle) and slightly hyperdense to surrounding subcutaneous fat (*). Multiple small secondary ducts are visualized as thin, wispy enhancing strands within the parenchyma (R, retromandibular vein).

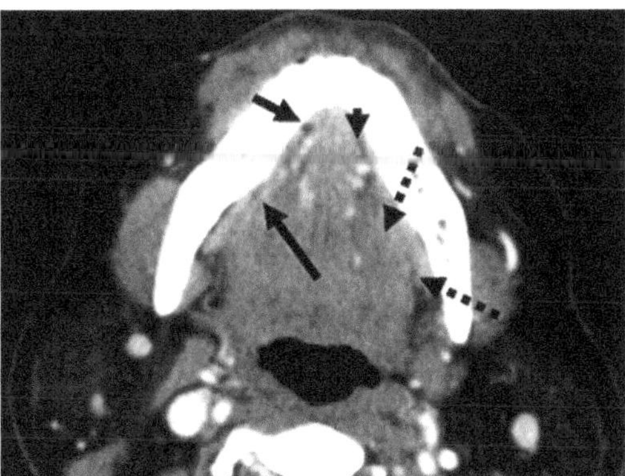

Fig. 19. Axial contrast-enhanced CT. The right Wharton's duct is mildly dilated with thickening and enhancement of the ductal walls (*long arrow*). Note the dilated orifice (*short arrow*). Compare the right side to the normal left Wharton's duct at the orifice (*arrowhead*) and remaining segments of the duct as it traverses through the sublingual space and over the posterior edge of the mylohyoid (*dashed arrows*).

CT

CT examinations are used routinely in North America as the modality of choice for evaluation of the salivary parenchyma and ductal systems. Ultrasonography remains the modality of choice as the first-line noninvasive technique for assessing an acute sialoadenitis or parotitis (for a complete discussion of the applications of ultrasonography, see the article by Katz and colleagues elsewhere in this issue).

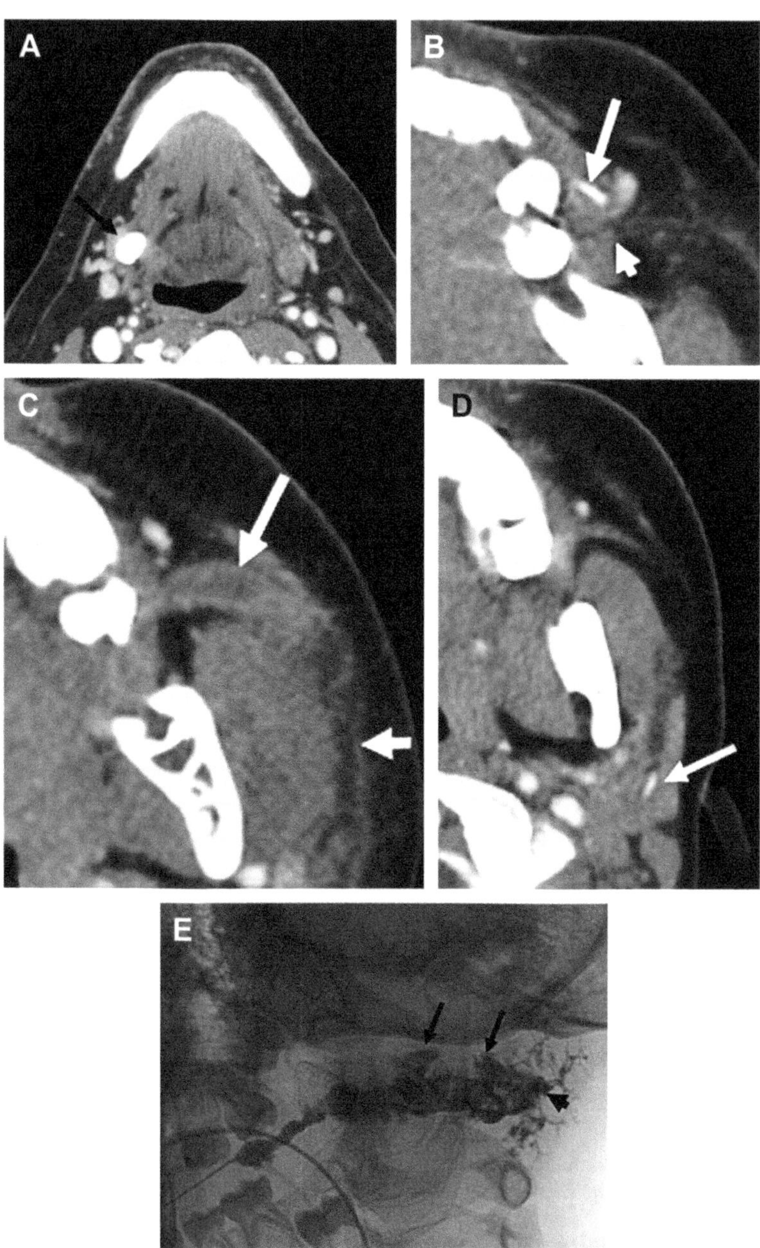

Conventional CT

CT examinations of the salivary glands are performed, in the author's institution, using helical or multidetector/multichannel techniques. Contiguous, axial, thin 2-mm slices are typically acquired from the skull base to the aortic arch as part of a neck examination and the images reformatted at 1 mm for display. On CT systems where multiplanar reformats are not possible or not ideal, axial images should be acquired parallel to the occlusal plane of the maxilla or the inferior border of the mandible to best visualize the course of Stensen's duct or Wharton's duct. Multiplanar reformats in appropriate systems are performed in the coronal and sagittal plane. The thin section technique is essential for visualization of the axial in-plane course of Stensen's duct or Wharton's duct (**Fig. 18**). On conventional contrast-enhanced CT, sialodochitis and some wall irregularities can be appreciated as increased thickening and enhancement of the ductal wall (**Fig. 19**).

Obstructions resulting from calcified sialoliths are evident as hyperdense nonenhancing masses having a typical Hounsfield unit in the range of bone, reflecting the calcified matrix components. Frequently there is associated dilatation of the duct. The location and size of sialoliths assist in predicting the sialoendoscopic approach; for example, a large stone at the mylohyoid turn with fibrosis may be extracted more efficaciously with laser lithotripsy than forceps in comparison to small clusters of stones near the orifice (**Fig. 20**).

Ductal obstruction is frequently associated with acute or chronic sialoadenitis. Acute sialoadenitis appears as increased enhancement of the gland on contrast-enhanced examinations, often with ductal dilatation (**Fig. 21**). The manifestation of chronic sialoadenitis due to the chronic inflammatory process and subsequent acinar atrophy is a smaller, "shrunken" gland, predominately of the superficial lobe (in parotid and submandibular glands) with relative increase in fat content (**Fig. 22**).

Ductal obstruction may more uncommonly result in the formation of sialoceles. A true siaocele appears as a focal cylindric or rounded dilatation of Stensen's duct, Wharton's duct, or a sublingual duct that may be an incidental finding or may present clinically as a palpable mass in the parotid or floor of the mouth (**Fig. 23**). False sialoceles are those sialoceles that have ruptured (**Fig. 24**).

Fig. 20. (*A*) Axial contrast-enhanced CT. The hyperdense ovoid mass (*arrow*) is a calcified sialolith located just at and inferior to the mylohyoid turn of the duct and involving the uncinate lobe of the submandibular gland. Note the absence of even a thin rim of ductal lumen surrounding the stone, suggestive of fibrotic adherence to the sidewalls. This stone measured 11 mm in greatest dimension making it amenable to endoscopic/laser fragmentation, shock wave lithotripsy, or an open intraoral approach. The fibrous adherence suggests that removal of the stone would leave a de-epithelialized duct segment after removal. (*B–D*) Axial contrast-enhanced CT images in a 5-year-old girl with symptoms of left parotid obstructive sialoadenitis. (*B*) The linear hyperdensity adjacent to the anterior facial vein (*long arrow*) is a displaced calcified sialolith that has penetrated through the wall of the duct (*arrowhead*). (*C*) Axial slice superior to B demonstrates dilation of the buccal (*long arrow*) and masseteric (*short arrow*) segments. (*D*) Axial contrast-enhanced CT obtained 2 months after the images shown in (*B–C*) shows that the sialolith has migrated to the hilum (*arrow*). (*E*) Conventional sialogram at an outside institution obtained approximately 4 days after the initial CT in (*B*) shows marked irregular dilation and severe sialodochitis of the masseteric and intraparenchymal segments. There is extravasation of contrast (*long arrows*) from weakened ductal walls that partially obscures the sialolith displaced by contrast injection during the sialogram (*arrowhead*).

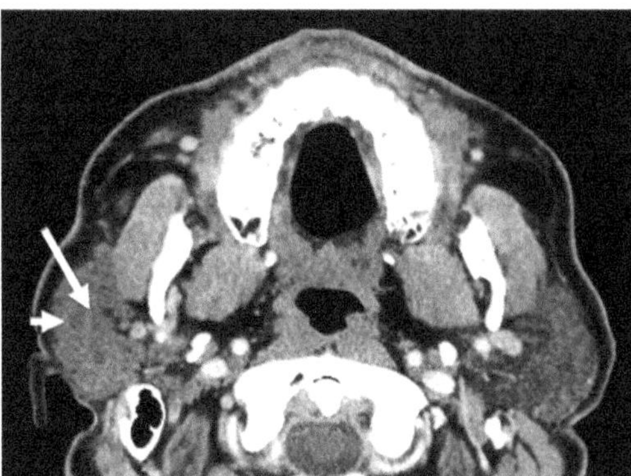

Fig. 21. Axial contrast-enhanced CT in adult male patient with symptoms of obstructive sialoadenitis illustrates the typical CT appearance of acute parotid obstructive sialoadenitis: hypderdensity of the parotid parencyhma, dilation of the intraparenchymal segment of Stensen's duct (*long arrow*), and other areas of secondary ductal dilation (*short arrow*) or early abscess formation.

CT Sialography

The combination of sialographic contrast of the ducts and the ability to evaluate the parenchyma in fine detail led to the development of CT sialography soon after CT techniques became widely available.[7–10] As with conventional sialography, a sialographic catheter is inserted into the orifice of the duct and the duct opacified with a contrast agent (**Fig. 25**). Images are acquired in the axial plane and, with multiplanar techniques, may be reformatted in orthogonal planes. The choice of contrast agent is important for CT sialography and should be performed with water-soluble, low-osmolar CT contrast agents (Omnipaque or Isovue) instead of Ethiodol. Although iodine concentrations are equivalent among the different radiographic contrast

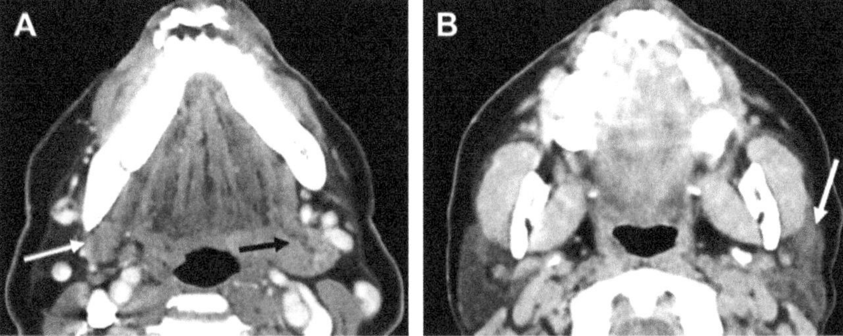

Fig. 22. Axial contrast-enhanced CT in two different patients. (*A*) Chronic sialoadenitis in the right submandibular gland demonstrated as smaller, hypodense gland (*white arrow*) reflecting fatty atrophy. The left submandibular gland (*black arrow*) is asymmetrically enlarged (accounting for patient rotation) and hyperdense with a dilatated hilum and duct reflecting an acute sialoadenitis. (*B*) Chronic sialoadenitis with acinar atrophy in the parotid glands may appear as a more hyperdense and smaller gland (*arrow*) due to fibrosis of the normal adipose tissue.

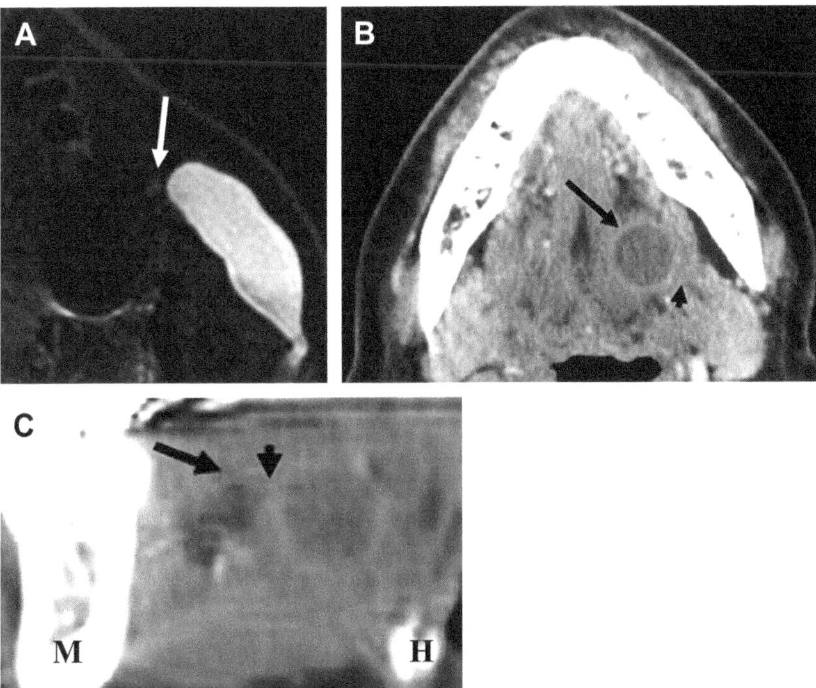

Fig. 23. (*A*) Axial STIR MR image shows a fusiform-shaped hyperintense mass in a patient presenting with a relatively acute onset of a left cheek swelling. The mass is a sialocele identified by smooth dilation of the masseteric segment of left Stensen's duct resulting from stricture and obstruction in the buccal segment (*arrow*). (*B*) Axial contrast-enhanced CT of a sialocele in a patient with a suspected mass in the floor of the mouth. The sialocele is seen as a circular rim-enhancing mass at the posterior aspect of the left sublingual space (*long arrow*); the dilated proximal segments of Wharton's duct are seen posterior to the mass (*arrowhead*). Sagittal reformats (*C*) reveal that the sialocele is contiguous with the distal segment of Wharton's duct (*arrow*) and the focal stricture at the anterior lip of the mass (*arrowhead*). H, hyoid; M, mandible.

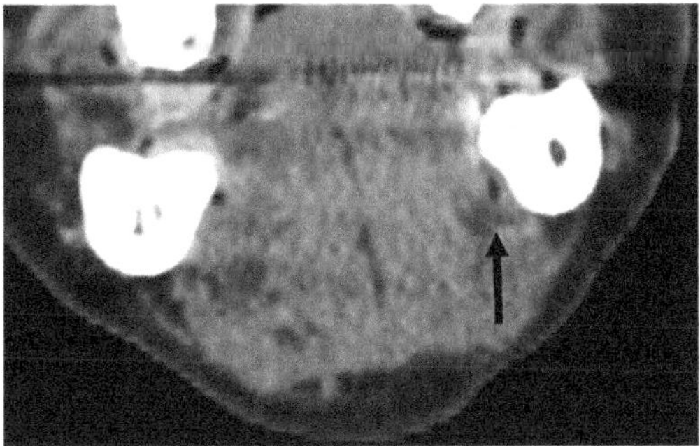

Fig. 24. Coronal contrast-enhanced CT in a patient with a false sialocele. The well-circumscribed fluid collection (*arrow*) in the sublingual space does not have a hyperdense or enhancing rim reflecting rupture of the submandibular ductal wall. The lack of dental pathology (not shown) differentiates this from a sublingual pheglmon of odontogenic origin.

agents, the lower viscosity of Ethiodol compared with the CT agents results in higher density of contrast material that may potentially obscure the duct and surrounding structures, especially with thin section technique. CT sialography, however, for all its potential advantages over conventional sialography, is not routinely performed. The intravenous administration of contrast done with a conventional CT examination typically provides adequate visualization of the main duct and, furthermore, the inability to dynamically visualize filling of the ducts with hand pressure of the syringe in CT sialography may lead to overfilling of the ducts and subsequent rupture.

MRI

The introduction of MRI in the early 1980s significantly enhanced the radiographic diagnosis of salivary gland disorders. The superior tissue contrast with MRI permits excellent discrimination of the parenchyma and ductal structures, and the use of fluid-sensitive pulse sequences allows for noninvasive sialography. MRI examinations of the salivary glands are best performed at higher field strengths (>1.0 T), as ductal structures are not well visualized at low field strengths (eg, as typically used in the majority of open magnetic resonance [MR] systems). In the author's institution, evaluation of ductal obstruction are conducted at 1.5 T or 3.0 T using standard T1- and T2-weighted pulse sequences before and after the administration of gadolinum contrast and with fat-suppression techniques. Images are obtained with contiguous thin sections (3 mm) acquired in the axial plane, again oriented along the occlusal plane of the maxilla or the inferior border of the mandible. Heavily T2-weighted images with fat suppression (short tau inversion recovery [STIR]) provide excellent visualization of fluid within the ducts and are sensitive to even small obstructions or strictures (ie, approximately 1 to 3 mm at 1.5 T). Newer pulse sequences that are fluid sensitive and allow 3-D volume acquisitions are used for MR sialography (discussed later).

The normal parotid glands are T1 isointense to mildly hyperintense to muscle (without fat suppression) and mild to moderately T2 hypointense. On T2-weighted sequences, Stensen's duct is mildly hyperintense to the adjacent buccal space and masseter muscle. Asymmetric hypertensity in the duct in symptomatic patients without dilatation may reflect slow flow or relative sialoparesis. On STIR images, the

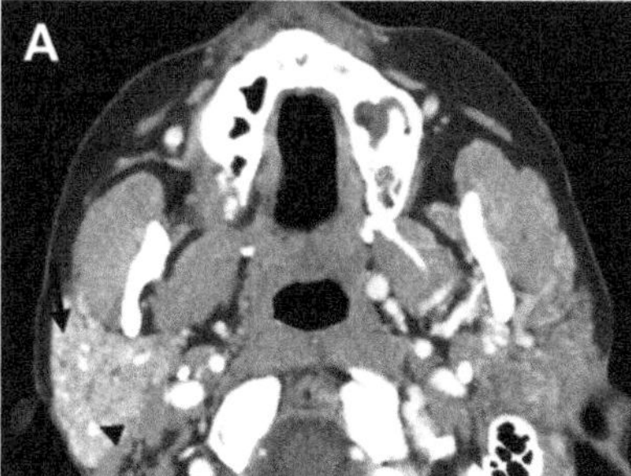

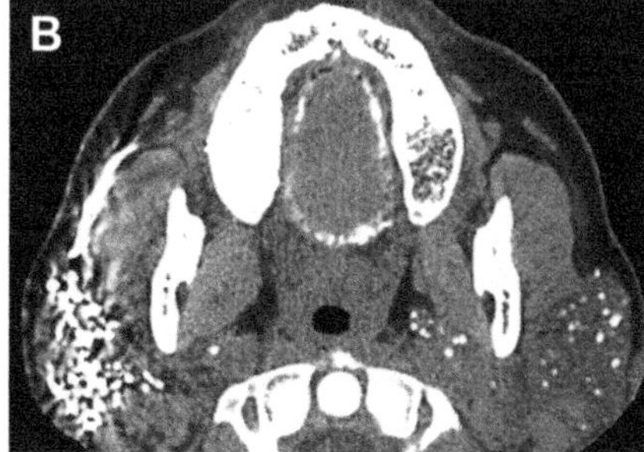

Fig. 25. (*A*) Axial image of CT sialogram of the right parotid gland using a water-soluble CT contrast agent (Isovue). Note the granular appearance of acinar enhancement (*arrow*) and contrast within secondary ducts (*arrowhead*).(*B*) Axial CT in a different patient immediately after conventional sialogram using Ethiodol as the contrast agent. Note that the greater viscosity of Ethiodol results in significant beam hardening artifact seen as streak artifact in the subcutaneous tissue and multiple focal black defects around the opacified secondary ducts.

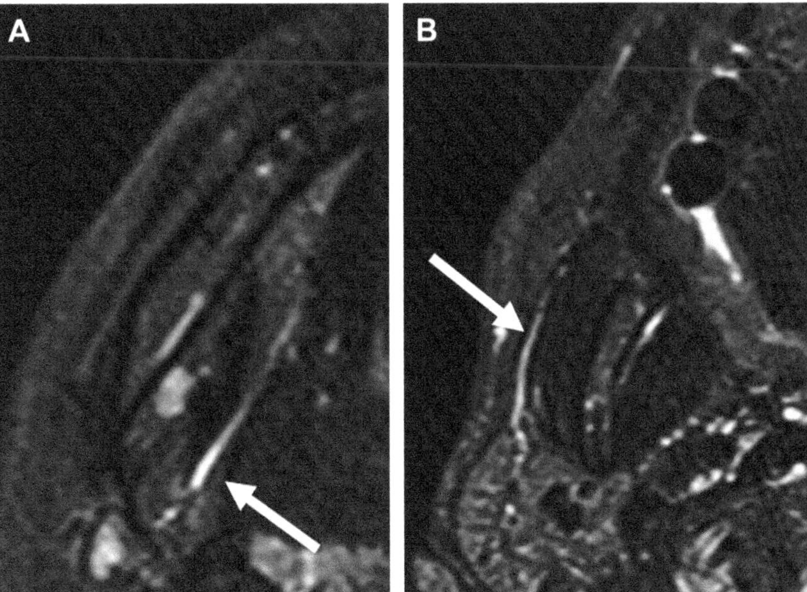

Fig. 26. Axial STIR MRIs in two different patients illustrate the normal hyperintense fluid signal of salivary ducts (*A*) in the submandibular duct as it exits the uncinate lobe (*arrow*) and enters the sublingual space and (*B*) in the masseteric segment of the parotid duct (*arrow*).

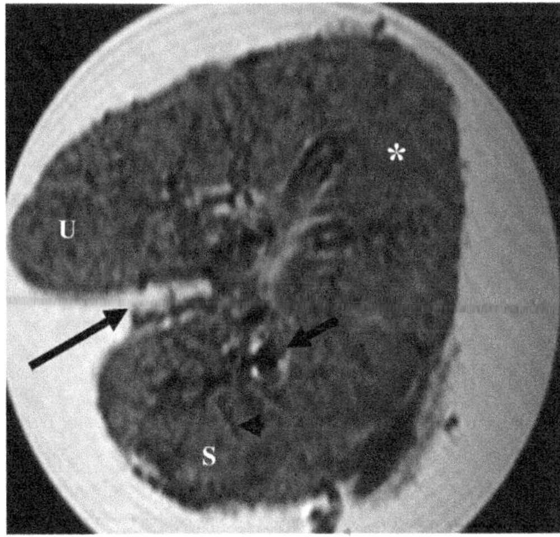

Fig. 27. Sagittal T2-weighted image of a normal human submandibular gland obtained at 9.4 T. The cleft for the mylohyoid muscle (*long arrow*) separates the smaller deep or uncinate lobe (U) from the larger superficial lobe (S). Note the secondary ducts emerging from the hilum, seen end on (*short arrow*), and the multiple branching tertiary ducts (*arrowhead*). Ductal arborization is more extensive in the superficial lobe. The granular appearance of the parenchyma (*) is due to the capability at this field strength to visualize the acinar units.

ducts are uniformly hyperintense (**Fig. 26**). The submandibular glands, due to their relatively decreased fat content compared with the parotid glands, are isointense to mildly hypointense to muscle on T1-weighted images and mildly hyperintense on T2-weighted images. The C-shaped configuration of the submandibular gland and the relationship of the main duct and secondary ducts is most readily appreciated on MRI obtained with very high resolution at high field strength (9.4 T; **Fig. 27**).

Although MR provides superior soft tissue contrast, ductal obstruction due to calcified sialoliths, fibrin, or mucous plugs cannot be differentiated, nor can they be differentiated from air. This is due to the similar magnetic susceptibility profile of mineralized tissue, fibrous tissue, and air in MR irrespective of the tissue weighting (T1 or T2) or the pulse sequence used. The magnetic susceptibility effects, in addition, overestimate the size of a calcified sialolith, from approximately 10% to 30%, depending on the pulse sequence used (**Fig. 28**). Susceptibility effects are reduced with spin-echo pulse sequences (eg, often used for most T1- and T2- weighted images in the head and neck) compared with gradient-echo techniques (more commonly applied to brain imaging). Overestimation of the size of a calcified sialolith may have an impact on sialoendoscopic treatment planning in terms of forceps or basket retrevial versus lithotripsy or sialoadenectomy; however, the overestimation error typically results in a favorable outcome when encountering a smaller obstruction than planned. Despite size errors in MRI of sialolithiasis, the advantage of MR tissue contrast permits

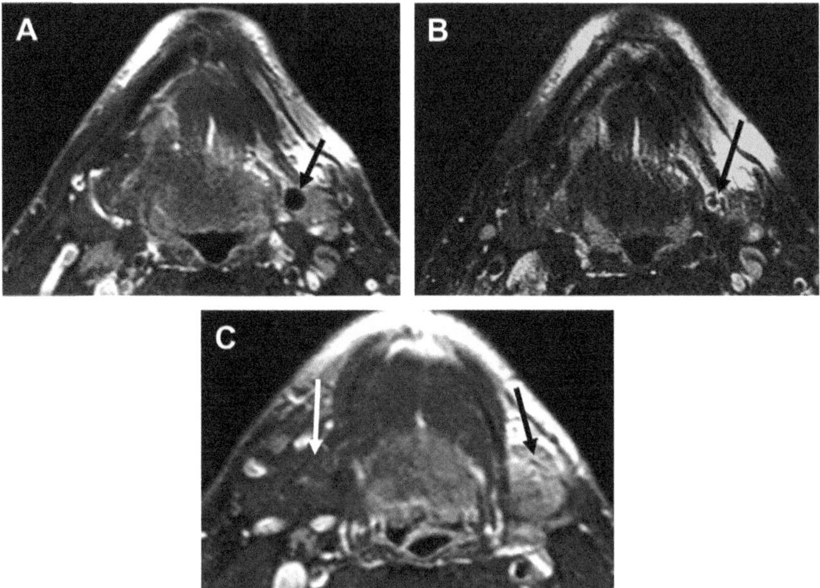

Fig. 28. (*A*) Axial T1-weighted MR with fat suppression through the submandibular glands shows the susceptibility artifact of a sialolith seen as a dark signal void in the uncinate portion of the left submandibular gland (*arrow*). (*B*) On axial STIR images in the same patient, the surrounding inflammatory response with fluid folding around the stone is apparent (*arrow*). (*C*) Axial, T1-weighted, contrast-enhanced images more inferiorly through the submandibular glands show the diffusely increased enhancement of the left submandibular gland superficial lobe (*black arrow*) indicative of acute sialoadenitis. Compare with the normal right submandibular gland (*white arrow*).

improved delineation of surrounding inflammatory responses to the sialolith (see **Fig. 28**). Moreover, the extent of the accompanying sialoadenitis is accurately assessed using the standard combinations of T1 weighting, T2 weighting, and contrast enhancement (see **Fig. 28**).[11,12]

Magnetic Resonance Sialography

MR sialography uses noninvasive methods to characterize the ductal architecture of the parotid and submandibular glands. Although cannulation of the duct with infusion of a MR contrast agent produces a MR sialogram, this is not performed as the wide availability of fluid-sensitive sequences obviates ductal cannulation. MR sialography using fluid-sensitive techniques was first described in 1996 by Lomas and colleagues[13] using RARE sequences that use long echo times such that nearly all of the tissue contrast is produced by static fluid as found in ducts. Subsequent efforts capitalized on improvements in 2-D and 3-D multislab imaging techniques for fluid-sensitive sequences (CISS, HASTE, EXPRESS) to better delineate the secondary and tertiary ductal architecture.[14–16] All of these sequences derive their contrast from the intrinsic hyperintensity of static fluid on heavily T2-weighted images; the differences in sequences arise primarily in the ability to resolve the main duct at more severe turns and the ability to resolve secondary and teriatry ductal structure. Regardless of the relative advantages or disadvantages of each sequence, comparison of MR sialography with conventional sialography in several studies demonstrates that MR sialographic techniques are generally as accurate as conventional sialography in detecting obstructions, stenosis, and stricture of the main duct.[16–18] In addition, the application of small surface coils increases the conspicuity of smaller obstructions and secondary and teritary ducts.[18–21] The more recent advances of 3-D volumetric techniques and the ability to reformat images with maximum intensity projection (MIP) permits the ability to generate virtual endoscopy views from the MR data.[22,23]

MR sialography at the author's institution is performed at 1.5 T and 3.0 T using conventional T1- and T2-weighted sequences with and without contrast, using a standard circular polarized transmit-receive coil or multichannel phased-array head coils.

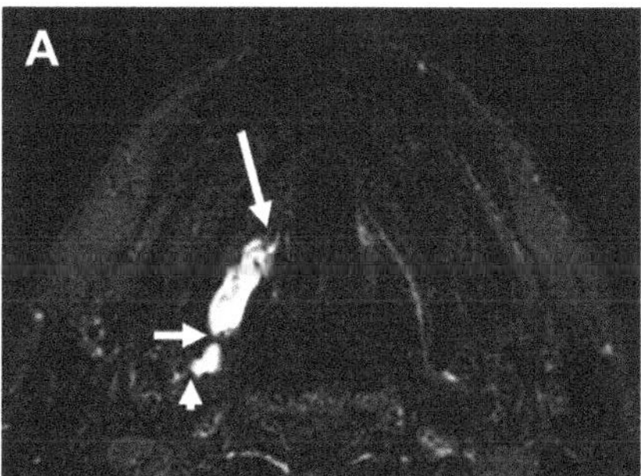

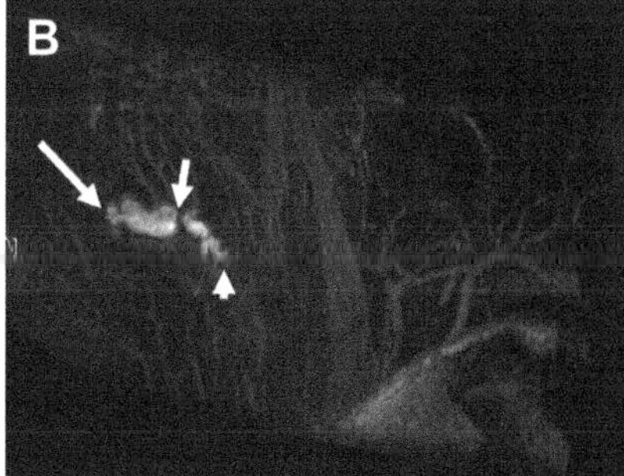

Fig. 29. (*A*) Axial SPACE images from a MR sialogram of the right submandibular gland in a patient with acute obstructive sialoadenitis. There is a small stone proximal to the orifice (*long arrow*) with dilation extending along the remaining sublingual segment of the duct and a significant stricture just proximal to the mylohyoid turn (*short arrow*). An additional stone at the mylohyoid turn (*arrowhead*), although relatively small, completely obstructs the remaining segment of the duct. (*B*) Sagittal MIP reconstruction of the image in (*A*). The MIP reconstructions generate the typical sialographic view in a 3-D volume that may better display, for endoscopic surgeons, the relationship between the obstructions caused by the stone and the associated areas of stenosis or stricture.

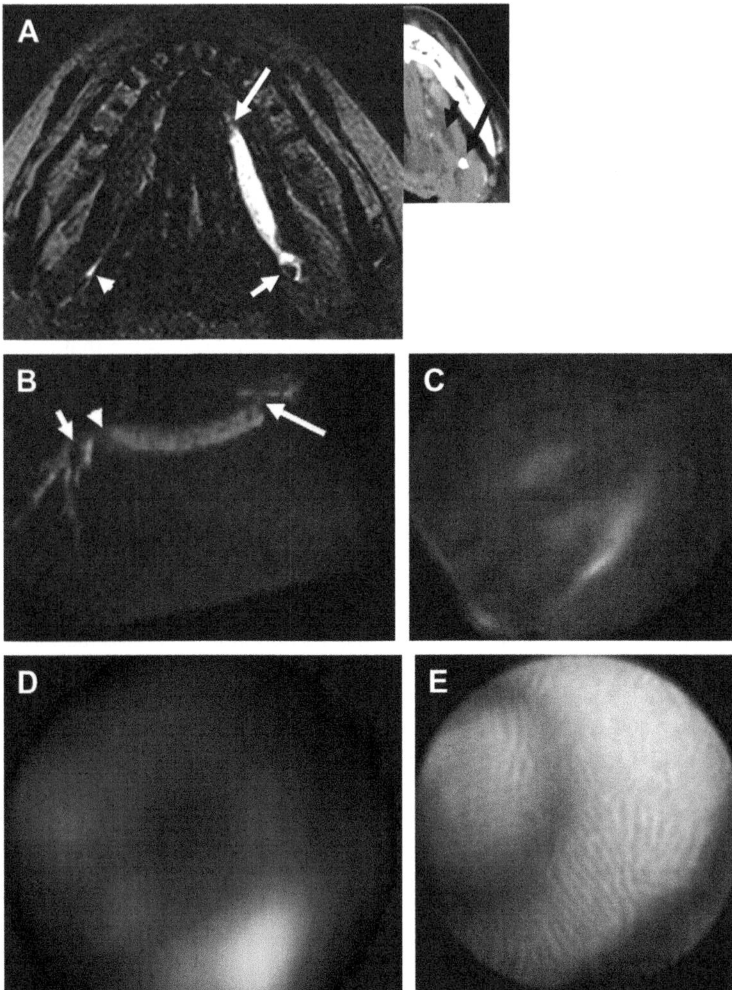

Fig. 30. (*A*) Axial SPACE image from a MR sialogram of the left submandibular gland in a patient with acute obstructive sialoadenitis. There is a significant stricture proximal to the orifice (*long arrow*) and significant dilation of the remaining sublingual segments. As is commonly found, there is a calcified sialolith at the mylohyoid turn (*short arrows*). (*Inset*) The calcification of the stone (*long black arrow*) and the dilation of the sublingual segments (*short black arrow*) are appreciated on the contrast-enhanced CT in the same patient. Compare the dilation and fluid content of the left submandibular duct to the normal right side (*arrowhead*). (*B*) Sagittal MIP reconstruction demonstrates more clearly the stricture near the orifice (*long arrow*), the stone and surrounding fluid (*short arrow*). Just distal to the stone is an area of stenosis (*arrowhead*). (*C*) Virtual MR endoscopic view of the stenosis in B, shown at the point of the arrowhead. The depression at the center of the image is the stenosis. This virtual endoscopic view was post-processed using a combination of log and spline function modeling which accentuates the 3-D effect of the fluid and thickened walls in the duct surrounding the stenosis. (*D*) Virtual MR endoscopic view of the stone seen in A and B. The dark circular area at the center of the image is the stone. The white-orange area around the stone is the surrounding hyperintense signal fluid and thickened ductal walls seen in A and B. (*E*) Intraoperative sialoendoscopic view of the same patient showing the stone at the center of the duct and the surrounding ductal walls.

Axial STIR images are acquired for better detection of ductal obstructions. 3-D SPACE images (Siemens Medical Corp, Erlangen, Germany) are acquired to generate multiplanar reformatted sialographic views of the ductal architecture (**Fig. 29**). The SPACE sequence is a single slab 3-D (turbo spin-echo) fluid-sensitive sequence that permits high-resolution 3-D reformats of the ductal system by virtue of the isotropic acquisition. The high resolution combined with 3-D techniques results in MR sialograms that not only provide accurate mapping of obstructions (**Fig. 30**A, B) but also are sufficiently sensitive to detect small strictures and stenoses (**Fig. 31**) or graft patency (**Fig. 32**). Finally, these 3-D techniques are capable of rendering virtual endoscopic views (see **Fig. 30**C–E). At present, however, virtual MR endoscopy is limited due to the inability of currently available software packages to generate accurate endoscopic views of small or mildly dilated ducts. Although these limitations may be offset by improvements in software and the use of small surface coils, the small clinical population available renders the routine application of virtual MR endoscopy impractical.

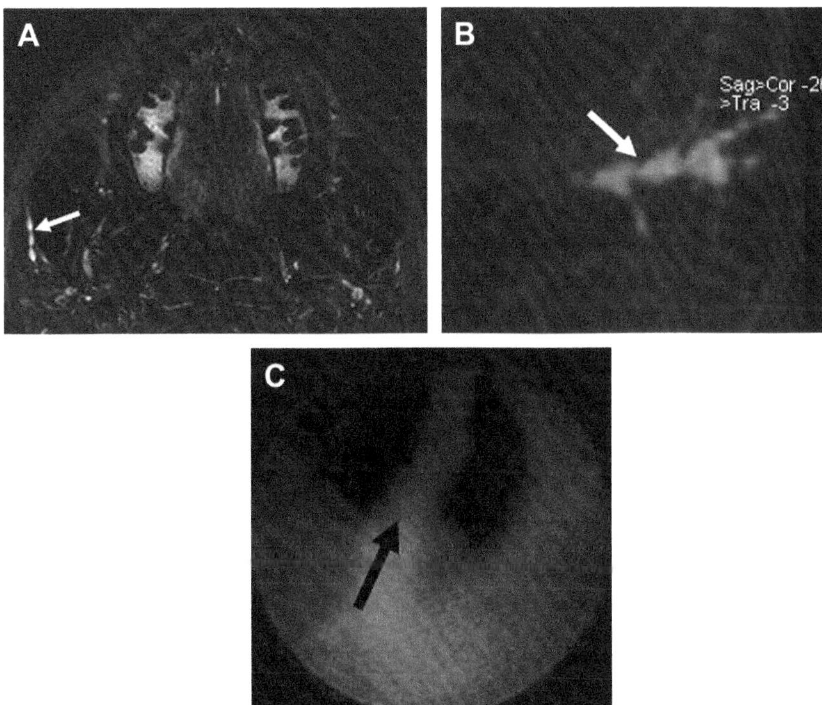

Fig. 31. (*A*) Axial SPACE image from a MR sialogram in a patient with symptoms of mild obstructive sialoadenitis. The string-of-beads appearance (*arrow*) in the intraparenchymal segment of right Stensen's duct is a classic appearance of sialodochitis. (*B*) Sagittal MIP reconstruction of right Stensen's duct reveals the stenoses to consist of a repeating pattern of arrowhead-shaped constrictions: this particular configuration is suggestive of synchia rather than areas of stricture (which would demonstrate a beaded appearance). Thus, rather than considering a balloon approach, these images suggest forceps reduction may be necessary. (*C*) Intraoperative sialoendoscopic view of the same patient confirms the presence of vertical synchia (*arrow*).

COMPARISON OF TECHNIQUES

Conventional sialography, contrast-enhanced CT, and MR sialography all may be used to preoperatively assess the salivary ductal system before sialoendscopy. **Table 1** lists the advantages and disadvantages of each technique.

Although conventional sialographic techniques confer many advantages over CT and MRI, the invasiveness of the procedure and exposure to ionizing radiation (with doses that may exceed those of CT) compels the development of alternative noninvasive and nonionizing or dose-reducing ionizing radiation techniques. Contrast-enhanced CT, despite limitations in current techniques, holds promise with the continuing development of multidetector systems with high spatial resolution, improvements in contrast resolution, and multiplanar reformat capabilities. Virtual CT endoscopy for the airways and gastrointestinal tract is now a widely available technique; however, virtual CT endoscopy of the salivary ducts has not gained wide acceptance due to the small ductal dimensions that impart insufficient air-tissue contrast for generation of virtual endoscopic views. Nevertheless, improvements with multidetector systems and segmentation algorithms in the near future should make CT-based virtual sialoendoscopy a reality. Finally, in MRI, the increasing use of high field-strength systems, coupled with the use of surface, mutltichannel phased array, or dual-tuned (multinuclear) coils and improvements in static-dynamic fluid imaging with newer pulse sequences should position MR sialoendoscopy as the modality of choice for the future.

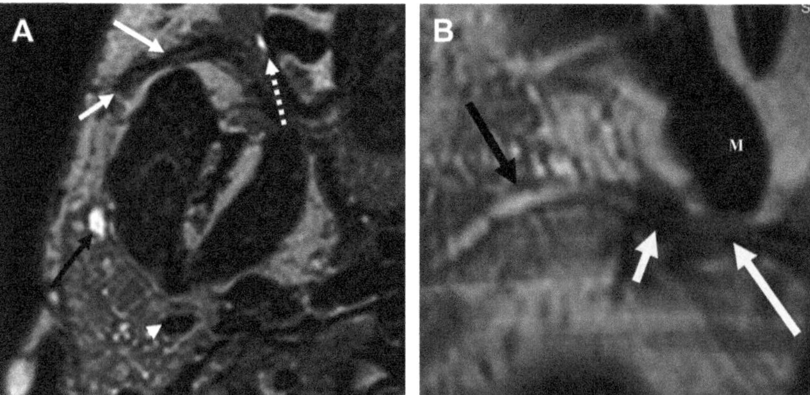

Fig. 32. (*A*) Axial SPACE image from a MR sialogram in patient after vein graft of the right parotid duct. The vein graft is seen as the relatively hypointense tubular structure extending from the buccinator muscle to the masseteric segment (*long white arrow*). Note this has the same appearance as the retromandibular vein (*arrowhead*). The anastomosis is seen at the junction of the buccal and masseteric segments (*short white arrow*). The remaining masseteric and intraparenchymal segments of the parotid duct are seen as mildly dilated hyperintense areas (*long black arrow*), incompletely visualized in this single plane. Although no hyperintense fluid signal is seen in the vein graft due to greater compliance of the vein walls and supine position of the patient, fluid is seen in the buccal mucosal interface (*dashed white arrow*) indicating patent flow from the vein graft. (*B*) Sagittal MIP reconstruction shows the parotid duct (*long black arrow*), anastamosis (*short white arrow*), and vein graft (*long white arrow*) with patent lumen. M, masseter muscle. This patient was additionally examined after lemon stimulation, which resulted in bilateral parotid flow but no obstructive symptoms.

Table 1
Comparison of conventional sialography, contrast-enhanced CT, and magnetic resonance sialography

	Conventional Sialography	Contrast-Enhanced CT	Magnetic Resonance Sialography
Invasive procedure	Yes	No[a]	No
Ionizing radiation	Yes	Yes	No
Visualize all segments of duct in one plane	+	±	±
Relationship of duct to surrounding structure/ regional anatomy	–	+	+
Detection of calcified sialoliths	+	+	±
Detection of fibrin/mucous plugs	+	±	±
Visualization of stricture, stenosis, kinks	+	±	±
Availability	Widely available	Widely available	Moderately available
Cost	Relatively low	Moderate–high	High

[a] Excluding venipuncture for intravenous administration of contrast.
Abbreviations: +, yes; –, no; ±, incompleate visualization.

REFERENCES

1. O'Hare AE. Sialography: past, present, future. CRC Crit Rev Clin Radiol Nucl Med 1973;4(1):87–139.
2. Buckenham TM, George CD, McVicar D, et al. Digital sialography: imaging and intervention. Br J Radiol 1994;67(798):524–9.
3. Gmelin E, Hollands-Thorn B, Rinast E. Digital subtraction sialography. Laryngol Rhinol Otol (Stuttg). 1987;66(8):444–6.
4. Lightfoote JB, Friedenberg RM, Smolin MF. Digital subtraction ductography. AJR Am J Roentgenol 1985;144:635–8.
5. McGurk M, Escudier MP, Brown JE. Modern management of salivary calculi. Br J Surg 2005;92:107–12.
6. Nahlieli O, Shacham R, Yoffe B, et al. Diagnosis and treatment of strictures and kinks in salivary ducts. J Oral Maxillofac Surg 2001;59:484–90.
7. McGahan JP, Walter JP, Bernstein L. Evaluation of the parotid gland. Comparison of sialography, non contrast computed tomography and CT sialography. Radiology 1984;152:453–8.
8. Stone DN, Mancuso AA, Rice D, et al. Parotid CT sialography. Radiology 1981; 138:393–7.
9. Som PM, Biller HF. The combined CT-sialogram. Radiology 1980;135:387–90.
10. Szolar DH, Groell R, Preidler K, et al. Three-dimensional processing of ultrafast CT sialography for parotid masses. AJNR Am J Neuroradiol 1995;16:1889–93.
11. Yousem DM, Kraut MA, Chalian AA. Major salivary gland imaging. Radiology 2000;216:19–29.
12. Shah G. MR imaging of salivary glands. Neuroimaging Clin N Am 2004;14(4): 777–808.

13. Lomas DJ, Carroll NR, Antoun GJN, et al. MR sialography. Radiology 1996;200: 129–33.
14. Jäger L, Menauer F, Holzknect N, et al. Sialolithiasis: MR sialography of the submandibular duc—an alternative to conventional sialography and US. Radiology 2000;216:665–71.
15. Murakami R, Baba Y, Nishimura R, et al. MR sialography using Half-Fourier Acquisition Single Shot Turbo Spin Echo (HASTE) sequences. AJNR Am J Neuroradiol 1998;19:959–61.
16. Becker M, Marchal F, Becker C, et al. Sialolithiasis and salivary ductal stenosis: diagnostic accuracy of MR sialography with three-dimensional extended phase conjugate-symmetry rapid spin-echo sequence. Radiology 2000;217:347–58.
17. Kalinowski M, Heverhagen JT, Rehberg E, et al. Comparative study of MR sialography and digital subtraction sialography for benign salivary gland disorders. AJNR Am J Neuroradiol 2002;23:1485–92.
18. Varghese JC, Thornton F, Lucey BC, et al. A prospective comparative study of MR sialography and conventional sialography of salivary duct disease. AJR 1999;173:1497–503.
19. Fischbach R, Kugel H, Ernst S, et al. MR sialography: initial experience using a T2-Weighted fast SE sequence. J Comput Assist Tomogr 1997;21(5):826–30.
20. Ohbaysashi N, Yamada I, Yoshino N, et al. Sjögren syndrome: comparison of assessments with MR sialography and conventional sialography. Radiology 1998;209:683–8.
21. Takagi Y, Sumi M, Van Cauteren M, et al. Fast and high-resolution MR sialography using a small surface coil. J Magn Reson Imaging 2005;22(1):29–37.
22. Morimoto Y, Tanaka T, Yoshioka I, et al. Virtual endoscopic view of salivary gland ducts using MR sialography data from three dimension fast asymmetric spin-echo (3D-FASE) sequences: a preliminary study. Oral Dis 2002;8(5):268–74.
23. Morimoto Y, Tanaka T, Kito S, et al. Utility of three dimension fast asymmetric spin-echo (3D-FASE) sequences in MR sialographic sequences: model and volunteer studies. Oral Dis 2005;11(1):35–43.

Clinical Ultrasound of the Salivary Glands

Philippe Katz, MD[a,*], Dana M. Hartl, MD, PhD[b], Agnès Guerre, MD[a]

KEYWORDS

• Sialitis • Ultrasound • Color Doppler • Sialolithiasis • Tumors

Since the 1980s, ultrasound (US) has been shown to be a highly sensitive means of evaluating the major salivary glands. Because of technological advances and the superficial location of the major salivary glands, most regions are now accessible by high-resolution transducers. Only a small portion of the deep lobe of the parotid gland may be hidden by the acoustic shadow of the mandible.[1] Linear transducers with high frequencies between 7.5 and 16 MHz are used. In large lesions, transducers with a lower frequency may be used to completely visualize the lesion.

Salivary gland US should always be performed on both sides; many lesions occur bilaterally. If a tumor is suspected, the cervical lymph nodes should examined as well. Color Doppler may be useful to investigate inflammatory lesions and tumors. Color Doppler is performed by comparing the vessel density with a normal reference gland or by comparing the vessel density of the tumor with the normal parenchyma. The peak systolic flow is generally measured, but the correction for the angle of the Doppler beam may be difficult to calculate in some cases. In Sjogren's syndrome, for example, the systolic peak velocity after salivary stimulation (with lemon juice) is often double the peak velocity in the resting state.

ULTRASONOGRAPHIC ANATOMY

All salivary glands are homogeneous echogenic organs. The normal sizes of the salivary glands have been evaluated.[2] The parotid gland measures on average 46 mm in its vertical dimension and 37 mm in its horizontal dimension, with a thickness of 7 mm anteriorly and 22 mm posteriorly. The submandibular gland measures approximately 33 × 35 × 14 mm. There does not seem to be any gender-related differences, but the size of the glands increase significantly with body weight.[2]

[a] Salivary Glands Functional Explorations Institut, 7, Rue Theodore de Banville, 75017 Paris, France

[b] Department of Otolaryngology Head & Neck Surgery, Institut Gustave Roussy, 39 rue Camille Desmoulins, 94805 Villejuif Cedex, France

* Corresponding author.

E-mail address: drkatz.philippe@gmail.com (P. Katz).

Otolaryngol Clin N Am 42 (2009) 973–1000
doi:10.1016/j.otc.2009.08.009
oto.theclinics.com

Parotid Gland

The parotid gland is located in the retromandibular fossa. Anatomically, the superficial lobe and deep lobe are separated by the plane of the facial nerve. On US, the nerve cannot be visualized and thus the anatomic lobes cannot be distinguished. Some refer to the caudal portion of the parotid gland as the superficial lobe, but we prefer referring to structures visualized around or within the gland for orientation, which avoids confusion with the anatomic definition of the parotid lobes. In most cases, the retromandibular vein is visualized without difficulty; however, normal intraglandular salivary ducts and the main duct (Stensen's duct) are generally not seen, even with high-frequency transducers. A dilated Stensen's duct may be visualized, running superficially along the masseter muscle through the corpus adiposum buccae and then turning medially through the buccinator muscle. In this anterior region, accessory salivary tissue can often be seen. The echostructure is usually homogeneous and the echogenicity comparable to that of the thyroid gland. Lymph nodes can be seen within the gland, and are located in the anatomic superficial lobe.

On US, the parapharyngeal space is only rarely visualized with sufficient quality. The internal carotid artery, the internal jugular vein and the posterior belly of the digastric muscle are not always seen. Because of acoustic absorption and dispersion, the deep part of the parotid gland is often difficult to visualize (**Fig. 1**).

Submandibular Gland

The submandibular gland is located anterior and caudal to the parotid gland. Sometimes the salivary tissues of both glands can be found adjacent to each other without any intervening facia, but their echostructure is different: the submandibular gland is more hypoechoic than the parotid gland. The other anatomic structures in the submandibular region are the mandible, the mylohyoid muscle, the anterior belly of the digastric muscle, and the facial vessels.[3] The facial artery runs posterior to or even within the submandibular gland. On a typical oblique section of the submandibular gland, the palatine tonsil can also be visualized as hypoechoic area in a cranioposterior position relative to the submandibular gland. Normally, the submandibular glands have a triangular shape with a posterior base. Normal intraglandular ducts are only rarely visualized. After stimulation with lemon, they may be more easily

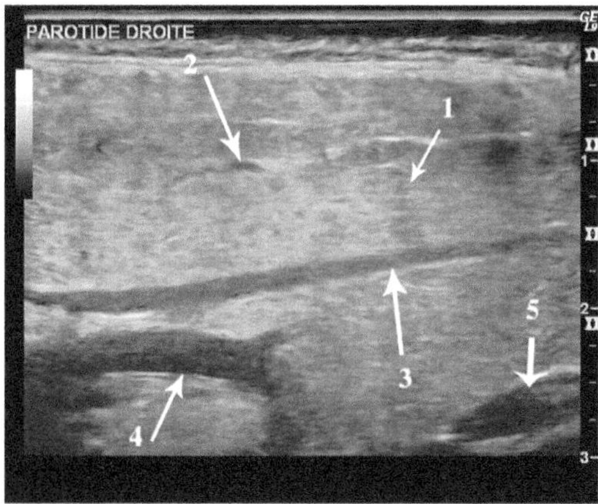

Fig. 1. Longitudinal sonogram of a normal parotid gland. 1: parenchyma, 2: small duct, 3: retromandibular vein, 4 and 5: external carotid artery.

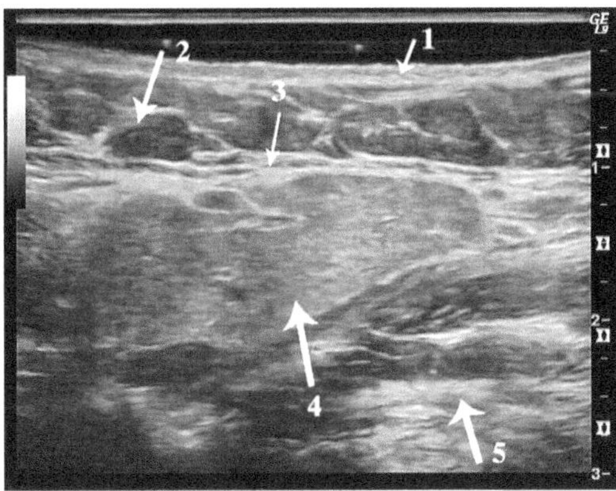

Fig. 2. Transverse sonogram of right normal submandibular gland. 1: skin, 2: fat, 3: fascia, 4: parenchyma, 5: mylohyoid muscle.

seen. The main submandibular duct (Wharton's duct) originates from the deep portion of the gland and ascends anteriorly to the caruncula in the floor of the mouth. The main duct can be differentiated from the lingual vessels by color Doppler (**Fig. 2**).

Sublingual Gland

The sublingual glands are localized in the floor of the mouth, cranial to the mylohyoid muscle, medial to the mandible and lateral to the geniohyoid muscle. In some cases the salivary tissue can even extend posteriorly to the submandibular gland.[4] The sublingual glands have multiple small excretory ducts that are not visible with US. The glands appear more echogenic than the hypoechoic muscles of the floor of the mouth (**Fig. 3**).

SALIVARY GLAND INFECTIONS OR *SIALITIS*

Infection of a salivary gland is called *sialitis*, which can be further divided into infection of the gland itself, or *sialadenitis*, and infection of the salivary duct or ducts, termed *sialodochitis*. This section will cover the most common infections.

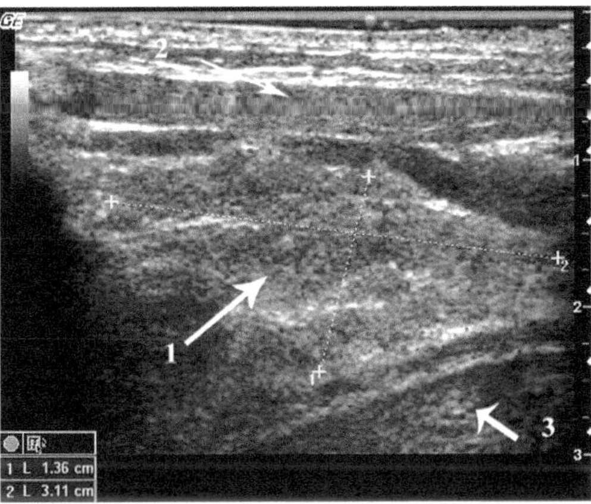

Fig. 3. Transverse sonogram of right normal sublingual gland. 1: parenchyma, 2: anterior belly digastric muscle, 3: floor of the mouth.

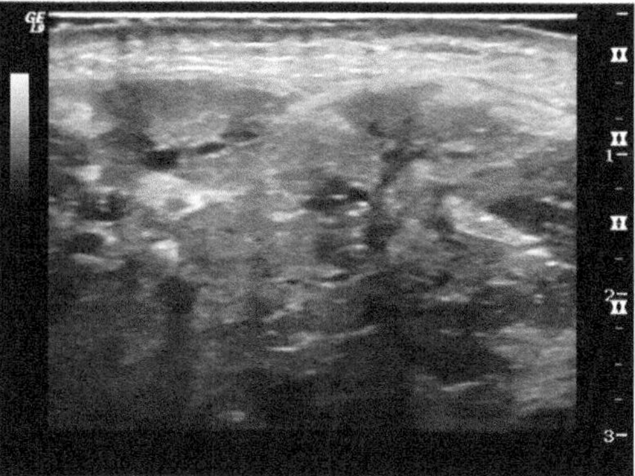

Fig. 4. Longitudinal ultrasound of a parotid gland. Unilateral heteroechogenic aspect of the parenchyma with duct dilatation and swelling of the gland.

Viral Sialadenitis

Endemic parotitis or the mumps, caused by a paramyxovirus, is the most frequent acute infection, even in the era of systematic vaccination. Usually, the clinical presentation is sufficient for a definitive diagnosis.[5] In 75% of cases both parotid glands are enlarged. Cervical lymph nodes are also always enlarged. On US, the parotid glands are enlarged with a more rounded shape, a convex lateral surface, and a hypoechoic structure.[6,7] Sometimes the salivary ducts are enlarged and visible. Color Doppler demonstrates diffuse hypervascularization.

Bacterial Sialadenitis

Acute bacterial parotitis

Normally the saliva within the salivary glands is sterile. Bacterial infection can originate in several ways. The most common origin is retrograde infection via the oral cavity, bacteria infecting the gland by way of the salivary duct. Less common origins include extracapsular spread of temporomandibular joint infections and hematogenous septicemia.

Acute bacterial parotitis is as common in adults as in children. Clinical presentation is typically unilateral, with sudden pain and swelling and increased pain at each meal (salivary colic, even in the absence of lithiasis). The examination of the ostium reveals

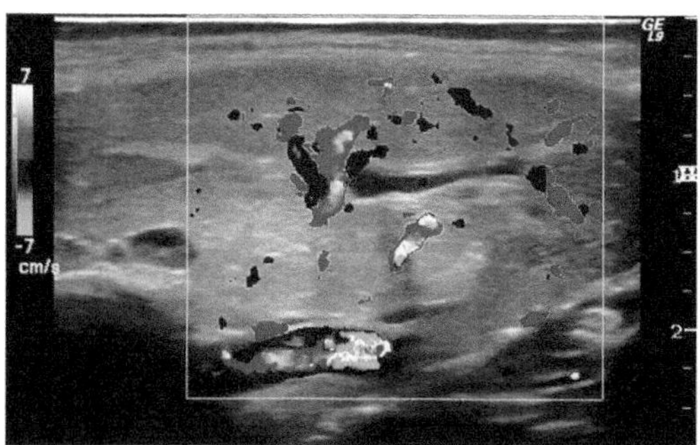

Fig. 5. Longitudinal ultrasound of parotid gland. Color Doppler reveals hyperemia. Acute sialoadenitis.

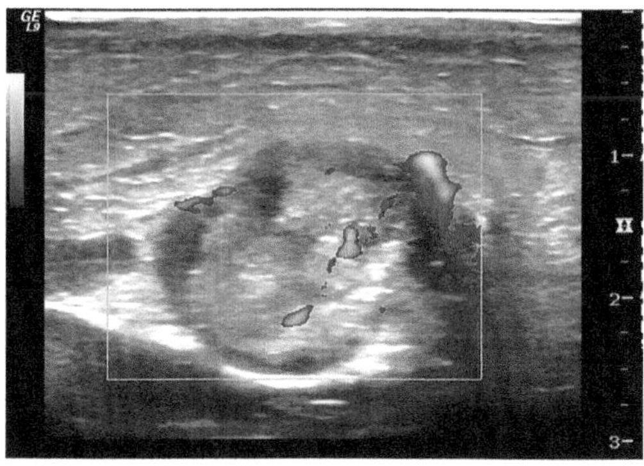

Fig. 6. Transverse sonogram and Doppler of a left parotid. Typical aspects of parotid abscess.

cloudy saliva or pus. Sialadenitis in adults is associated in approximately 50% of cases with sialolithiasis.

US is the only radiographic examination indicated, revealing salivary duct dilatations, hypoechoic parenchyma, and enlarged intraglandular lymph nodes (**Fig. 4**). Hypervascularization because of the inflammation is visible on color Doppler (**Fig. 5**). The main goal of US in inflammatory diseases is to rule out lithiasis or other ductal obstructions.[8,9] In severe infections, intraglandular liquid spaces, implying abscess formation, may be observed and are more frequent in diabetic patients. Air may also be seen,[10] as well as moving, echoic debris within an abscess.[11] US guidance is particularly useful for needle aspiration or drainage of the abscess (**Fig. 6**).

Acute bacterial submandibulitis

Acute bacterial submandibulitis occurs suddenly, with submandibular pain and swelling. Pus and debris may be seen at the Wharton's duct ostium in the floor of the mouth. US is essential for diagnosis (**Fig. 7**). The gland is heterogeneous with dilatation of the salivary ducts and increased vascularization on Doppler (**Fig. 8**). US is also necessary in this case to rule out an associated lithiasis.

Pediatric chronic bacterial parotitis

Chronic bacterial parotitis in children is a relatively common disease. Occurring at age 2 or 3, more rarely at a younger age, this sialadenitis presents initially like an acute viral

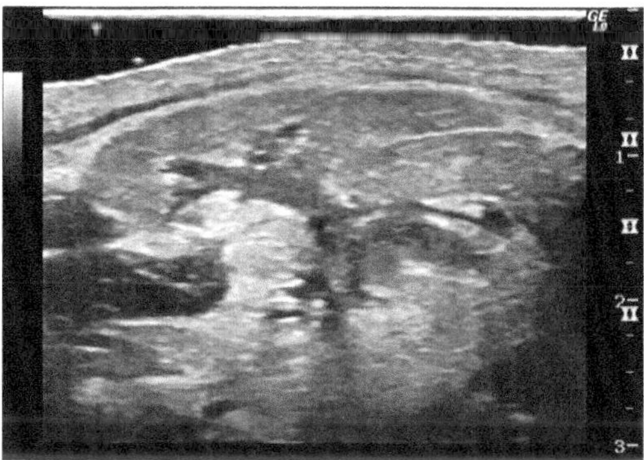

Fig. 7. Transverse ultrasound of left submandibular gland. Hypoechogenic parenchyma and ducts dilatation. Acute submandibularis.

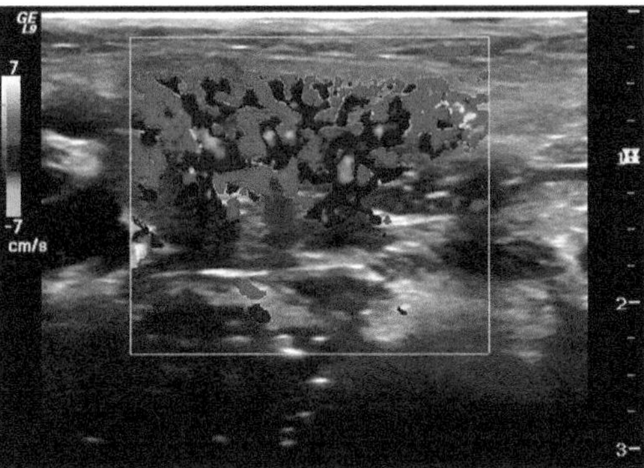

Fig. 8. Transverse color Doppler of left submandibular gland with hyperemia, acute submandibularis.

infection. Then it evolves unilaterally or bilaterally with episodes of acute pain and swelling and enlarged cervical lymph nodes.

US is indicated as soon as the first symptoms occur. Images are typical and pathognomonic.[12–14] Multiple hypoechoic, cystoid areas and 2- to 3-mm vacuoles in the parotid glands are caused by the destruction of the glandular tissue by the chronic infection, and can take on a milary aspect on US (**Figs. 9** and **10**). Focal destruction of the glandular tissue can also cause salivary duct ectasia, which can be visualized on US. Small hyperechoic calcifications, which are not lithiases but a reaction to the inflammation, may also be seen. The Doppler shows hypervascularization of the gland and of the intra- and extraglandular lymph nodes (**Fig. 11**).

Chronic parotitis in adults

In chronic inflammation, the glandular modifications seen on US are often less prominent than in acute diseases. An atrophic hypoechoic gland may be seen, but the size of the gland is variable. Sometimes ductal ectasia is found (**Fig. 12**); however, sialography is superior to US for visualizing chronic inflammatory obstructions of the salivary ducts.

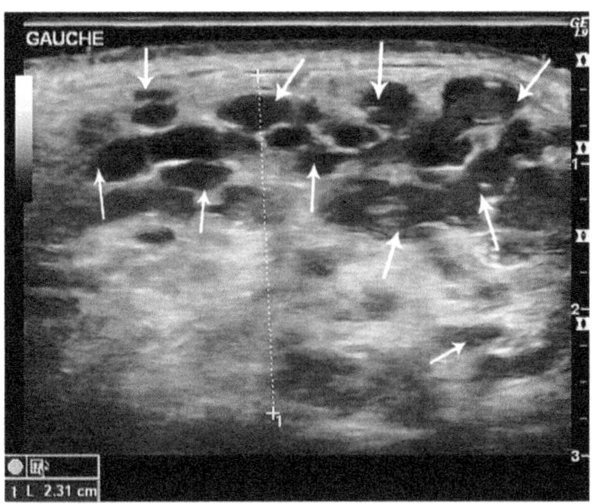

Fig. 9. Longitudinal sonogram of left parotid in a 6-year-old boy. Heteroechogenic structure with many hypoechogenic nodules (*arrows*). Typical aspects of chronic parotidis.

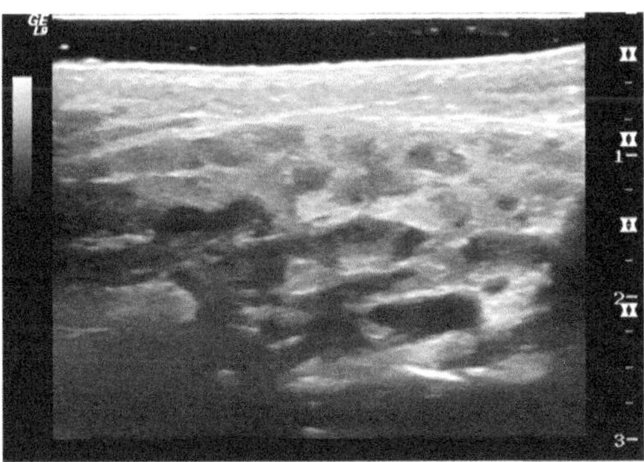

Fig. 10. Longitudinal sonogram of right parotid on an 8-year-old girl. Heteroechogenic structure with moderate hypoechogenic nodules. Moderate chronic parotidis.

Adult chronic parotitis may occur in a patient having suffered from chronic or acute parotitis as a child or with a history of acute parotitis, or in the context of a systemic disease such as Sjogren's syndrome. It can also be secondary to a stricture or stenosis of a salivary duct, itself secondary to an acute infection.

US shows partial destruction of the gland, which is heterogeneous with hypoechoic regions representing destroyed parenchyma and hyperechoic regions of sclerosis. Dilatation of the salivary ducts with strictures or stenosis is always found, with strictures along Stensen's canal creating a "string of pearls" image. Ductal ectasia may also be present. Lymph nodes are visible within the gland and in the cervical regions. Doppler may or may not show hypervascularization, according to whether inflammation is present or not.

Tuberculous parotitis

Tuberculosis of the salivary glands is rare, with parotitis mimicking a malignant tumor. Moderate pain, or no pain at all, may be present. On US, there are heterogeneous, hypoechoic, poorly-defined lesions, with regional lymphadenopathy (**Fig. 13**). The lymph nodes themselves have poorly defined margins as well (**Fig. 14**).[15] US-guided fine-needle aspiration (FNA) cytology is diagnostic showing specific granulomatous lesions with giant cells and necrosis.

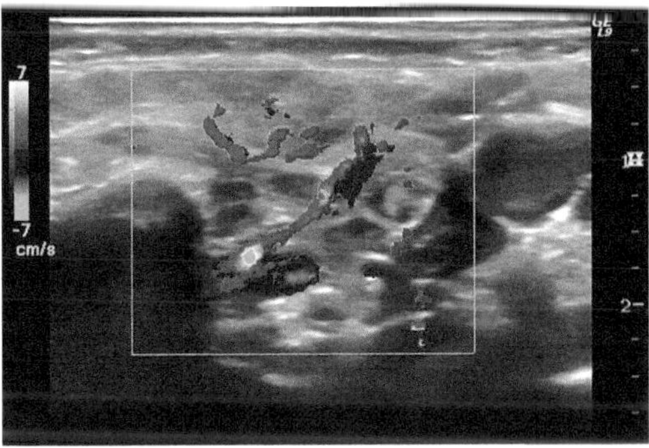

Fig. 11. Transverse color Doppler of left parotid gland in a 5-year-old girl. Moderate hyperemia with two big hypoechogenic lymph nodes posteriorly.

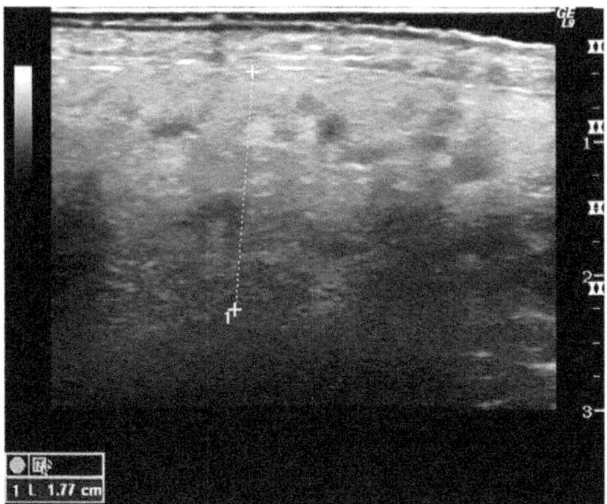

Fig. 12. Longitudinal sonogram of left parotid on an adult. Heteroechogenic structure with small hypoechogenic nodules. Chronic parotidis.

Idiopathic Dilatation of the Salivary Ducts

This problem is attributable to a stricture or stenosis located at the level of the sphincter of the main salivary duct that causes a dehiscence of the wall of the duct. The dilatation resembles a hernia of the main salivary duct, occurring during meals. As the disease progresses, pain can also occur, giving rise to a salivary colic, and bilateralization generally occurs. At this stage, the duct can be seen and palpated under the skin of the cheek.[15] It occurs most often in Stensen's duct of the parotid gland, primarily in females.

US confirms the diagnosis, showing a major dilatation of the duct with a diameter of up to 1 cm, all along the duct (**Fig. 15**). The stenosis is generally well visualized, and may be located anywhere along the canal (**Fig. 16**). No lithiasis is visible (**Figs. 17** and **18**). The glandular tissue may be hypotrophic with other dilated ducts. Signs of infection are often associated with the disease because of the stagnation of saliva within the gland. Doppler shows hypervascularization along the wall of the duct and also at the level of the stenosis.

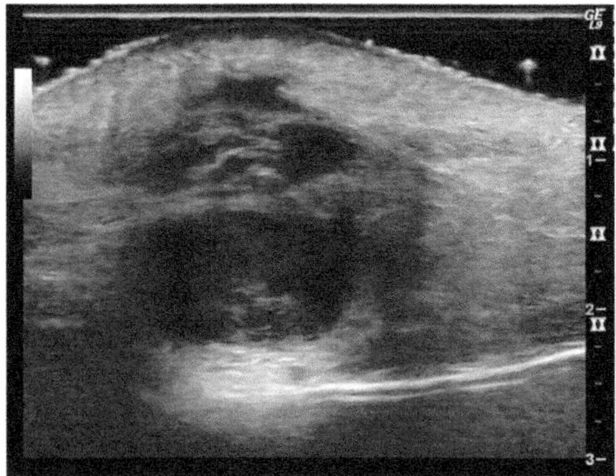

Fig. 13. Longitudinal sonogram of parotid on an adult. Big lesion inside the parenchyma badly delimitate with heteroechonic aspect mimic a tumor: tuberculosis.

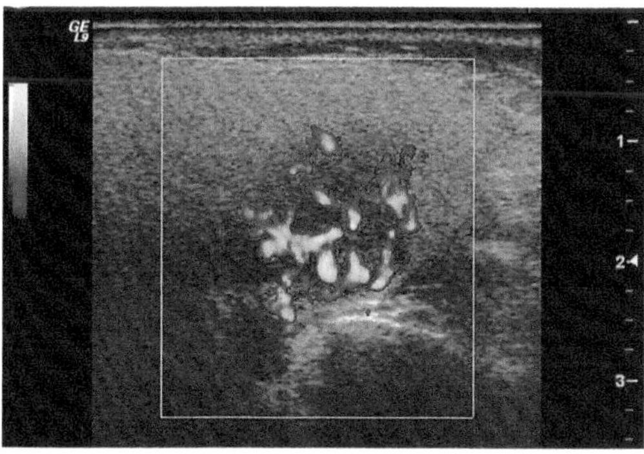

Fig. 14. Color Doppler of parotidis tuberculosis. Hyperemia inside the lymph nod.

Sialodochitis with Sialolithiasis

It is now generally acknowledged that lithiasis formation can be found during early childhood, around the age of 1 year, but even earlier in some cases (our youngest case was a 2-month-old girl). A genetic predisposition has also been shown, with more that 300 families identified. In our experience of 3500 cases of lithiasis over a 20-year period, we have observed that only one type of major salivary gland is involved per patient, uni- or bilaterally; we have never observed lithiasis in different types of glands (parotid and submandibular, for example) in the same patient. Submandibular and parotid lithiases show the same composition, but with different proportions of calcium and phosphate.[15]

More than 80% of salivary concretions are localized in the submandibular gland or in Wharton's duct. Approximately 15% of cases of sialolithiasis occur in the parotid gland or in Stensen's duct.[16] Sublingual lithiasis is rare.[17]

Salivary calculi usually cause symptoms only if an obstruction of the ductal system occurs.[18] For therapeutic purposes it is important to differentiate lithiasis of the main duct from those of the intraglandular ducts.[19] Typical locations for lithiasis are at the anterior bend of Wharton's duct and at the confluence of the intraglandular ducts. Sometimes intraoral transducers are used to localize submandibular stones.[20] Lithiasis of the parotid system is often located in the ducts in the periphery of the gland or deep in the parenchyma.

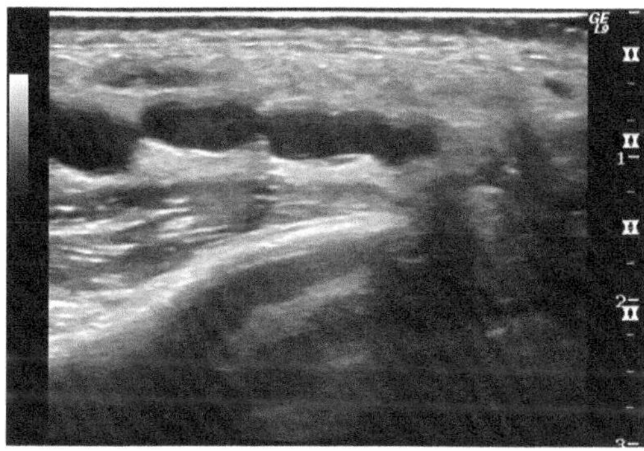

Fig. 15. Transverse sonogram of left parotid. Excretory duct dilatation with stenosis.

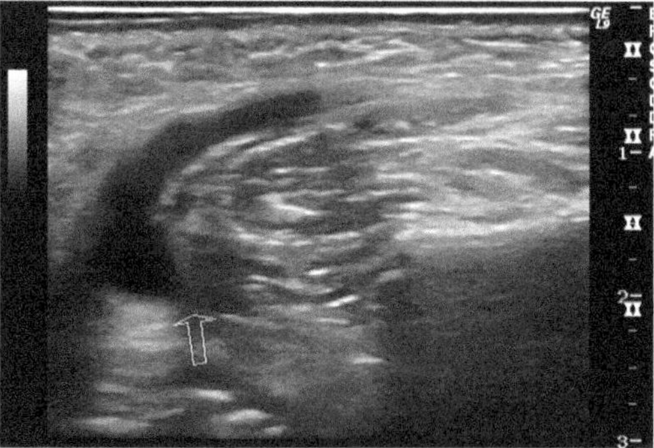

Fig. 16. Transverse sonogram of a left parotid. Stenosis on Stensen's duct (*arrow*).

Sonographically, lithiasis typically appears as a bright curvilinear echo complex with posterior shadowing (**Figs. 19** and **20**).[21] In lesions smaller than 2 mm, this shadow may be missing (**Fig. 21**).

In symptomatic sialolithiasis, a concomitant dilatation of the ductal system or inflammation is often visualized (**Fig. 22**). Intraglandular duct ectasia presents as multiple tubular hypoechoic structures, whereas the dilated main duct is located in an extraglandular position and has a more linear shape. Inflammatory changes render the gland diffusely hypoechoic and with more rounded, globular margins. Color Doppler shows hypervascularization.

The accuracy of US in the assessment of sialolithiasis is approximately 90%.[22] It is possible to differentiate calcified lymph nodes and phleboliths in facial veins from sialolithiasis. Approximately 20% to 40% of the salivary lithiases are not opaque on plain films, but most of these stones are visible on US. Salivary stimulation (lemon or vitamin C) leads to more prominent intraglandular ducts. This facilitates the visualization of small lithiases and the echogenic lithiases contrast better with the dilated hypoechoic ducts.

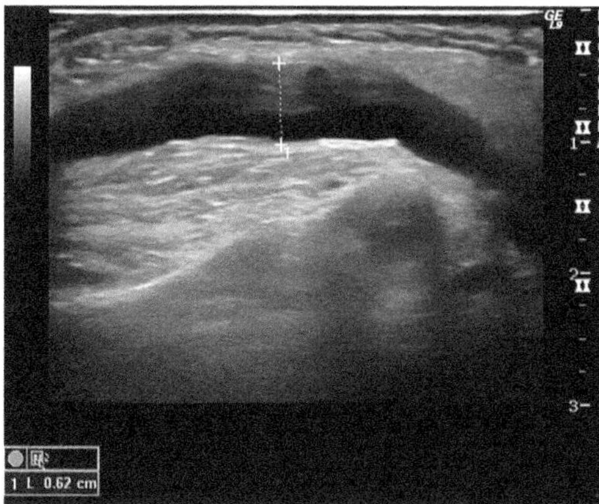

Fig. 17. Transverse sonogram of parotid. Important dilatation of the Stensen's duct.

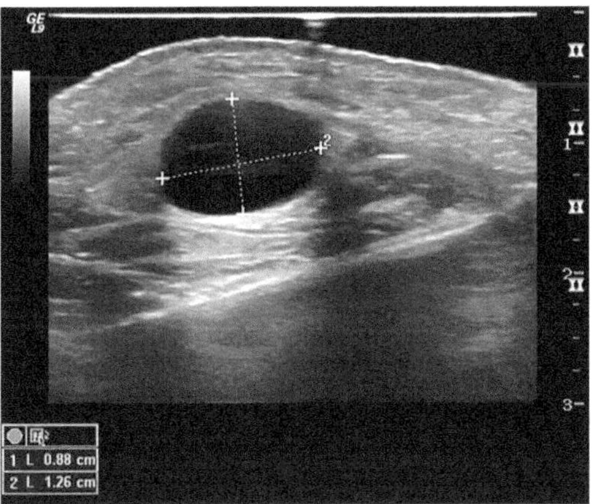

Fig. 18. Longitudinal sonogram of parotid gland. Wide dilatation of the duct.

In experienced hands, US is the primary method for detecting salivary calculi. Computed tomography, MRI,[23] or sialography can be reserved for those patients with inconclusive sonographic results or for patients with negative sonographic results and a typical clinical presentation of ductal obstruction.

Sialosis

The term of *sialosis* designates all the chronic diseases of the salivary glands that are not infections or tumors. This includes nutritional, dystrophic, and systemic diseases affecting the salivary glands. Most of these diseases are characterized by a hyperplasia of the salivary gland or glands, termed *sialomegaly*, and with deficit in salivary secretion.

Sialoadenosis

Often diabetes, alcoholism, and anorexia nervosa are clinically evident.[24] US shows enlarged glands with a hyperechoic structure and no focal lesions. Because of the

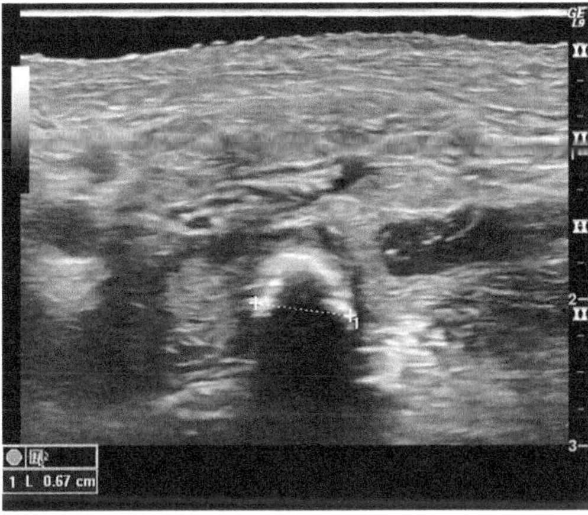

Fig. 19. Transverse ultrasound of right submandibular gland. Heteroechogenic aspect of the gland with a white hyperechogenic structure inside the pelvis. Silalolithiasis (6.7 mm diameter).

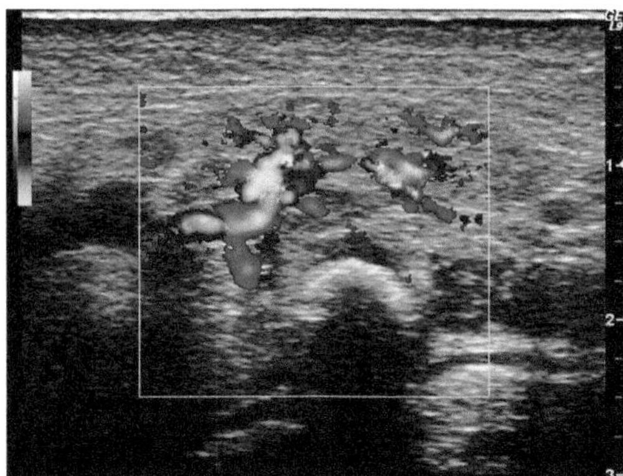

Fig. 20. Same gland as in Fig. 19 with color Doppler showing hyperemia.

high echogenicity, the deep portions of the parotid glands are usually not visualized (**Fig. 23**). Sometimes low-frequency transducers have to be applied to delineate the glands completely. Hypervascularization, as often found in acute inflammation, should be ruled out by demonstration of normal or subnormal color Doppler saturations (**Fig. 24**). In these bilateral painless enlargements of the glands it is important to rule out tumors and ductal obstructions. This can be performed by demonstration of a homogeneous glandular structure.

Systemic Sialosis

Sjogren's syndrome

Sjogren's syndrome (SS) is an autoimmune disease with chronic inflammation of the major salivary glands, the lacrimal glands, and arthritis. The exocrine glands are infiltrated by lymphocytes and plasma cells. The incidence of Sjogren's disease in women is seven to nine times higher than in men. Usually, patients present with a sicca complex. Often the antinuclear antibodies (ANAs) are positive, especially the subsets Anti-Ro/SSA, Anti-La/SSB. Definitive diagnosis is made by biopsy of the minor salivary glands of the lips.

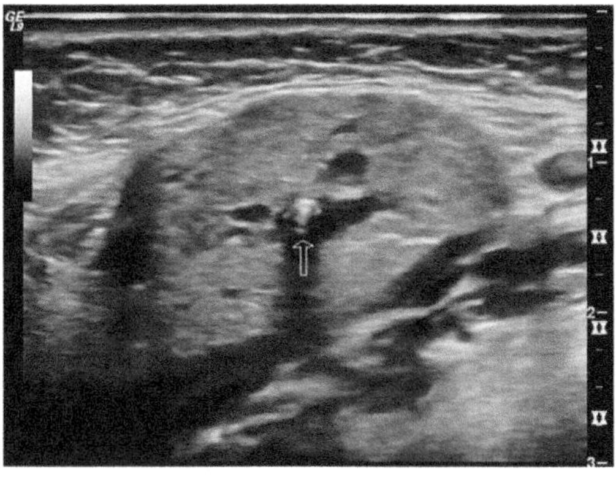

Fig. 21. Transverse ultrasound of right submandibular gland. Small lithiasis inside the pelvis less than 1 mm (*arrow*).

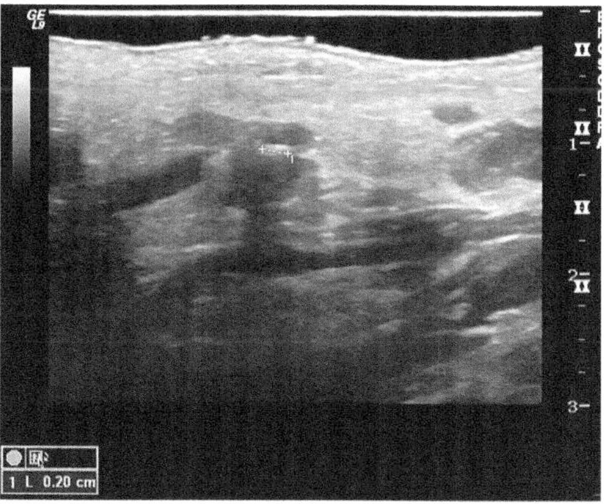

Fig. 22. Longitudinal sonogram of parotid gland. Hyperechogenic signal inside the pelvis with duct dilatation all around: sialolithiasis.

In SS, usually all of the major salivary glands are involved. In the acute stage, swelling and hypoechoic transformations are found.[25,26] Often the glands are heterogeneous because of inflammation, enlarged lymph nodes, and myoepithelial hyperplasia (**Fig. 25**). The peripheral ductal system may be dilated; furthermore, multiple small cysts are found.[27] The sonographic changes correlate with histological involvement(**Fig. 26**).[26] With time, the glands become small, hypoechoic, heterogeneous, and difficult to delineate (**Fig. 27**).

Color Doppler shows hypervascularization in the acute inflammatory stage[28]; however, when the salivary production is impaired owing to chronic fibrotic changes, the arterial blood flow reaction caused by stimulation is diminished.[29] Salivary stimulation causes a significant elevation of the arterial blood flow. In SS, the maximum systolic flow velocity is often doubled.[30]

An important issue in SS is to rule out malignant lymphoma, which has an increased incidence in this disease; however, in a heterogeneous gland it is difficult to rule out small lesions through imaging. For hypoechoic lesions larger than 2 cm and for rapidly growing lesions, a biopsy should be performed.

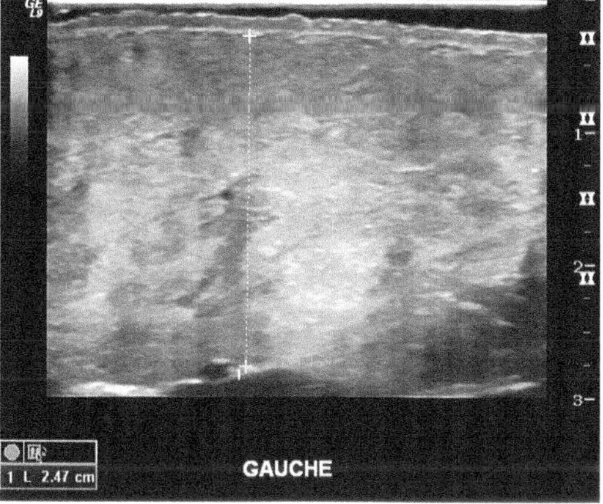

Fig. 23. Longitudinal sonogram of left parotid. Enlarged homogeneous gland, increased volume, lightly hyperechogenic. Anorexia syndrome.

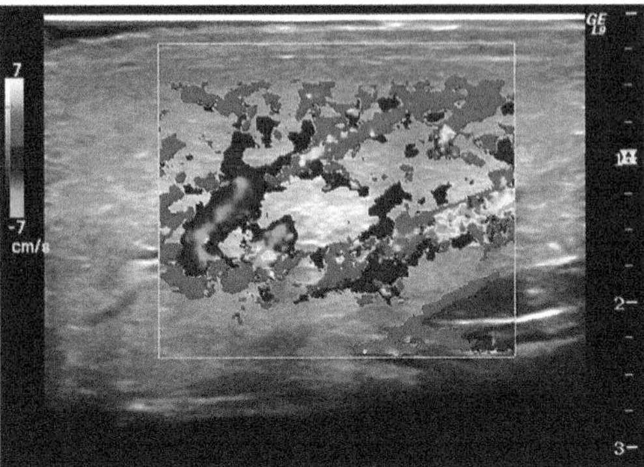

Fig. 24. Same gland as in Fig. 23 with the color Doppler showing hypervascularization and inflammation.

Kimura's disease

Kimura's disease, a non-neoplastic-hyperplastic multinodular lymph node disease, occurs predominately in the Asian population.[31] Often the cervical lymph nodes and the nodes in the salivary glands are involved. No specific, distinguishable sonographic signs have been described, however.

SALIVARY GLAND TUMORS

Benign Tumors of the Glandular Epithelium

Pleomorphic adenoma

Pleomorphic adenoma is the most frequent tumor of the salivary tissue (24%–71%).[15,32,33] In approximately 80% of cases the tumor is located in the superficial part of the parotid gland. In approximately 10% of cases the deep part of the parotid gland is involved. Rarely, the lesion protrudes into the parapharyngeal space ("iceberg" tumors). Histologically, the lesion is composed of epithelial, myoepithelial, and mesenchymal tissue.

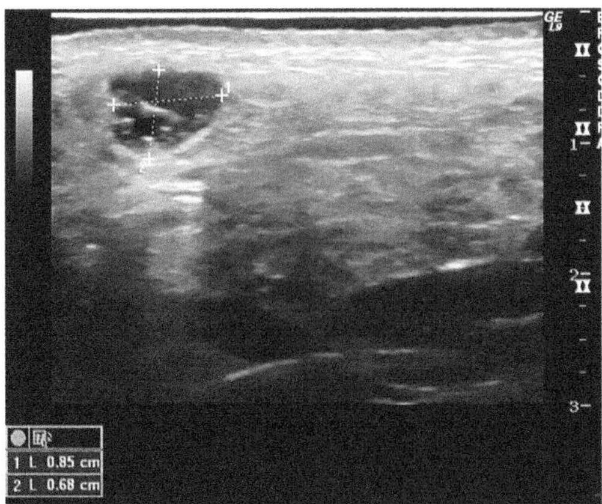

Fig. 25. Longitudinal sonogram of parotid gland. Heteroechogenic structure like chronic parotidis with a big lymph node inside the parenchyma: Sjogren's syndrome.

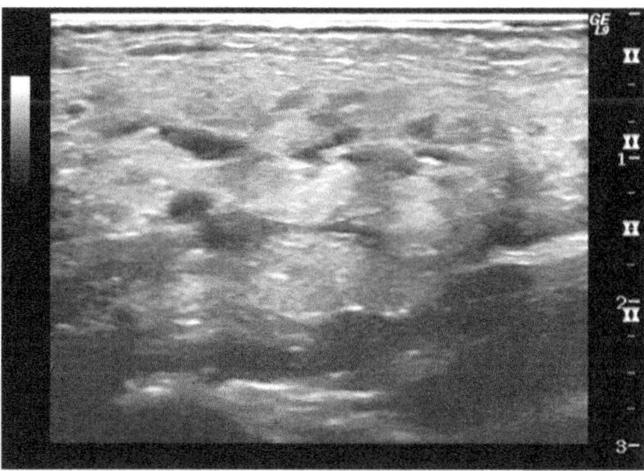

Fig. 26. Longitudinal sonogram of parotid gland. Lightly hyperechogenic structure of the parenchyma with ducts dilation hypoechogenic: Sjogren's syndrome.

Sonographically, the tumor is well circumscribed and usually is homogeneous and hypoechoic. A well-defined, lobulated margin is regarded as typical (**Figs. 28** and **29**).[34] When calcifications are found in parotid tumors, pathology reveals a pleomorphic adenoma in most cases, although some malignancies also commonly show calcifications.[35] Color Doppler most often demonstrates moderate vascularization. A predominately peripheral flow pattern has been described.[36] Maximum systolic flow most often is below 25 cm/s (**Figs. 30** and **31**).[34] Pleomorphic adenoma of the submandibular gland occurs in approximately 10% of cases (**Figs. 32** and **33**).

Pleomorphic adenoma is usually a slowly growing lesion. Surgery is recommended. Malignant transformation has been reported in up to 5% of cases. Rapid growth of a formerly stable parotid mass is suspicious for carcinoma ex pleomorphic adenoma. Blurry, ill-defined borders are suspicious for malignancy.

Cystadenolymphoma (Warthin's tumor)

Papillary cystadenoma lymphotosum (Warthin's tumor) is the second most frequent salivary gland tumor. On palpation these tumors are usually soft and compressible, unlike pleomorphic adenomas. The tumors are most often located in the caudal part of the parotid gland and may be bilateral. Cystadenolymphomas of the submandibular gland are rare.

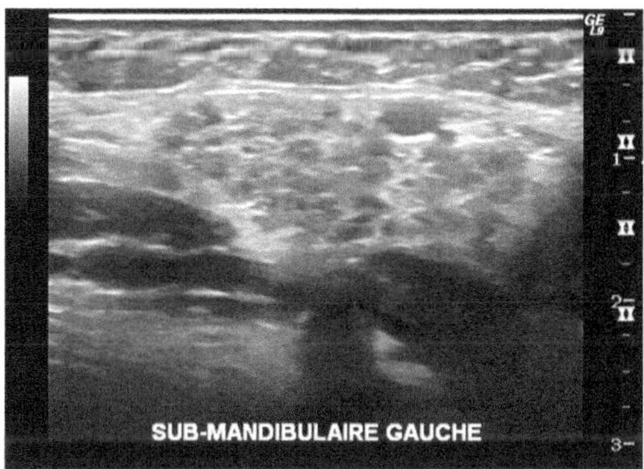

Fig. 27. Transverse ultrasound of left submandibular gland. Typical aspect of Sjogren's syndrome, with many hypoechogenic nodules inside the parenchyma.

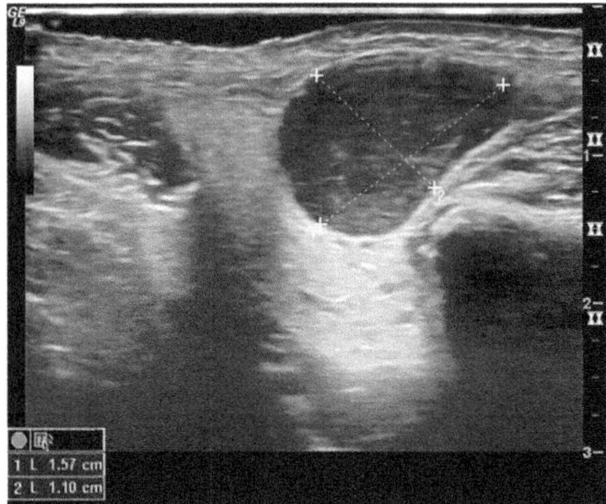

Fig. 28. Transverse sonogram of right parotid gland. Homogeneous hypoechogenic tumor well delimitate inside the parenchyma. Histology demonstrated pleomorphic adenoma.

On pathology, the tumors are composed of epithelial and lymphatic tissue. Cystic parts within a solid lesion are regarded as typical for Warthin's tumor (**Figs. 34** and **35**).[36–38] Often they present with an ovoid shape. On US the lesion is usually more heterogeneous than pleomorphic adenomas (**Fig. 36**)[35,38] and have well-defined borders. These tumors are multicentric in up to 30% of cases.[36] Recurrent tumors are not unusual. Nuclear medicine studies after salivary stimulation show a higher uptake than the normal parenchyma; therefore, this tumor can be diagnosed relatively specifically. If large cystic lesions are present, however, the technetium scan may be negative.[39] Oncocytoma may also show a strong tracer uptake on scintigraphy and be mistaken for a cystadenolymphoma.

Malignant Epithelial Tumors

Mucoepidermoid carcinoma

Mucoepidermoid carcinoma is the most frequent malignant tumor of the salivary glands. These tumors are differentiated pathologically into two main groups:

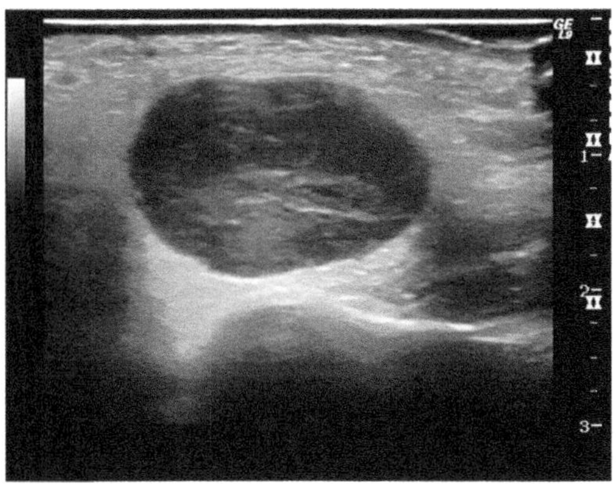

Fig. 29. Longitudinal sonogram of gland parotid gland. Aspect homogeneous hypoechogenic of a tumor. Fine needle aspiration cytology (FNAC) diagnosed a pleomorphic adenoma.

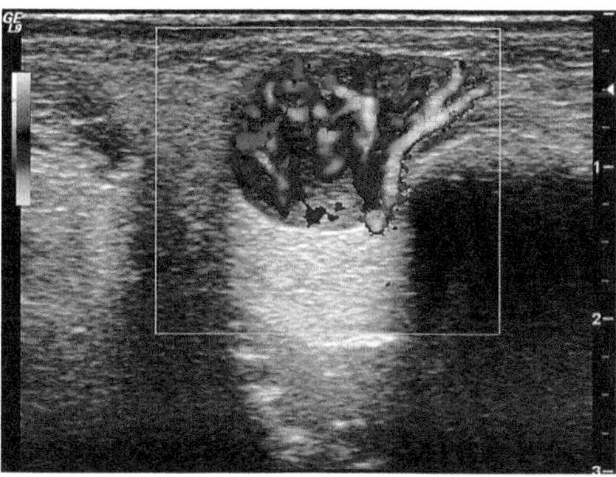

Fig. 30. Transverse sonogram of right parotid gland. Color Doppler inside a well-deliniated hypoechogenic tumor. Hypervascularization inside a pleomorphic adenoma.

carcinoma with a high grade of malignancy and tumors with a low grade of malignancy. Malignant tumors smaller than 2 cm in diameter usually have a homogeneous structure and present with smooth borders; therefore, especially low-grade malignant tumors are often incorrectly diagnosed as benign lesions by imaging.[32] High-grade malignant tumors and larger lesions mostly show irregular borders and a typical heterogeneous echo pattern. Frequently, irregular zones of necrosis are found. These tumors are most often correctly assessed as malignant tumors by US.

In larger lesions, the main drawback of US is its incapacity to completely delineate the tumor. Infiltrations of the parapharyngeal space, the base of the skull, or the mandible are not accessed by US.

Adenoid cystic carcinoma

Adenoid cystic carcinoma is also sometimes misdiagnosed as a benign lesion (**Fig. 37**). The typical perineural infiltrations are usually not detected by US. Acinus cell carcinoma, squamous cell carcinoma, undifferentiated carcinoma, or adenocarcinoma are less frequent.

In malignant tumors, color Doppler usually shows a higher degree of vascularization as compared with the normal parenchyma or with benign tumors. High systolic values

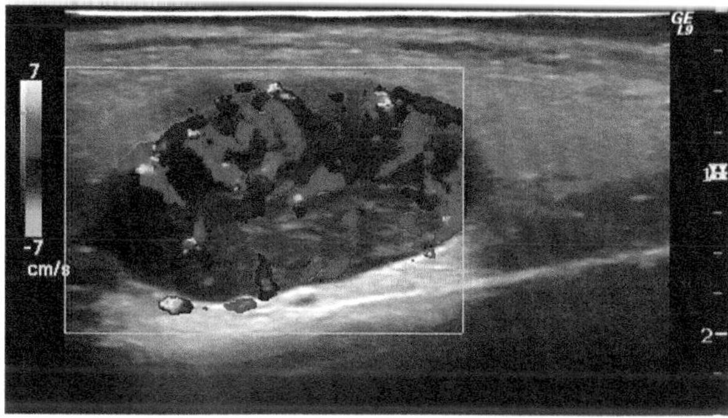

Fig. 31. Longitudinal sonogram of gland parotid gland. Color Doppler inside a well-deliniated hypoechogenic tumor. Hypervascularization inside a pleomorphic adenoma.

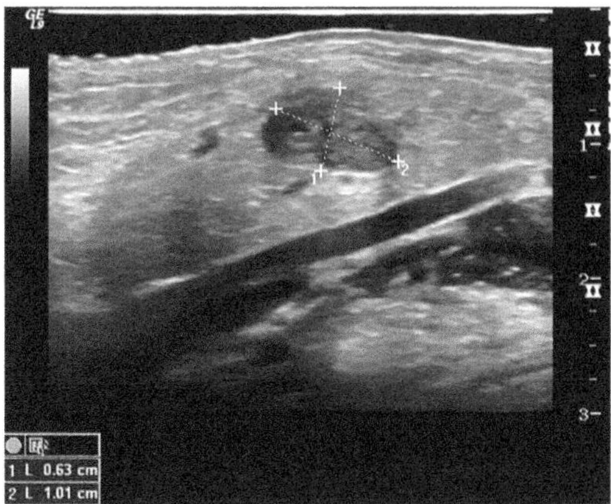

Fig. 32. Transverse ultrasound of right submandibular gland. Hypo to isoechogenic tumor inside the gland well delineated: pleomorphic adenoma.

and a chaotic pattern of tumor vessels are suspicious for malignancy, even when gray-scale imaging suggests a benign lesion[34]; however, up to now, color Doppler of salivary gland tumors is a method under clinical investigation. No criteria are known to definitively differentiate between benign and malignant tumors.

Nonepithelial Tumors

Lymph node metastases within the parotid gland

Intraglandular lymph node metastases most often present as multiple, round, well-defined lesions (**Fig. 38**). Lymph node metastases of the parotid gland are most commonly caused by malignant melanoma, squamous cell carcinoma, or metastatic carcinoma of the lung or breast. Malignant lymphoma (non-Hodgkin's lymphoma) may also involve the salivary glands. Most often, multiple hypoechoic, well-defined lesions are present. Color Doppler usually shows hypervascularization.

Lipomas

Lipomas are rare salivary gland tumors. Both CT and MRI reveal a specific morphology by demonstration of fat-equivalent tissue; therefore, whenever a lipoma is suspected clinically or on US, one of these investigations should be performed.

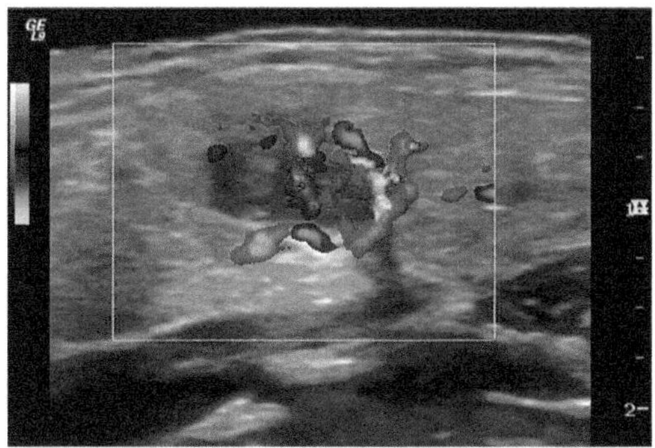

Fig. 33. Same gland with the color Doppler, see the hypervascularization inside the tumor.

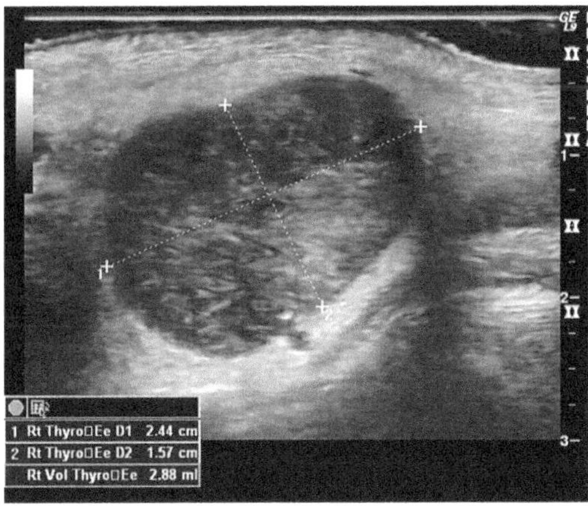

Fig. 34. Transverse sonogram of right parotid gland. Hypo to isoechogenic lesion with several cystic areas, but well deliniated. FNAC reported papillary cystadenoma lymphotosum or Whartin's tumor.

On US, these relatively soft, fat-containing tumors typically have an ovoid shape, sharp outlines, and are moderately compressible. Compared with the parotid parenchyma, pure fat-containing lipomas are moderately hypoechoic lesions.[40–42] Typically, a striated, feathered echogenicity is found (**Fig. 39**). Fibrolipomas are only slightly hypoechoic with regard to the parotid tissue. Lipoblastomas usually reveal cystic components. On color Doppler, lipomas show no or very little Doppler signal.

Liposarcomas are rare tumors in the salivary gland region. The diagnosis should be considered in fast-growing echogenic tumors.

Neurogenic tumors

Neurogenic tumors (schwannomas, neurofibromas) in the cervical soft tissue present as spindle-shaped lesions with a connection to the originating nerve. However, the facial nerve is not visible in the parotid gland; therefore, the specific diagnosis is rarely established on US. Neurogenic tumors often present with cystic areas. Usually moderate vascularization is present in color Doppler. Malignant schwannomas have been described.

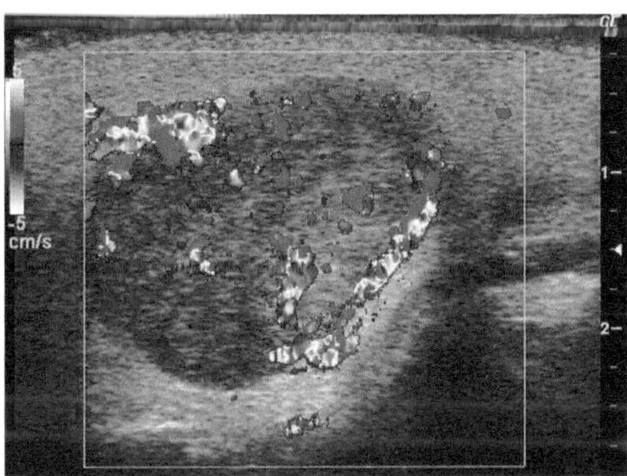

Fig. 35. Same tumor with color Doppler seeing lightly hyperemia.

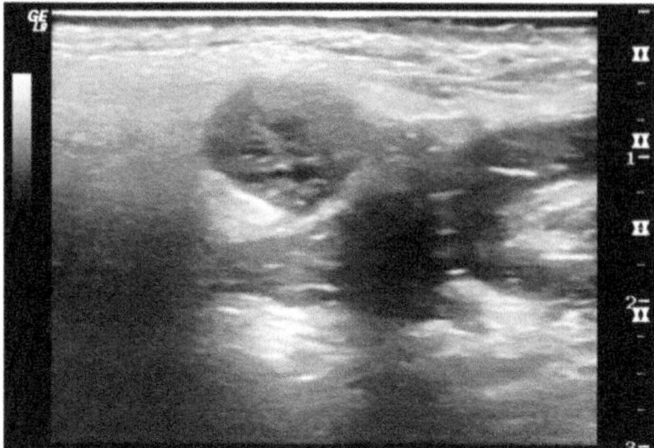

Fig. 36. Longitudinal sonogram of gland parotid gland. Hypo to isoechogenic lesion with several cystic areas but well delimitate. FNAC reported papillary cystadenoma lymphotosum.

Hemangiomas and lymphangiomas

In children, hemangiomas are the most frequent tumors of the salivary gland regions.[43] The diagnosis is usually made by clinical findings. Imaging is needed in deep-seated lesions, when the overlying skin is normal, or when the lesion encroaches on vital structures. On US, hemangiomas usually appear as hyperechoic, ill-defined lesions, or as hypoechoic lesions with a typical lobular pattern (**Figs. 40** and **41**).[44] Hemangiomas are compressible. Color Doppler shows hypervascularity, which is defined as more than five color structures per square centimeter. Pulsed Doppler shows a peak systolic flow of up to 90 cm/s. The diastolic flow is also increased with spectral broadening and a low resistive index (RI: 0.4–0.7).[43]

In most cases, spontaneous involution occurs in adolescence; however, when significant complications, such as bleeding, compression of vital structures, or coagulopathy are present, they are treated surgically or by embolization. In these therapeutic cases, CT or MRI is indicated to delineate the lesion completely.

Approximately 75% of lymphangiomas occur in the neck. Usually they are located in the posterior compartment. Histologically, a combination of cystic hygroma, cavernous, capillary, and vascular-lymphatic malformations may be present within

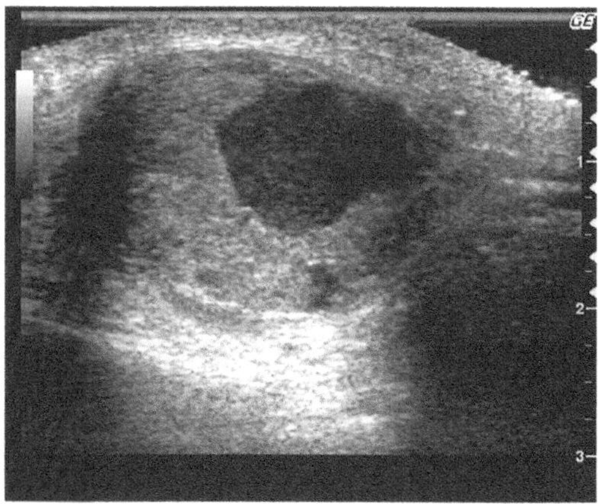

Fig. 37. Longitudinal sonogram of gland parotid gland. Heterogeneous tumor inside the parenchyma, with a hypoechogenic cyst. Histology was adenoid cystic carcinoma.

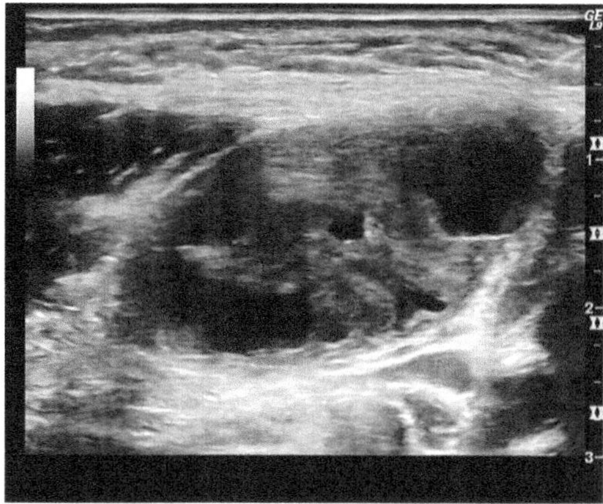

Fig. 38. Lymph node metastases to the salivary gland.

a single lesion. On US, they are predominantly cystic lesions with septae of variable thickness (**Fig. 42**). The echogenic components correspond to clusters of atypical lymphatic vessels, which are too small to be seen owing to the spatial resolution of US.[45] When hemorrhage or infection is present, the cysts contain floating debris. On color Doppler, lymphangioma appears avascular or hypovascularized (**Fig. 43**). Lymphangiomas are often surgically treated. In macrocystic lymphangioma, sclerosing therapy can be performed under US guidance.[46]

Dermoid cysts

Occasionally dermoid tumors are found in the salivary gland region. Usually these dysontogenetic cysts are localized in the midline in the floor of the mouth. These tumors can be echogenic owing to the high acoustic impedance between fluid, fat, hair, and sebaceous material (**Fig. 44**).

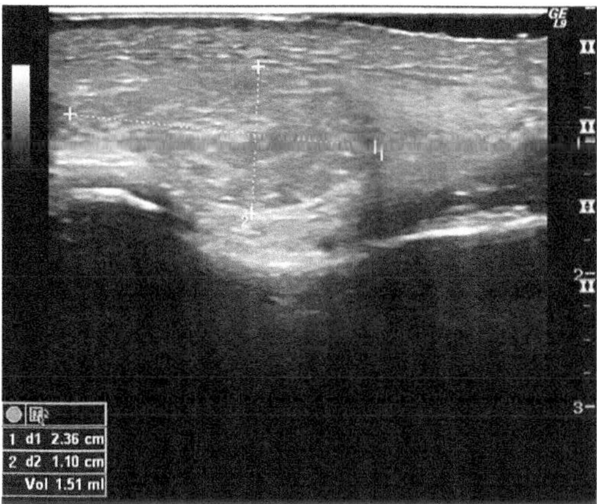

Fig. 39. Longitudinal sonogram of gland parotid gland. Moderately hypoechogenic lesion with smooth borders. Notice the fine hyperechogenic trabeculation inside the lesion, a typical aspect of lipoma.

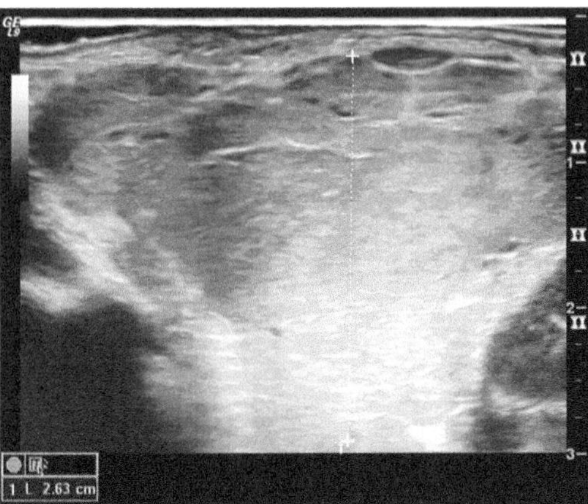

Fig. 40. Transverse sonogram of right parotid gland of a 6-month-old baby. Big lobulated hypoechogenic lesion inside the gland indicative of hemangioma.

Basal cell adenomas

Basal cell adenomas are rare. They generally involve minor salivary glands or accessory salivary tissue. Usually, a solid encapsulated lesion is found[47] (**Fig. 45**).

PSEUDOTUMORS

Masseter Muscle Hypertrophy

Unilateral hypertrophy of the masseter muscle is often misdiagnosed.[48] Hypertrophy of the masseter muscle can be assumed if the masseter measures more than 14 mm in its short-axis diameter at rest.

First Branchial Cleft Cysts

Cysts of the first branchial cleft, which are usually located in the parotid parenchyma, can be echogenic; they may mimic a solid tumor.[49] Most often these lesions are strictly homogeneous, and sometimes floating echoic cholesterol crystals may be

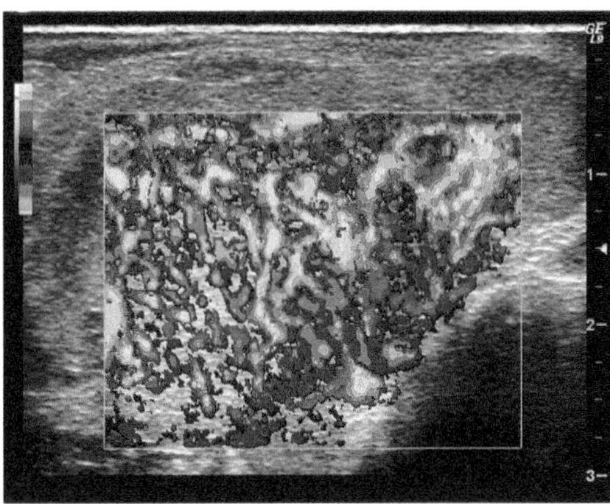

Fig. 41. Same patient as in Fig. 40 with the color Doppler: see the important hypervascularization inside the lesion.

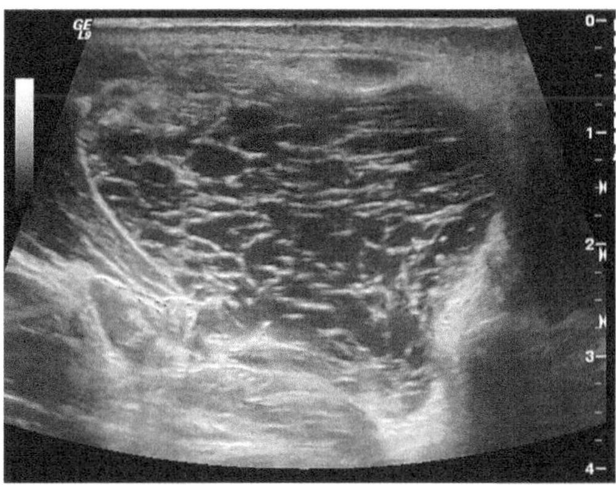

Fig. 42. Transverse sonogram of right parotid gland. Very big hypoechogenic lesion located at the bottom of the parotid gland with fine hyperechogenic cluster typical of lymphangioma.

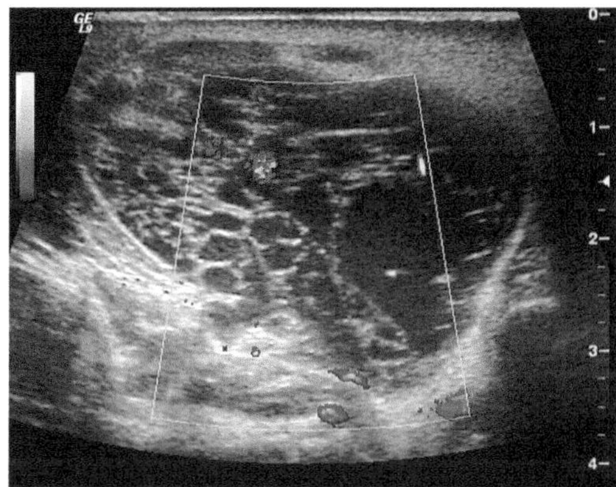

Fig. 43. Same patient as in Fig. 42 with color Doppler. See the hypovascularization of the lesion.

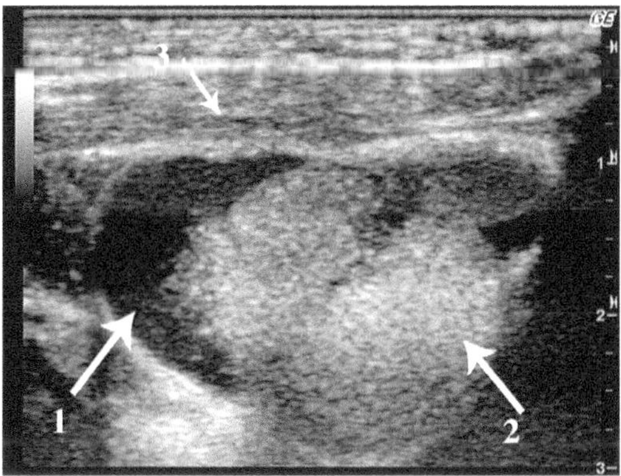

Fig. 44. Transverse sonogram of the floor of the mouth with a dermoid cyst. 1: hypoechogenic part of the cyst, 2: hyperechogenic part of the cyst, 3: anterior belly of digastric.

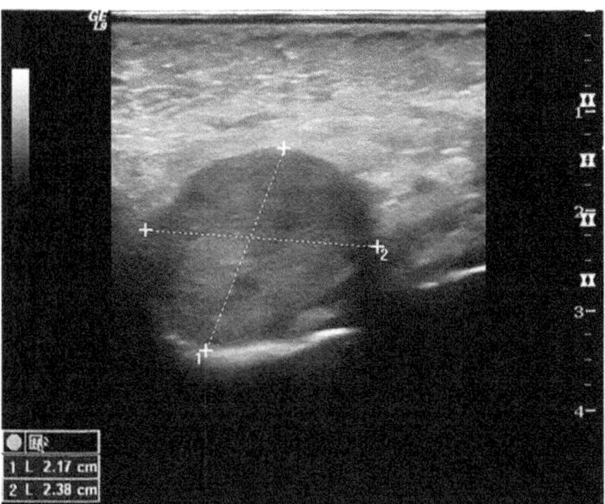

Fig. 45. Transverse sonogram of right cheek. Huge lesion at the internal face of the cheek, lightly hypoechogenic, encapsulated. Cytology was a basal cell adenoma.

mobilized by palpation. Color Doppler should be used to evaluate the intrinsic vascularization.

Retention Cysts (Ranulae)

These benign lesions generally occur following trauma involving the floor of the mouth. These retention cysts (ranulae) of the sublingual gland can appear hypoechoic.[50] The cyst is always very well delineated in the floor of the mouth (**Figs. 46** and **47**).

Chronic Sclerosing Sialdenitis

Chronic sclerosing sialdenitis (Kuttner's tumor) generally involves the submandibular gland. These hypoechoic pseudotumors should be investigated carefully to visualize the ductal structures of the lesion, which are typical for Kuttner's tumor.

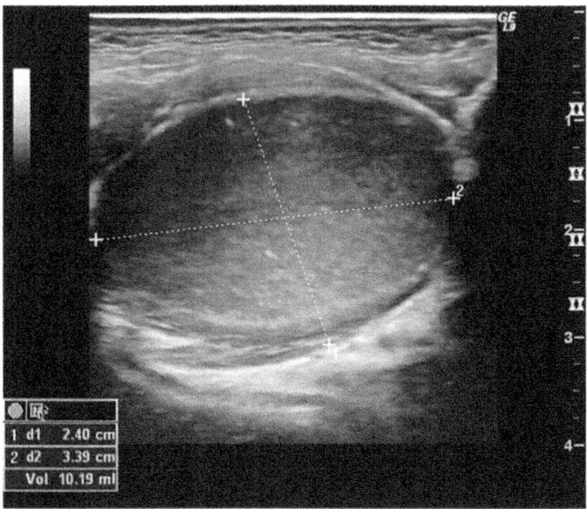

Fig. 46. Transverse sonogram of right floor of the mouth. Huge hypoechogenic lesion very well deliniated and encapsulated located under the Wharton's canal: a ranula.

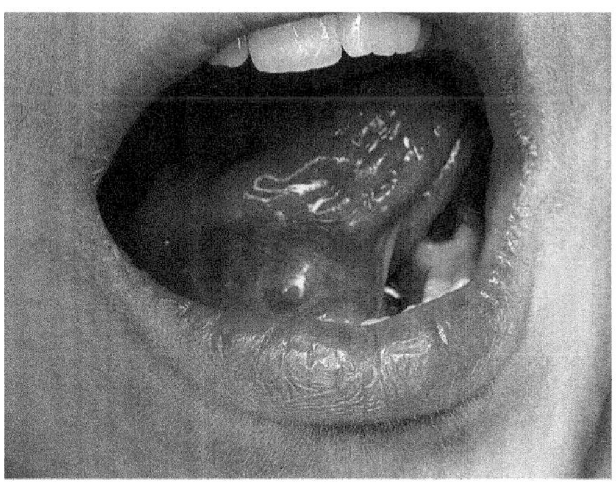

Fig. 47. Clinical aspects of the ranulae.

AIDS-related Lymphoepithelial Cysts

Depending on the clinical presentation, a mixture of multiple cystic and solid lesions may be caused either by lymphoepithelial cysts in AIDS or by sarcoidosis. In benign lymphoepithelial lesions in AIDS, gray-scale US shows a broad range of findings. Usually the parotid glands are enlarged with multiple cystic or hypoechoic lesions, but mixed lesions and septae can also be detected. Color Doppler shows a variety of avascular or hypervascularized lesions.[51–54] In most cases the cervical lymph nodes are enlarged. In these patients it is difficult to exclude malignant lymphoma by imaging.

SUMMARY

In most clinical situations, US is the first-line imaging method in the evaluation of the major salivary glands. In inflammation and infection, US differentiates obstructive and nonobstructive sialoadenitis. In sialolithiasis, US can differentiate intraductal from intraglandular lithiasis and visualize radiotransparent lithiasis. Concomitant obstruction and inflammation can be evaluated. In Sjogren's syndrome, US correlates with histological grade.

US is very sensitive in detecting tumors and lymph nodes. Superficial tumors can be delineated, whereas large or deeply located tumors usually require MRI. The specificity of US in differentiation of tumors is limited, but US is important for guiding FNA. Pseudotumors, such as tuberculosis, sarcoidosis, Kuttner's tumor, and intraglandular lymphadenopathy, should be distinguished from true neoplasms. With progress in ultrasound technology such as elastography, US distinction between benign and malignant tumors may be possible in the near future.

REFERENCES

1. Katz P. Nouvel apport de l'échographie en pathologie maxillo-faciale [Salivary glands, new approach by sonography]. Inf Dent 1990;72:2593–8.
2. Dost P, Kaiser S. Ultrasonographic biometry in salivary glands. Ultrasound Med Biol 1997;23:1299–303.
3. Gritzmann N, Fruhwald F. Sonographic anatomy of the tongue and floor of the mouth. Dysphagia 1988;2:196–202.

4. Yasumoto M, Nakagawa T, Shibuya H, et al. Ultrasonography of the sublingual space. J Ultrasound Med 1993;12:723–9.
5. Tarantino L, Giorgio A, de Stefano G, et al. Ultrasonography in the diagnosis of post-pubertal epidemic parotitis and its complications. Radiol Med 2000;99:461–4.
6. Schurawitzki H, Gritzmann N, Fezoulidis J, et al. Value and indications for high-resolution real-time sonography in nontumor salivary gland diseases. Rofo 1987;146:527–31.
7. Schwerk WB, Schroeder HG, Eichhorn T. High-resolution real-time sonography in salivary gland diseases. I. Inflammatory diseases. HNO 1985;33:505–10.
8. Ching AS, Ahuja AT, King AD, et al. Comparison of the sonographic features of acalculous and calculous submandibular sialadenitis. J Clin Ultrasound 2001; 29:332–8.
9. Kessler A, Strauss S, Eviatar E, et al. Ultrasonography of an infected parotid gland in an elderly patient: detection of sialolithiasis during the acute attack. Ann Otol Rhinol Laryngol 1995;104:736–7.
10. Curtin JJ, Ridley NT, Cumberworth VL, et al. Pneumoparotitis. J Laryngol Otol 1992;106:178–9.
11. Nusem-Horowitz S, Wolf M, Coret A, et al. Acute suppurative parotitis and parotid abscess in children. Int J Pediatr Otorhinolaryngol 1995;32:123–7.
12. Shimizu M, Ussmuller J, Donath K, et al. Sonographic analysis of recurrent parotitis in children: a comparative study with sialographic findings. Oral Surg Oral Med Oral Pathol Oral Radiol Endod 1998;86:660–5.
13. Nozaki H, Harasawa A, Hara H, et al. Ultrasonographic features of recurrent parotitis in childhood. Pediatr Radiol 1994;24:98–100.
14. Rubaltelli L, Sponga T, Candiani F, et al. Infantile recurrent sialectatic parotitis: the role of sonography and sialography in diagnosis and follow-up. J Radiol [Br] 1987;60:1211–4.
15. Katz P, Heran F. Pathologies des glandes salivaires [Salivary gland pathologies]. Encyclopédie Médico-chirurgicale (Elsevier, Masson, SAS, Paris), radiodiagnostic cœur-poumon 2007;32-800-A-30.
16. Gritzmann N, Hajek P, Karnel F, et al. Sonography in salivary calculi: indications and status. Rofo 1985;142:559–62.
17. Traxler M, Gritzmann N. Sonographic detection of salivary calculi of the sublingual gland. Rontgenblatter 1986;39:328–9.
18. Zenk J, Constantinidis J, Kydles S, et al. Clinical and diagnostic findings of sialolithiasis. HNO 1999;47:963–9.
19. Yoshimura Y, Inoue Y, Odagawa T. Sonographic examination of sialolithiasis. J Oral Maxillofac Surg 1989;47:907–12.
20. Brown JE, Escudier MP, Whaites EJ, et al. Intra-oral ultrasound imaging of a submandibular duct calculus. Dentomaxillofac Radiol 1997;26:252–5.
21. Gritzmann N. Sonography of the salivary glands. Am J Roentgenol 1989;153:161–6.
22. Bartlett LJ, Pon M. High-resolution real-time ultrasonography of the submandibular salivary gland. J Ultrasound Med 1984;3:433–7.
23. Becker M, Marchal F, Becker CD, et al. Sialolithiasis and salivary ductal stenosis: diagnostic accuracy of MR sialography with a three-dimensional extended phase conjugate-symmetry rapid spinecho sequence. Radiology 2000;217:347–58.
24. Herrlinger P, Gundlach P. Hypertrophy of the salivary glands in bulimia. HNO 2001;49:557–9.
25. Ariji Y, Ohki M, Eguchi K, et al. Texture analysis of sonographic features of the parotid gland in Sjogren's syndrome. Am J Roentgenol 1996;166:935–41.

26. Salaffi F, Argalia G, Carotti M, et al. Salivary gland ultrasonography in the evaluation of primary Sjogren's syndrome. Comparison with minor salivary gland biopsy. J Rheumatol 2000;27:1229–36.
27. Bradus RJ, Hybarger P, Gooding GA. Parotid gland: US findings in Sjogren syndrome. Work in progress. Radiology 1988;169:749–51.
28. Steiner E, Graninger W, Hitzelhammer J, et al. Color-coded duplex sonography of the parotid gland in Sjogren's syndrome. Rofo 1994;160:294–8.
29. Chikui T, Yonetsu K, Izumi M, et al. Abnormal blood flow to the submandibular glands of patients with Sjogren's syndrome: doppler waveform analysis. J Rheumato 2000;127:1222–8.
30. Ariji Y, Yuasa H, Ariji E. High frequency color Doppler sonography of the submandibular gland: relationship between salivary secretion and blood flow. Oral Surg Oral Med Oral Pathol Oral Radiol Endod 1998;86:476–81.
31. Ahuja AT, Loke TK, Mok CO, et al. Ultrasound of Kimura's disease. Clin Radiol 1995;50:170–3.
32. Koischwitz D, Gritzmann N. Ultrasound of the neck. Radiol Clin North Am 2000; 38:1029–45.
33. Hausegger KW, Krasa H, Pelzmann W, et al. Sonography of the salivary glands. Ultraschall Med 1993;14:68–74.
34. Schick S, Steiner E, Gahleitner A, et al. Differentiation of benign and malignant tumors of the parotid gland: value of pulsed Doppler and color Doppler sonography. Eur Radiol 1998;8:1462–7.
35. Shimizu M, Ussmuller J, Hartwein J, et al. A comparative study of sonographic and histopathologic findings of tumorous lesions in the parotid gland. Oral Surg Oral Med Oral Pathol Oral Radiol Endod 1999;88:723–37.
36. Gritzmann N, Turk R, Wittich G, et al. Hochauflosende sonographie nach operation von cystadenolymphomen der glandula parotis. Rofo 1996;145:648–51 [in German].
37. Klein K, Turk R, Gritzmann N, et al. The value of sonography in salivary gland tumors. HNO 1989;37:71–5.
38. Yoshiura K, Miwa K, Yuasa K, et al. Ultrasonographic texture characterization of salivary and neck masses using two-dimensional gray-scale clustering. Dentomaxillofac Radio 1997;26:332–6.
39. Miyake H, Matsumoto A, Hori Y, et al. Warthin's tumor of the parotid gland on Tc-99 m pertechnetate scintigraphy with lemon juice stimulation. Tc-99m uptake, size, and pathologic correlation. Eur Radiol 2001;12:2472–8.
40. Gritzmann N, Schratter M, Traxler M, et al. Sonography and computed tomography in deep cervical lipomas and lipomatosis of the neck. J Ultrasound Med 1988;7:451 60.
41. Gritzmann N. The diagnosis of salivary gland lipoma. Rofo 1989;151:419–22.
42. Chikui T, Yonetsu K, Yoshiura K, et al. Imaging findings of lipomas in the orofacial region with CT, US, and MRI. Oral Surg Oral Med Oral Pathol Oral Radiol Endod 1997;84:88–95.
43. Toma P, Rossi UG. Pediatric ultrasound. II. Other applications. Eur Radiol 2001; 11:2369–98.
44. Yang WT, Ahuja A, Metreweli C. Sonographic features of head and neck hemangiomas and vascular malformations: review of 23 patients. J Ultrasound Med 1997;16:39–44.
45. Sheth S, Nussbaum AR, Hutchins GM, et al. Cystic hygromas in children: sonographic-pathologic correlation. Radiology 1987;162:821–4.
46. Dubois J, Garel L, Abela A, et al. Lymphangiomas in children: percutaneous sclerotherapy with an alcoholic solution of zein. Radiology 1997;204:651–5.

47. Raffaelli C, Amoretti N, Parlotti B. Salivary glands. In: Bruneton JN, editor. Applications of sonography in head and neck pathology. Berlin/Heidelberg/New York: Springer; 2002. p. 91–136.
48. Traxler M, Ertl U, Ulm C, et al. Sonographic diagnosis of the unilateral benign hypertrophic masseter muscle. Z Stomatol 1991;88:23–6.
49. Calderazzi A, Falaschi F, Esposito S, et al. First branchial arch cysts. A diagnostic assessment. Radiol Med 1989;77:420–2.
50. Horiguchi H, Kakuta S, Nagumo M. Bilateral plunging ranula. A case report. Int J Oral Maxillofac Surg 1995;24:174–5.
51. Mandel L. Ultrasound findings in HIV-positive patients with parotid gland swellings. J Oral Maxillofac Surg 2001;59:283–6.
52. Martinoli C, Pretolesi F, Del Bono V, et al. Benign lymphoepithelial parotid lesions in HIV-positive patients: spectrum of findings at gray-scale and Doppler sonography. Am J Roentgenol 1995;165:975–9.
53. Goddart D, Francois A, Ninane J, et al. Parotid gland abnormality found in children seropositive for the human immunodeficiency virus (HIV). Pediatr Radiol 1990;20:355–7.
54. Gritzmann N, Rettenbacher T, Hollerweger A, et al. Sonography of the salivary glands. Eur Radiol 2003;13:964–75.

Technology of Sialendoscopy

Urban W. Geisthoff, Priv.-Doz. Dr. med.[a,b,*]

KEYWORDS

• Sialendoscopy • Sialoscopy • Technology • Salivary
• Treatment • Salivary

The diameter of salivary ducts sets a limit on the size of the instruments that can be used within them.[1] The miniaturization of endoscopes finally allowed sialendoscopy to begin in 1988 (**Fig. 1**).[2–6] Multiple considerations are needed to adapt endoscopes to the salivary ducts and glands, including compact outer diameter, highest number of pixels, durability, effective cleaning and sterilization, large working channel for various instruments, ergonomic handling, and flexible maneuverability inside the duct system.

TYPES OF ENDOSCOPES AND THEIR PROPERTIES

Different types of endoscopes have emerged to meet the demands listed previously: flexible sialendoscopes, rigid sialendoscopes, and semiflexible sialendoscopes (compact and modular). **Table 1** lists different models of sialendoscopes from the past and present. **Box 1** lists the addresses of different producers and distributors for material usable for sialendoscopy. Each type of endoscope has its own clinical properties.

Flexible Endoscopes

Flexible endoscopes are advantageous as it is possible to move them through ductal kinks and bends. Some of the flexible endoscopes can be steered, which is especially helpful when a certain branch has to be intubated (see **Fig. 1; Figs. 2–5**). Their use is atraumatic; however, a drawback is that only weak forces can be applied (eg, to surmount stenotic areas). Handling is often more difficult than for semirigid or rigid endoscopes. The success rate for normal stones seems to be lower than for semirigid

Urban Geisthoff consulted with Spiggle & Theis, Overath, Germany, and Gyrus ACMI, Tuttlingen, Germany for the development of instruments without any financial benefit, thus far.

[a] University of the Saarland, Medical Faculty, Kirrberger Str, D-66421, Homburg/Saar, Germany
[b] Department of Otorhinolaryngology, Holweide Hospital, Hospitals of the City of Cologne, Neufelder Strasse 32, D-51067 Cologne, Germany
* HNO, KHS Holweide, Neufelder Street 32, D-51067 Koeln, Germany.
E-mail address: http://www.geisthoff.de

Otolaryngol Clin N Am 42 (2009) 1001–1028
doi:10.1016/j.otc.2009.08.008 **oto.theclinics.com**

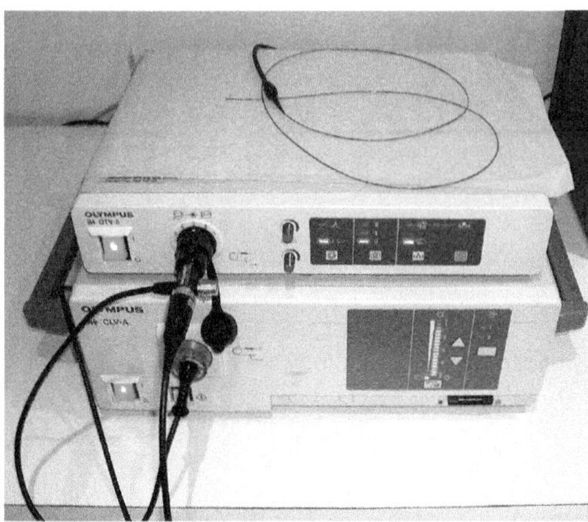

Fig. 1. Flexible endoscope (Olympus, Tokyo, Japan) used by Philippe Katz for the first salivary gland endoscopy in December 1988. (*Courtesy of* Dr Philippe Katz, Paris, France; with permission.)

endoscopes.[7] Flexible endoscopes are fragile and have a short lifespan and it is not possible to autoclave them.[8]

Rigid Endoscopes

Most clinical endoscopes rely on a fiberoptic system for image transmission. Rigid endoscopes, however, use a pure lens system with superb optical qualities and better resolution. These endoscopes have larger diameters but are more stable (**Fig. 6**). They can be autoclaved. The camera is fixed directly onto the ocular attached to the endoscope, resulting in a cumbersome handling.

Semirigid Endoscopes

Semirigid endoscopes are a compromise between flexible and rigid endoscopes. The long, flexible, optical fiber connection for light and image transmission enables the decoupling of the examination probe from the rigid eyepiece. This means that work with semiflexible endoscopes can be performed with great freedom of movement and minimal effort while maintaining excellent precision. A modular and a compact construction type of semirigid endoscopes exist.

Semirigid Compact Endoscopes

A typical therapeutic semirigid compact endoscope combines a fiber light transmission, a fiber image transmission, a working channel and an irrigation channel within one compact instrument (**Fig. 7**). The outer tube covers, stabilizes, and protects all of the components resulting in a minimum outer diameter of the whole system. **Fig. 8** shows the construction principle of the sheath of the examination probe of a semirigid compact endoscope and **Figs. 9–11** show enlarged the tips of such endoscopes.

Semirigid Modular Endoscopes

The optical fibers used for light and image transmission are combined into a single probe-like component (**Fig. 12**A, B). This can be used in combination with different sheaths (see **Fig. 12**C). Using a small single sheath creates a diagnostic endoscope. The gap between optical system and the sheath's outer wall is used as irrigation channel (**Fig. 13**). A combination with a large single lumen sheath or a double-lumen sheath creates enough space to introduce different instruments (**Fig. 14**).

In comparison with the compact versions, the ratio of the working channel to the total endoscope diameter is usually lower in modular endoscopes. The single therapeutic outer sheaths of modular endoscopes sometimes trap air, which can impair visualization by irrigating into the ducts. The modular systems, however, have two important advantages:

1. Economic advantage: only one optical system is necessary for a variety of procedures. The optical system is the most expensive part of the endoscope. By combining it with different sheaths, a versatile tool is created.
2. Hygienic advantage: compact endoscopes often have very thin irrigation channels. These are difficult to clean.[9] Plasma sterilization may not be sufficient for these narrow channels, gas sterilization is often not available, and autoclaving can damage the endoscope. The probe-like optical system of modular endoscopes is easy to clean and is normally suitable for plasma sterilization. The channels of the different sheaths generally have larger diameters and the sheaths themselves are normally autoclavable or single use only.

Outer Diameter, Shape, Material, Maneuverability

The outer diameter is of paramount importance for the introduction of the scope and its advancement inside the narrow duct system. The endoscopes with diameters of approximately 1.5 mm and larger are sometimes not thin enough to accommodate the ducts and might not advance the pathology. In such cases, other approaches, such as sonographically controlled procedures, should be taken into consideration.[10] Modular semiflexible endoscopes are produced with two different cross-sectional shapes: the round version conforms well with the round shape of the duct. The outer shape of a double tube uses the same perimeter of the duct for a lower cross-sectional area. The unused space between the two tubes, however, also has advantages: it can be used to flush fragments or debris with irrigation to clear the field of view. This space also allows for higher flow and passage of larger particles. For other large round endoscopes, it is sometimes necessary to interrupt endoscopy by removing the scope and massaging the gland to clear the duct system.

Some endoscopes are made from nitinol steel (see **Fig. 12**B; **Fig. 15**), which is more flexible than regular steel and can be advantageous when following a curved duct. A more rigid system, however, is often easier to steer. Again, outer diameter also plays an important role here.

An interesting feature of one compact semirigid endoscope series (Marchal model, Karl Storz) is a slight bend in the endoscope shaft near its distal tip (**Fig. 16**). This can make steering and selectively following branchings easier. The bend does reduce the usable diameter of the working channel, however, and prevents the use of straight, nonflexible instruments.

In most cases, the intraductal position of the endoscope tip can be easily seen by skin transillumination. Centimeter markings on the shaft, however, can help to assess exactly the tip's position (Erlangen model, Karl Storz) (**Fig. 17**).

Good maneuverability is also achieved by flexible, steerable, fine endoscopes. These endoscopes are mainly used for diagnostic purposes but do have a "working channel" in some models (Spiggle & Theis and Almikro) mainly for irrigation. Such models are of limited use for stone fragmentation and extraction as only fine baskets fit through the working channels. The use of laser fibers is limited as they are often not resistant to strong bending and break. The increase in combined endoscope

Table 1
Overview of different historic and current endoscopes

Author, Year, no. of Pixels, Additional Information	Type of Endoscope	Compact/Modular/ Steerable Flexible	Manufacturer/ Distributor	Outer Diameter/mm	Diameter of the Working Channel/mm	Diameter of the Irrigation Channel/mm
Gundlach 1990[4]	Flexible	Unknown	Richard Wolf	2	0.6	Only one channel
Königsberger 1990[5]	Flexible	Steerable	Karl Storz	Unknown	>0.8	
Katz 1991[2,3]	Flexible		Olympus (Tokyo, Japan)	0.8	None	
Arzoz 1994[20]	Rigid	Unknown	Karl Storz	2.3	1	Only one channel
Gundlach 1994[21]	Flexible			1.5	0.5	
Nahlieli 1994[22]	Rigid	Modular	Friatec (Mannheim, Germany)	2.9	None	2.9–2.7
Zenk 1994[23]	Flexible	Steerable		1.6	>0.4	
Iro 1995[24]	Flexible	Steerable		1.6	0.6	Only one channel
Ito 1996[25]	Flexible		Clinical Supply (Japan)	1.5	0.2	
Iro 1996[26]	Flexible	Steerable		1.5–2.0	>0.4	0.2
Arzoz 1996[27]	?		Karl Storz	2.1	1.0	
Yuasa 1997[28]	Flexible		Medical Science (Tokyo, Japan)	0.8	None	
Yuasa 1997[28]	Rigid		Medical Science	1.0	None	
Nahlieli 1997[29]	Rigid			2.0	1.0	
Nahlieli 1997[29]	Rigid			2.5	1.0	
Hopf 1998[30]	Flexible	Steerable	?	1.6	0.5	Only one channel
Marchal 1998[31]	?	?		0.9–1.6		
Nahlieli 1999[8]	Semirigid		Karl Storz	1.3	None	1.3–1.0
Nahlieli 1999[8]	Semirigid		Karl Storz	2.3 × 1.3	1.0	1.3–1.0
Kerr 2001[32]	Rigid		Richard Wolf	1.5	?	?

Marchal 2001[7]	Flexible	Nonsteerable		0.5–0.8	None	None
Marchal 2001[7]	Semirigid	Modular	Karl Storz	1.3	None	1.3–1.0
Marchal 2001[7]	Semirigid	Modular	Karl Storz	(2.67 mm^2)	0.8	+
Marchal 2001[7]	Semirigid	Modular	Karl Storz	(2.29 mm^2)	0.8	+
Chu 2003[33]	Rigid			3.1	+	
Zenk 2004[34] 6000 px	Semirigid	Compact	PolyDiagnost	1.1	0.4	+
Geisthoff 2007,[35] 2008,[15] 6000 px, a	Semirigid	Compact	Gyrus ACMI/ Spiggle & Theis	1.7	1.0	0.2
Nahlieli 2007,[12] Iro 2008,[18] 6000 px, a	Semirigid	Compact	Karl Storz	0.8	-	0.25
Nahlieli 2007,[12] Iro 2008,[18] 6000 px, a	Semirigid	Compact	Karl Storz	1.1	0.4	0.25
Nahlieli 2007,[12] Iro 2008,[18] 6000 px, a	Semirigid	Compact	Karl Storz	1.6	0.8	0.26
6000 px	Semirigid	Modular	PolyDiagnost	0.9, 1.1, 1.6, 2.0	One-joint working and irrigation channel also containing the optical system (0.53 mm)	
10,000 px (one version with opening angle of 70° and one of 120°)	Semirigid	Modular	PolyDiagnost	1.1, 1.6, 2.0	One-joint working and irrigation channel also containing the optical system (0.9 mm)	
30,000 px	Semirigid	Modular	PolyDiagnost	1.6, 2.0	One-joint working and irrigation channel also containing the optical system (1.2 mm)	
6000 px, a	Semirigid	Compact	Spiggle & Theis	0.9	None	0.26
6000 px, a	Semirigid	Compact	Spiggle & Theis	1.0	0.41	0.2
6000 px, a	Semirigid	Compact	Spiggle & Theis	1.2	0.62	0.2
6000 px, a	Semirigid	Compact	Spiggle & Theis	1.4	0.62	0.3
6000 px	Flexible	Steerable	Spiggle & Theis	1.3	One-joint working and irrigation channel of 0.35 mm	

Abbreviations: a, suitable for autoclave; px, pixels/number of fibers in the optical transmission system; ?, unknown; +, containing such a channel of unknown diameter; −, not containing such a channel.

Box 1
Companies selling or producing technology that might be used for sialendoscopy

- Almikro, Bad Krozingen, Germany (www.almikro.de)
- Balaton, Warsaw, Poland
- Boston Scientific, Natick, Massachusetts (www.bostonscientific.com)
- Cook Medical, Bloomington, Indiana (www.cookmedical.com)
- Gyrus ACMI, Southborough, Massachusetts (www.gyrusacmi.com) (formerly Gyrus ACMI/ Stuemer, Tuttlingen, Germany)
- Karl Storz, Tuttlingen, Germany (www.karlstorz.com)
- PolyDiagnost, Pfaffenhofen, Germany (www.polydiagnost.com)
- Richard Wolf, Knittlingen, Germany (www.richard-wolf.com)
- Sialo Technology, Ashkelon, Israel (www.sialotechnology.com)
- Spiggle & Theis, Overath, Germany (www.spiggle-theis.com)

approaches might give these instruments some more importance: a small, flexible, steerable endoscope is more likely to reach a stone in a curved duct system than a semirigid one. It can be used to mark the stone by the transillumination effect, so that it can be approached externally.[11–14] Maneuvering a flexible steerable endoscope, however, often requires more skill and experience than a semirigid one.[7]

Working Channel Diameter

The diameter of the working channel is of paramount importance for some therapeutic tasks. **Table 1** gives an overview of the diameters of instruments used in therapeutic endoscopies. It is important to realize the effect of the diameter on the stability of the instruments. For instruments, such as forceps, balloons, or baskets, the cross-sectional area of a 0.4-mm diameter instrument is one quarter that of a 0.8-mm diameter instrument. The cross-sectional area of the latter one is 0.64 the size of a 1-mm diameter instrument. The rate of success and the risk of material fatigue breakage of the instruments are directly correlated with cross-sectional area. Additionally, the

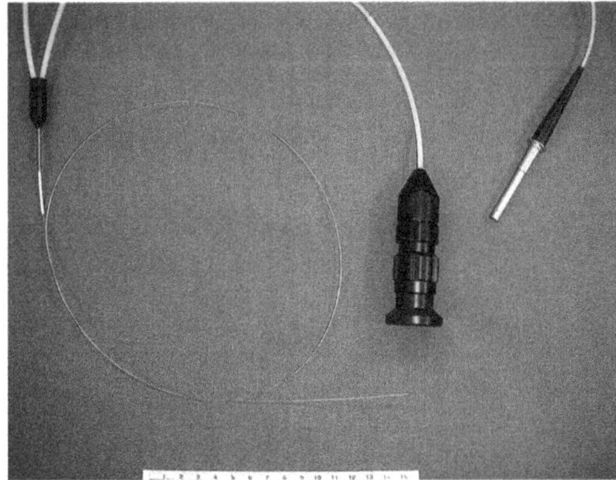

Fig. 2. Historic flexible endoscope without steering and without working channel similar to the one used by Katz in 1988. (*Courtesy of* Richard Wolf, Knittlingen, Germany.)

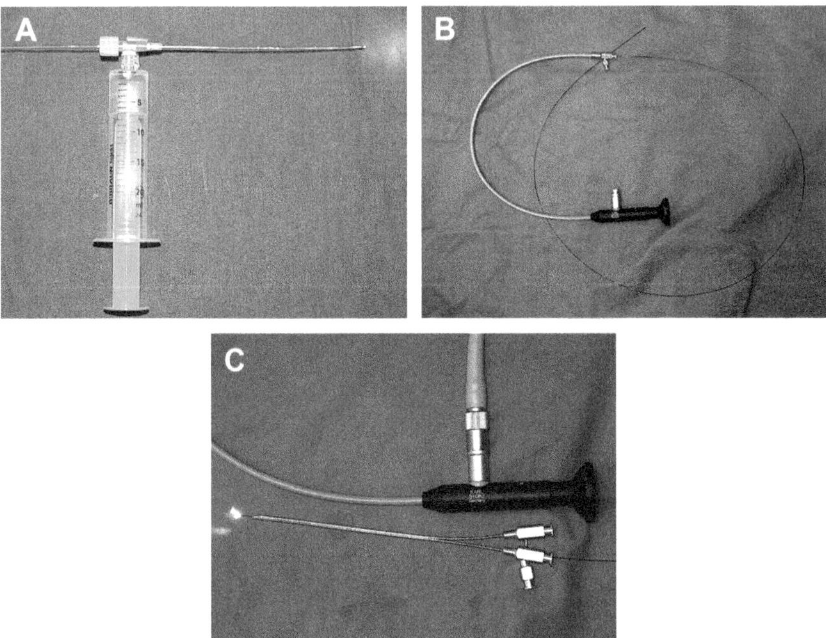

Fig. 3. (*A*) Self-made construction to allow irrigation for the endoscope shown in **Fig. 2**. (*B*) Modern flexible nonsteerable endoscope with 3000 fibers primarily sold for endoscopy of the lacrimal ducts and the eustachian tube. (*Courtesy of* Karl Storz, Tuttlingen, Germany.) (*C*) To allow steering of such a flexible endoscope, rigid outer sheaths can be used. A functionality similar to the mother-baby endoscopes used in gastroenterology results. These systems, however, are extremely fragile and expensive.

finer instruments are often more expensive. Alternatively, a large, stable instrument is of no use when it is too large to reach the relevant duct region. Sophisticated instruments in this respect are the so-called optical forceps, which are a combination of an outer sheath with an incorporated instrument (PolyDiagnost, Pfaffenhofen, Germany) (**Figs. 18** and **19**). These instruments allow the effective use of forceps in combination with a small overall diameter of the whole instrument. Minor drawbacks of this system

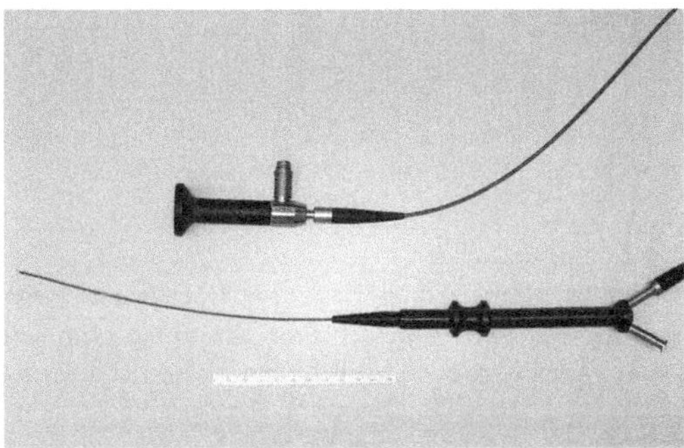

Fig. 4. Modern flexible steerable endoscope with 6000 fibers, an outer diameter of 1.5 mm, and a working channel of 0.4 mm. (*Courtesy of* Spiggle & Theis, Overath, Germany.)

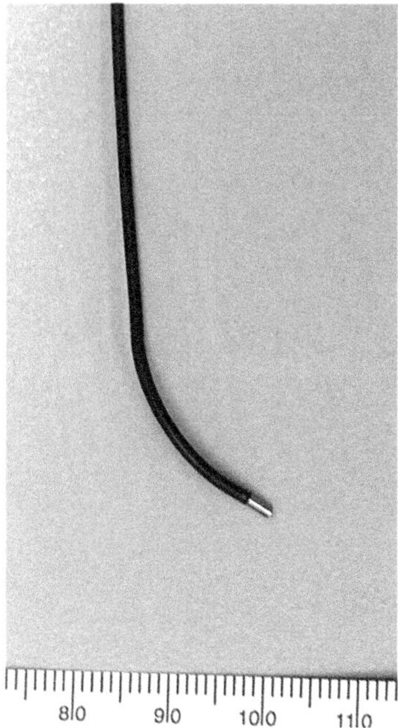

Fig. 5. The tip of the endoscope shown in **Fig. 2** can be bent to facilitate changing the direction of view, passing curves and kinks.

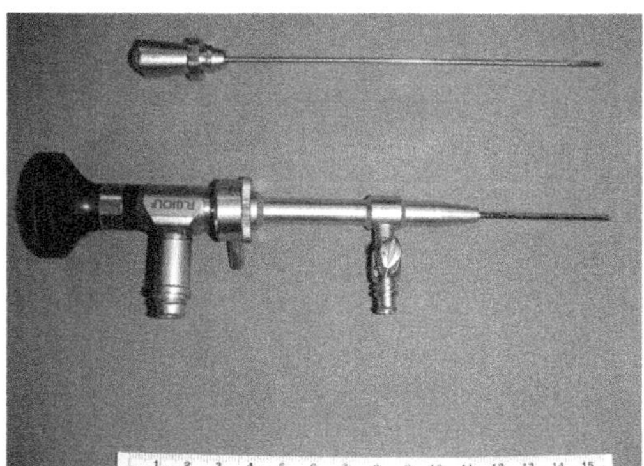

Fig. 6. Rigid endoscope together with a sheath that allows irrigation. (*Courtesy of* Richard Wolf, Knittlingen, Germany.) Endoscopes of this type are also used for arthroscopies or pediatric cystoscopies. No working channel is provided. One possibility for interventions is to remove the optics from the irrigation channel in the moment when the target has been reached. Afterwards, instruments can be introduced and operations be performed under haptic control.

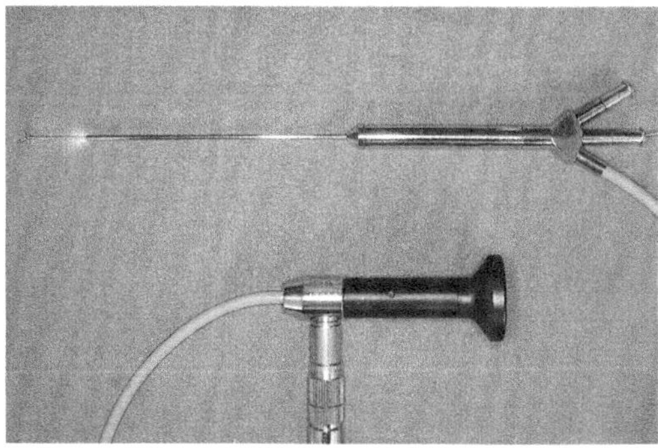

Fig. 7. Example of a compact semirigid endoscope (instrument according to Geisthoff, Spiggle & Theis, Overath, Germany). This therapeutic endoscope has a working channel of 1 mm, which also allows the introduction of quite stable forceps (as shown). The existence of the irrigation channel (diameter of 0.2 mm) can be noted by the second Luer lock tube at the back part of the endoscope. The endoscope has a large outer diameter of 1.7 mm; therefore, Seldinger's technique often has to be applied for insertion (see also article by Geisthoff on "Basic Technology of Sialendoscopy" elsewhere in this issue).

are that the forceps can impede vision during endoscope advancement. Additionally, a change of the instrument always means complete removal of the endoscope, a change-out of the instrument, and then its reinsertion.

Cleaning and Sterilization

Hygiene is an important issue and laws and regulations can differ from country to country. Manufacturers have different recommendations regarding their endoscopes. High-level cleaning for "semicritical" instruments might be sufficient for several sialendoscopic procedures, as the instruments only come into contact with intact mucous membranes or smaller fissures and are introduced through natural, unsterile orifices.[12] For some procedures, however, such as endoscopic biopsies or laser lithotripsies, sterilization is preferable. Sialendoscopes are fragile, sensitive instruments. Several manufacturers allow autoclaving some of their instruments (see **Table 1**). They warranty only a limited number of sterilization cycles, however. Experience shows

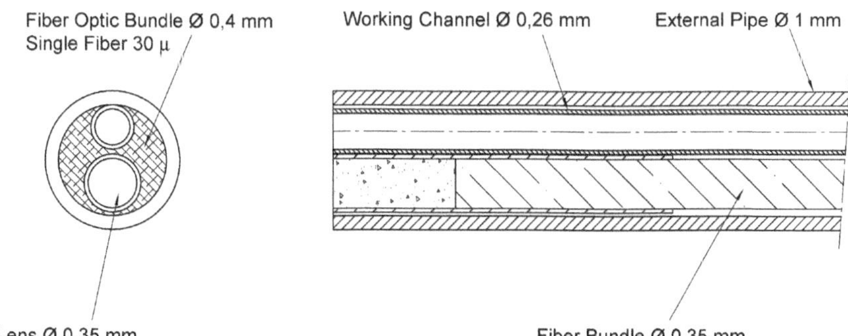

Fig. 8. Construction principle of a compact semirigid endoscope. One outer tube protects and stabilizes all internal components, including fiber optics and working and irrigation channels. In this case, the diagnostic endoscope contains only an irrigation and no true working channel. (*Courtesy of* Spiggle & Theis, Overath, Germany; with permission.)

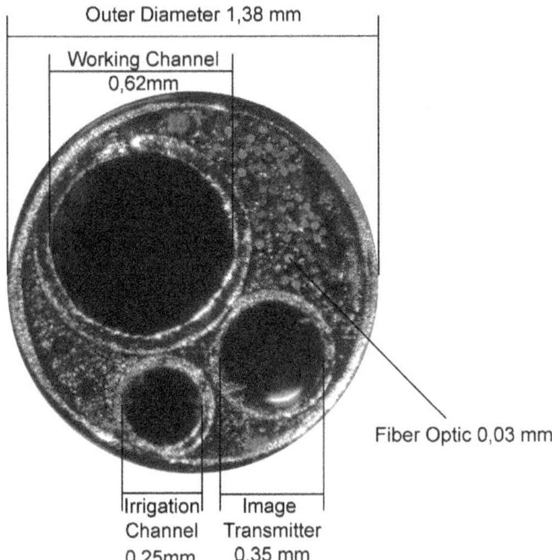

Fig. 9. Microscopic view of a tip of a therapeutic compact semirigid endoscope similar to the one shown in **Fig. 7**. The fibers of the image transmitter are covered by a lens, whereas the optical fibers for the light source are filling the gaps between the outer tube, the image transmitter, and the working and the irrigation channel. (*Courtesy of* Spiggle & Theis, Overath, Germany; with permission.)

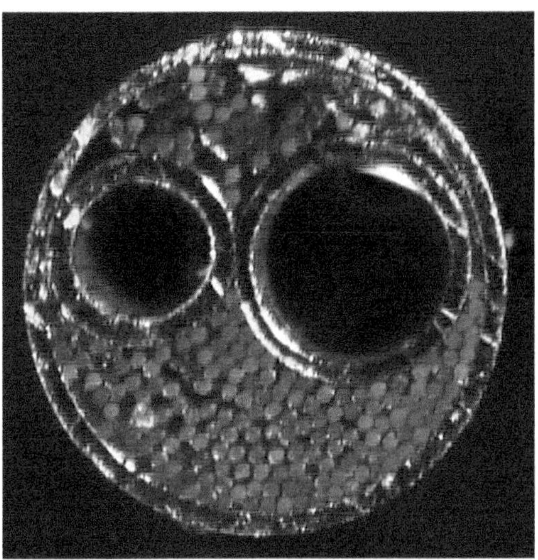

Fig. 10. Enlarged tip of a diagnostic semirigid endoscope as shown in **Fig. 8**. When comparing to **Figs. 7** and **9**, it can be clearly seen that there is only an irrigation but no working channel (outer diameter: 0.9 mm). (*Courtesy of* PolyDiagnost, Pfaffenhofen, Germany; with permission.)

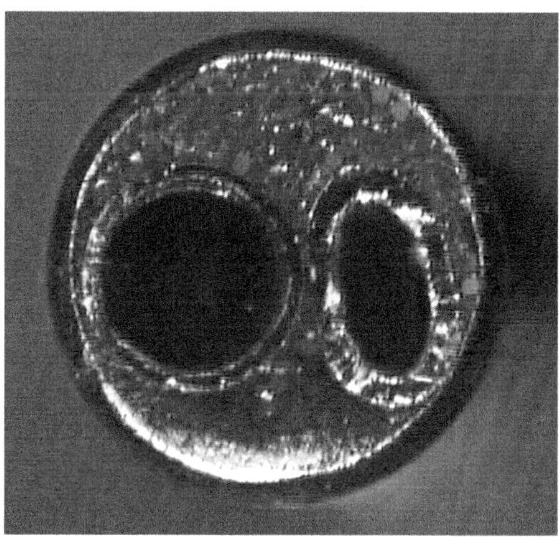

Fig. 11. Enlarged top of a diagnostic semirigid endoscope similar to the one shown in **Fig. 10**. The form of the irrigation channel is oval instead of round for further miniaturization (outer diameter: 0.7 mm). (*Courtesy of* PolyDiagnost, Pfaffenhofen, Germany; with permission.)

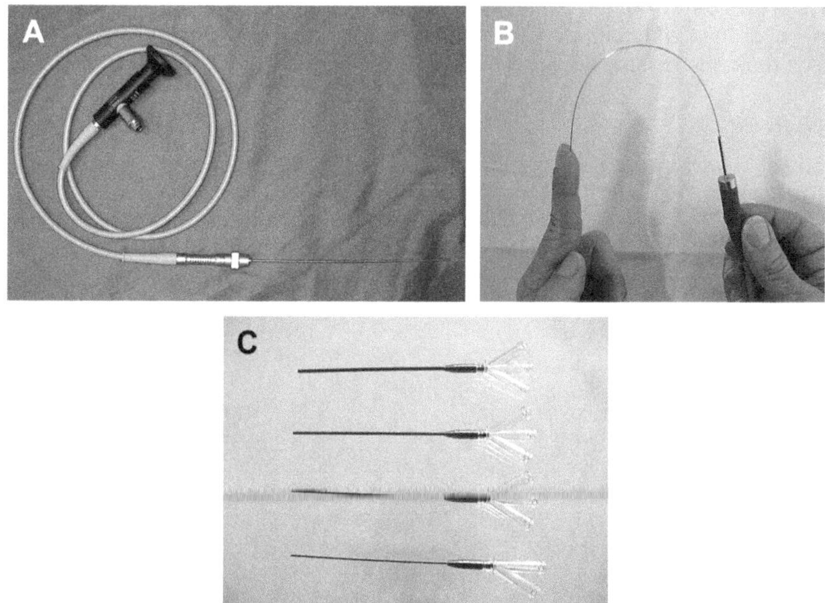

Fig. 12. (*A*) Probe-like optical system of a modular semirigid endoscope. The probe-like sheath includes the fibers for the light source and the image-transmission system (instrument according to Nahlieli, Karl Storz, Tuttlingen, Germany). (*B*) Probe-like optical system of a modular semirigid endoscope. The covering of this version is made from nitinol steel giving it high flexibility and low risk of breakage. (*Courtesy of* PolyDiagnost, Pfaffenhofen, Germany; with permission.) (*C*) Different sheaths with diameters of 0.9 mm, 1.1 mm, 1.6 mm, and 2.0 mm for the optical system shown in **Fig. 12**B. These sheaths are single use only; a version for autoclave also exists. A disadvantage of this system is that air is sometimes entrapped in the sheaths and can be annoying during the endoscopy. (*Courtesy of* PolyDiagnost, Pfaffenhofen, Germany; with permission.)

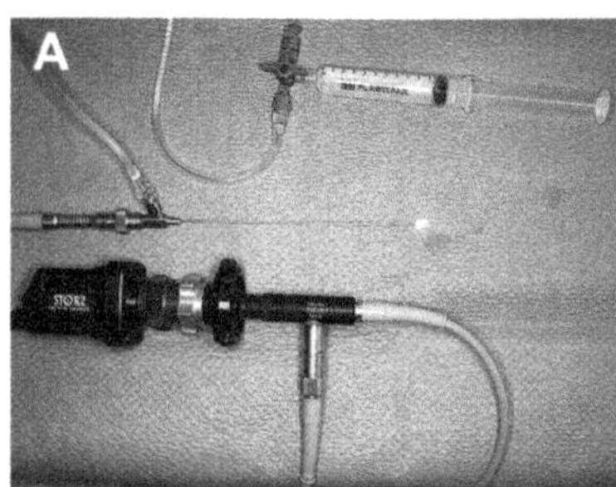
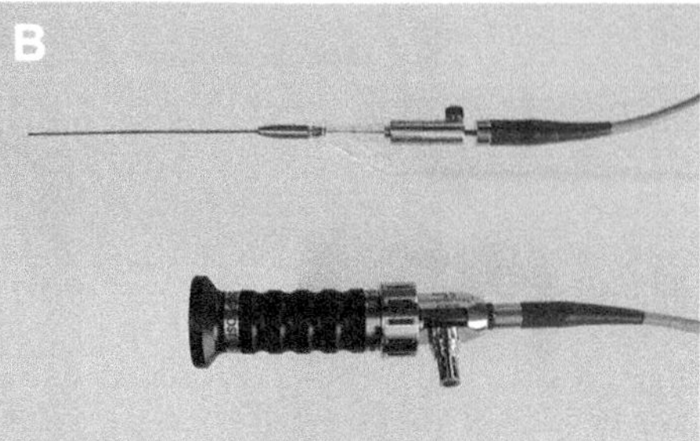

Fig. 13. (*A*) The combination of the optical system shown in Fig. 12A with one simple sheath results in a diagnostic endoscope with only one irrigation channel. (*From* Karl Storz, Tuttlingen, Germany; with permission.) (*B*) Combination of the optical system shown in Fig. 12B and a sheath with an outer diameter of 0.9 mm. A diagnostic endoscope with irrigation channel but without working channel results. (*Courtesy of* PolyDiagnost, Pfaffenhofen, Germany; with permission.)

a decreasing optical quality that results from an increasing number of autoclave procedures. Methods associated with lower temperatures, such as gas sterilization (ethylene oxide), plasma sterilization, or high-level sterilization (STERIS), are gentler. Gas sterilization is not available everywhere and is time consuming, with cycles even longer than 24 hours, depending on the temperature. The effectiveness of sterilization methods for small-diameter working and irrigation channels is controversial.[9]

Image Quality

In general, the image quality of available sialendoscopes has increased greatly in the past few years. Apart from some rigid endoscopes, all systems use optical fiber bundles for image transmission. The visual direction is straightforward (0°); the visual angle is normally approximately 70°. Dense packing of the fiber optics and a mean diameter of approximately 3- to 4-μm per fiber allow for higher-quality images. The

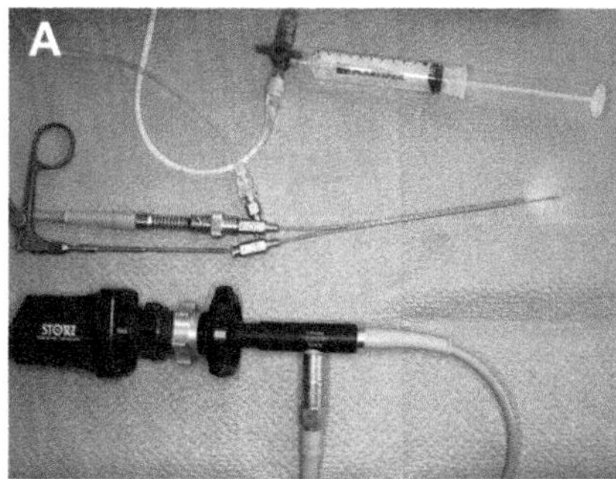
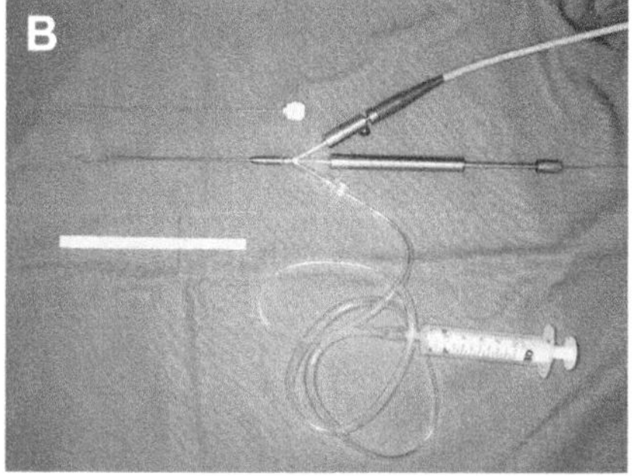

Fig. 14. (*A*) The combination of the same optical system shown in Fig. 12A with a double-tube–like sheath makes an interventional endoscope with irrigation and working channel. Different sizes of working channels for different tasks can be chosen, making this a versatile instrument. (*From* Karl Storz, Tuttlingen, Germany; with permission.) (*B*) When combining the optical system shown in Fig. 12B with a larger sheath, an interventional endoscope results. In this case, a sheath with an outer diameter of 1.1 mm was used; a 0.4-mm basket was introduced through the common working and irrigation channel. (*From* PolyDiagnost, Pfaffenhofen, Germany; with permission.)

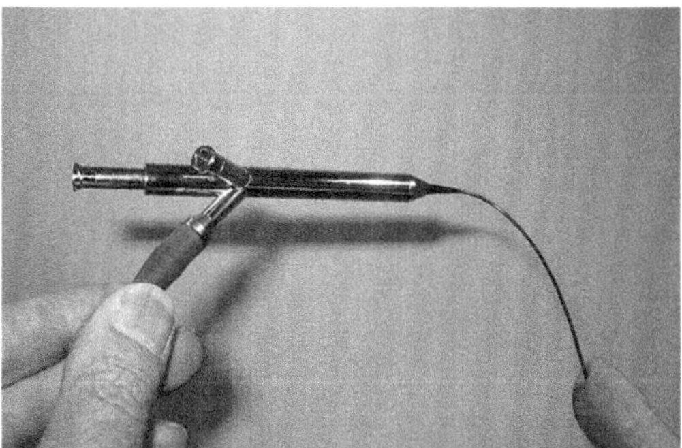

Fig. 15. Compact modular semirigid interventional endoscope made with outer tubing from nitinol steel. This gives a high flexibility and a lower risk of breakage. The flexibility is sometimes advantageous during interventions; sometimes more rigid instruments are better for steering. (*Courtesy of* PolyDiagnost, Pfaffenhofen, Germany; with permission.)

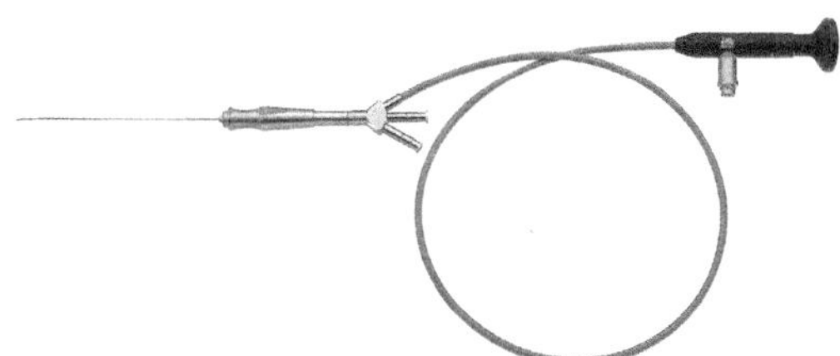

Fig. 16. Compact modular semirigid interventional endoscope according to Marchal with a slight curve at the distal tip. This bend can be advantageous when following a curve duct or trying to intubate a ductal branching. (*Courtesy of* Karl Storz, Tuttlingen, Germany; with permission.)

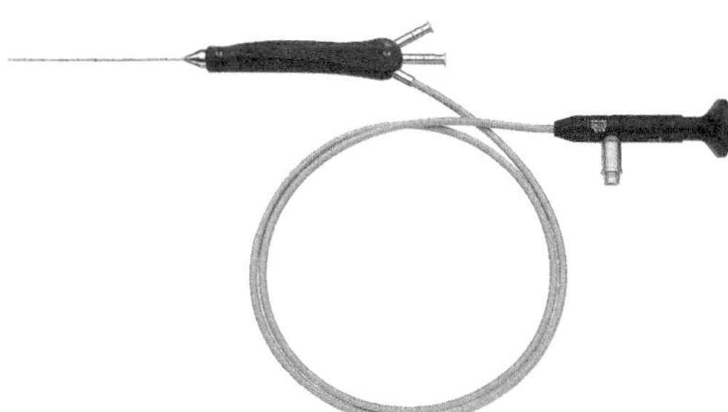

Fig. 17. Compact modular semirigid interventional endoscope, Erlangen type, with centimeter markings on the sheath. In addition to the transillumination effect, these markings can be helpful to assess the current position of the tip of the endoscope. (*Courtesy of* Karl Storz, Tuttlingen, Germany; with permission.)

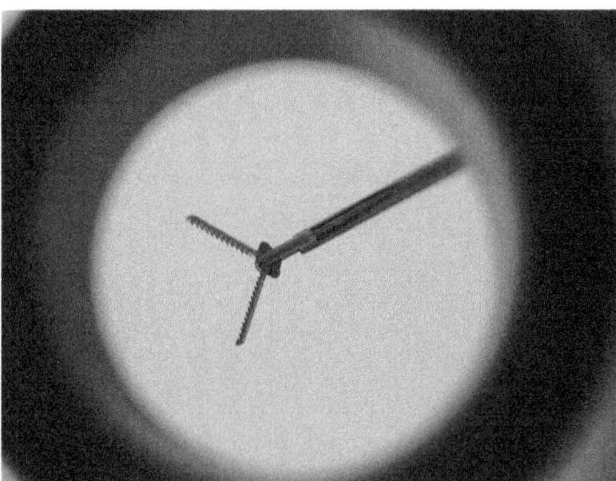

Fig. 18. Sheath for the flexible modular system, which contains a grasping forceps at its tip. The advantage of the system is its low outer diameter of 1.1 mm; disadvantages are that the vision can be impeded by the instruments and that a change of the instrument is always associated with a retraction of the whole system. (*Courtesy of* PolyDiagnost, Pfaffenhofen, Germany; with permission.)

resolution of the picture is mainly dependent on the number of pixels. This can be seen in the **Fig. 20**. Alternatively, an increased number of fibers also increases the total outer diameter. Therefore, a sensible compromise is the sign of a good endoscope. Most modern endoscopes provide a minimum of 6000 pixels. Even 3000 pixels, however, provide sufficient optical quality for most tasks, although the resolution provided by 3000 pixels is probably a lower limit.[15]

INSTRUMENTATION

A large variety of instrument types are made by different companies for endoscopes. The quality tolerance limits of different manufacturers can vary widely and it is wise to test that the instruments easily fit through the working channels of the individual endoscopes before buying them.

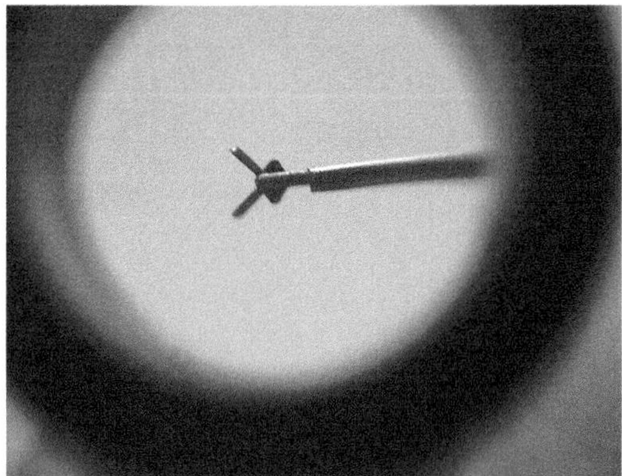

Fig. 19. Sheath for the flexible modular system from PolyDiagnost, which contains a biopsy forceps at its tip. See also legend to **Fig. 18**. (*Courtesy of* PolyDiagnost, Pfaffenhofen, Germany; with permission.)

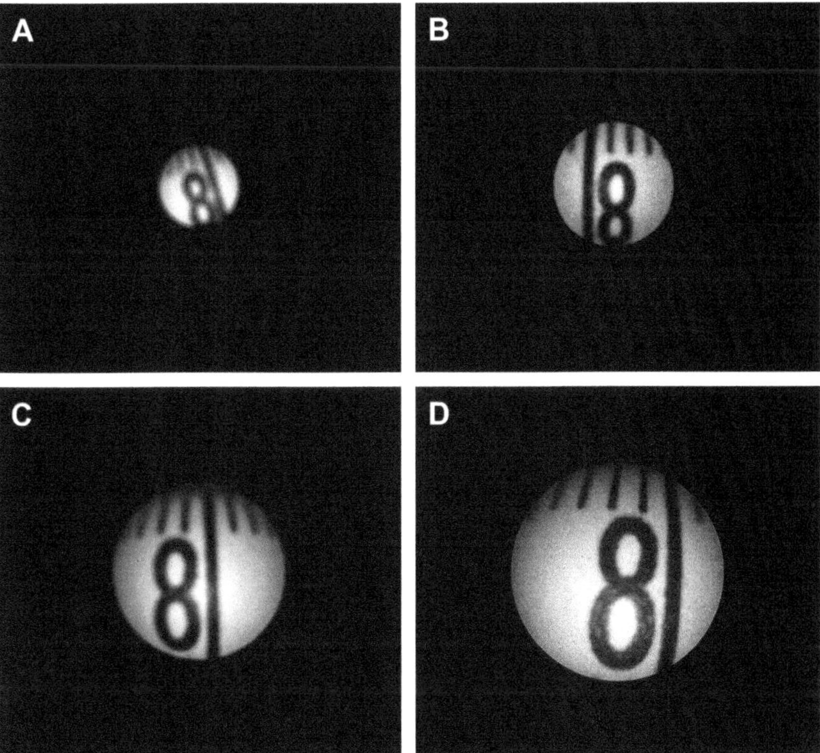

Fig. 20. Images of the same object using endoscopes with different numbers of fibers/pixels for image transmission: (*A*) 1600 pixels; (*B*) 3000 pixels; (*C*) 6000 pixels; (*D*): 10,000 pixels. The higher resolution can easily be seen. (*Courtesy of* Spiggle & Thess, Overath, Germany; with permission.)

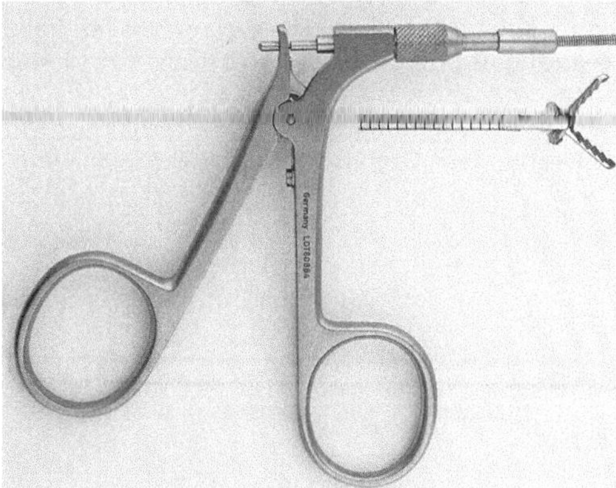

Fig. 21. Grasping forceps with serrated surface on the prongs and with a handle that allows determining the orientation of the prongs easily (forceps handle). (*Courtesy of* Spiggle & Theis, Overath, Germany; with permission.)

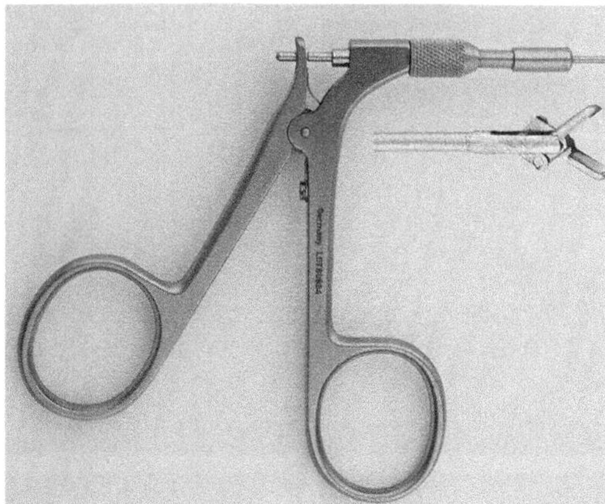

Fig. 22. Biopsy forceps with sharp cutting edges. (*Courtesy of* Spiggle & Theis, Overath, Germany; with permission.)

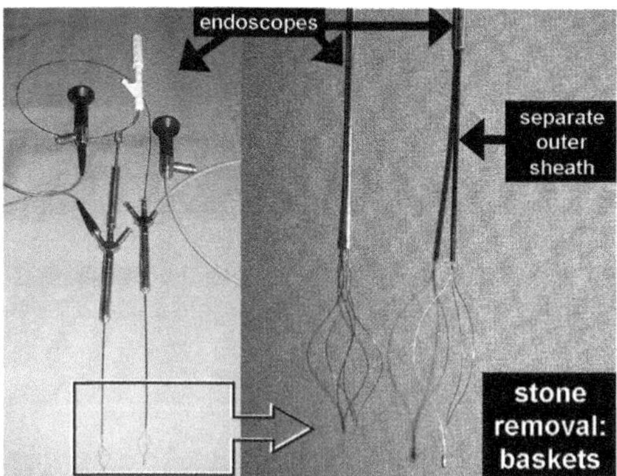

Fig. 23. Different types of baskets: the type on the right hand side has a separate outer sheath allowing opening it behind the stone. The type on the left hand side opens directly in front of the scope, reducing its possibilities. Alternatively, it has a smaller outer diameter, is autoclavable, and can be used with a one-hand spring mechanism, which is screwed to the working channel port of the scope. (*From* Geisthoff UW. Techniques for multimodal salivary gland stone therapy. Operative Tech Otolaryngol 2007;18:332–40; with permission.)

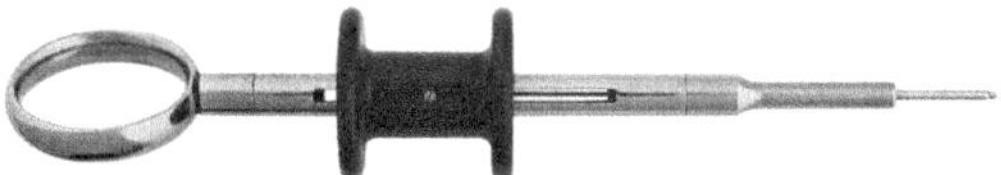

Fig. 24. One type of multiple handle versions used for baskets. This type of handle (draw roll handle) is less optimal for the use with forceps as it is difficult to determine the orientation of the prongs. (*Courtesy of* Spiggle & Theis, Overath, Germany; with permission.)

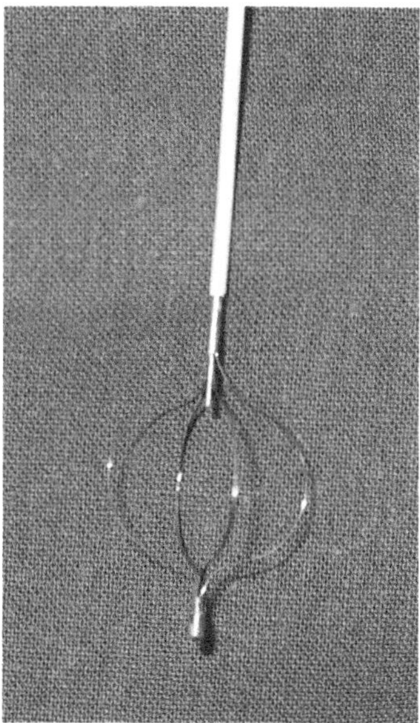

Fig. 25. Basket with an additional central separate channel for use with a laser fiber build for urologic purposes. (*Courtesy of* Cook Medical, Bloomington, Indiana.)

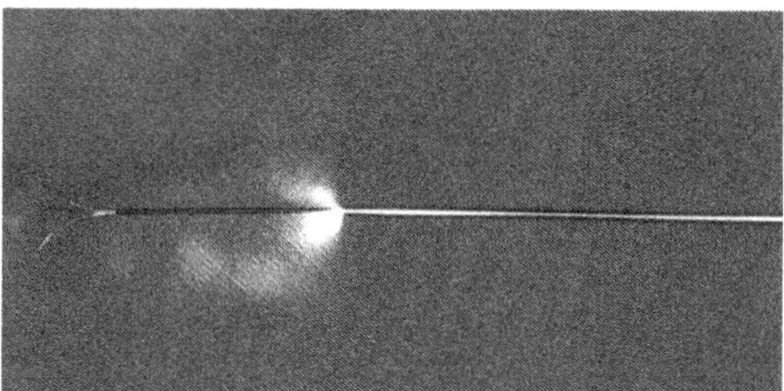

Fig. 26. A grasper is a mixture between a forceps and a basket. The risk of blockage is lower than for a basket; however, it is a lot weaker than a forceps. (*From* Karl Storz, Tuttlingen, Germany.)

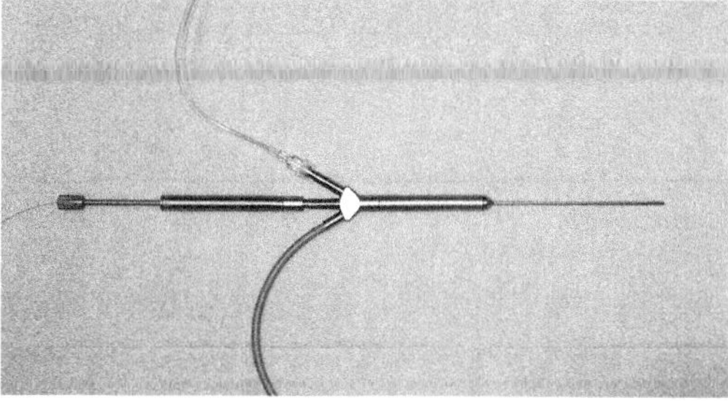

Fig. 27. Large therapeutic compact semirigid endoscope (Spiggle & Theis, Overath, Germany) with a laser fiber (MikoMed, Herne, Germany) inside its working channel. The fiber is hold in place by a shifter system originally made for the one-hand operation of baskets (PolyDiagnost, Pfaffenhofen, Germany). The shifter system is a comfortable solution to make sure that the fiber is not too far inside or outside the endoscope, that the fiber will not slip away unwontedly, and to allow one-hand operability.

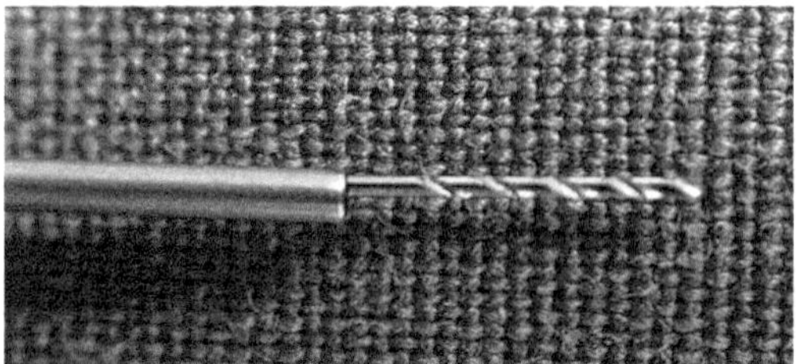

Fig. 28. Tip of an endoscope with a burr (PolyDiagnost).

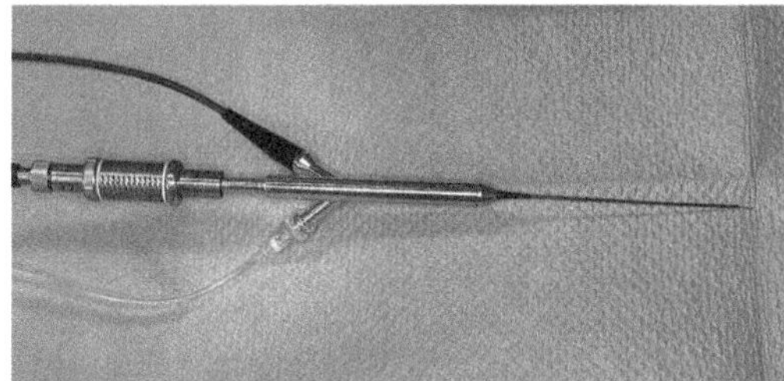

Fig. 29. Compact semirigid interventional endoscope made from nitinol together with a burr and a shifter system allowing advancement and retraction of the burr with the same hand steering the endoscope. A mechanical flexible transmission axle connects the endoscope to an electric motor (PolyDiagnost).

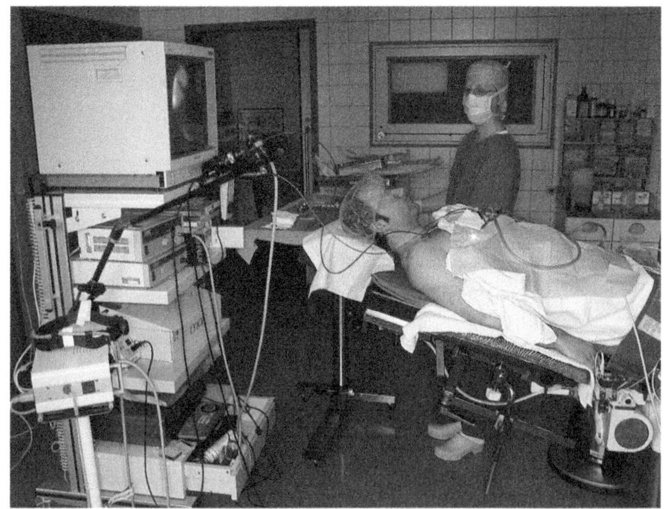

Fig. 30. Setup of an electric drilling system for endoscopically controlled fragmentation of stones. The endoscope is connected via a flexible transmission axle to the electric motor (PolyDiagnost).

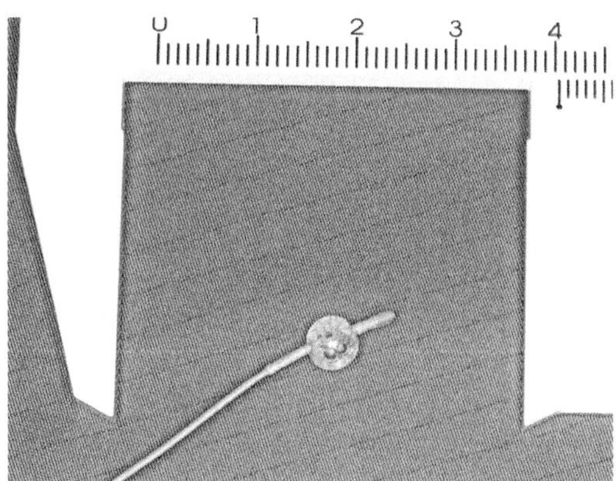

Fig. 31. Latex balloon for use in salivary ducts (Karl Storz). In the author's experience the efficacy of these types of balloons is limited and they are at high risk of rupturing when applying pressure.

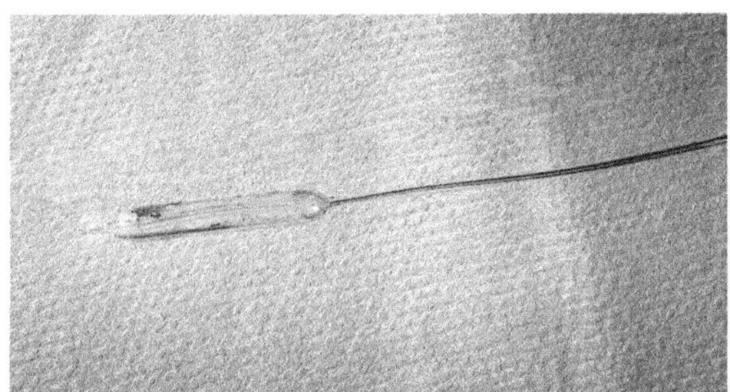

Fig. 32. High-pressure balloon for use in salivary ducts. Nondilated diameter: 2F; balloon length: 10 mm; nominal pressure: 10 bars (sialodilatation catheter with high-pressure balloon produced by Balton; distributed by Sialo Technology). Technically this is a compliant balloon; balloons used in interventional cardiology are mostly noncompliant and are probably better; however, they also are more expensive.

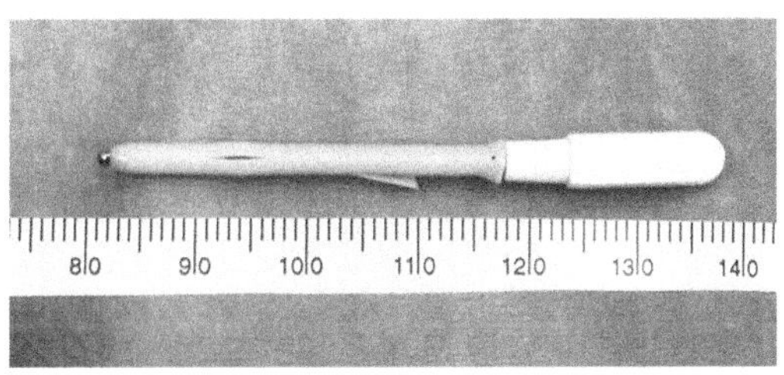

Fig. 33. Soft polyurethane drain for the stenting of salivary ducts (Sialo Technology).

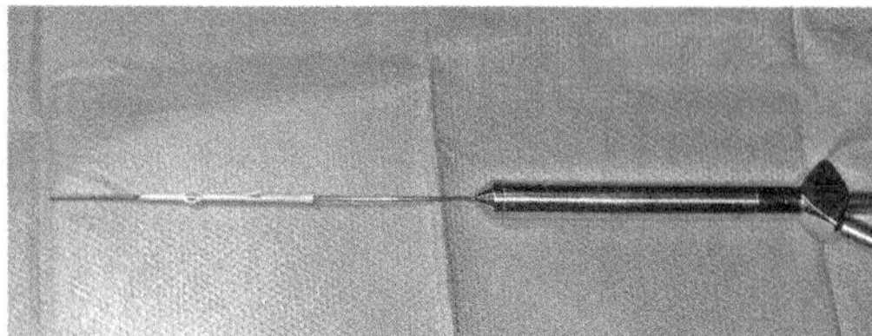

Fig. 34. Polyurethane drain (Sialo Technology) for the stenting of salivary ducts sled over a diagnostic compact semirigid endoscope (Spiggle & Theis) ready to be used.

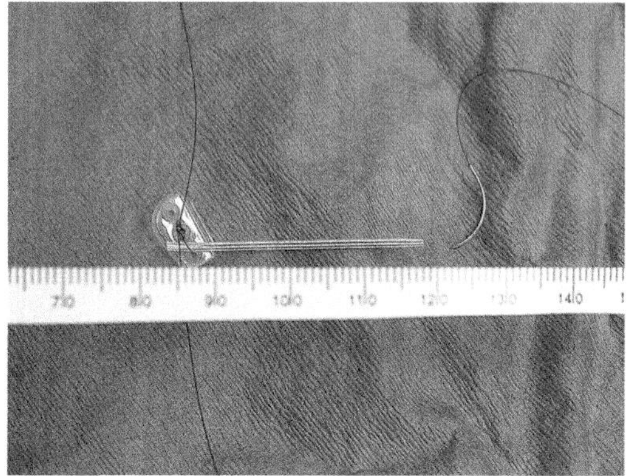

Fig. 35. Custom-made drain from an intravenous cannula. The large part at the fixation site has the function to prevent the dislocation of the tube-like drain into the duct in case that the sutures to the mucosa should loosen.

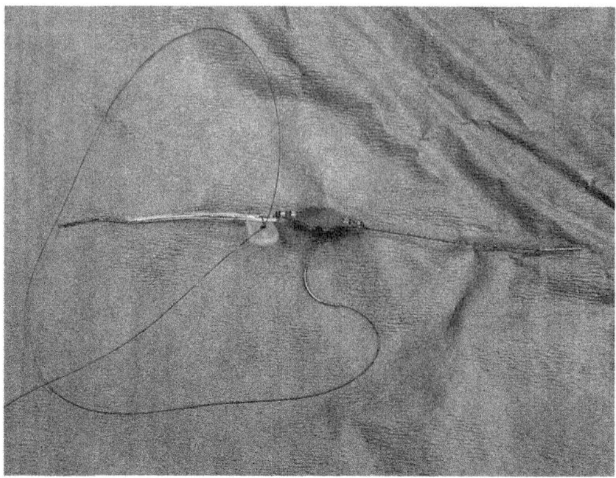

Fig. 36. The same custom-made drain on a probe ready for insertion into a salivary duct.

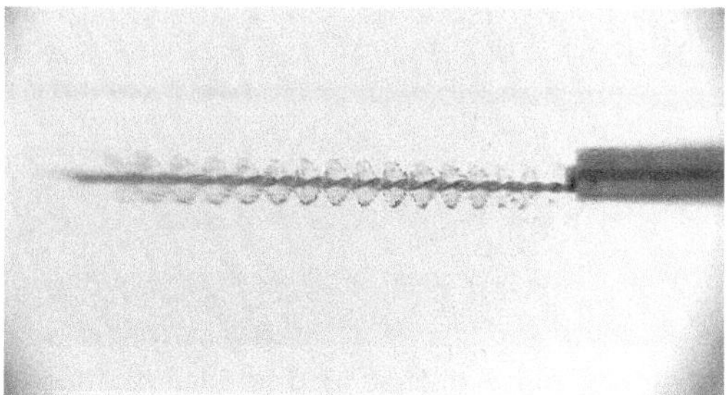

Fig. 37. Cytology brush (*Courtesy of* PolyDiagnost; with permission.) inside an endoscope. Originally made for endoscopies inside the mammary duct system these brushes might also be helpful for cytologic diagnostics inside the salivary duct system, which is not reachable by biopsy forceps.

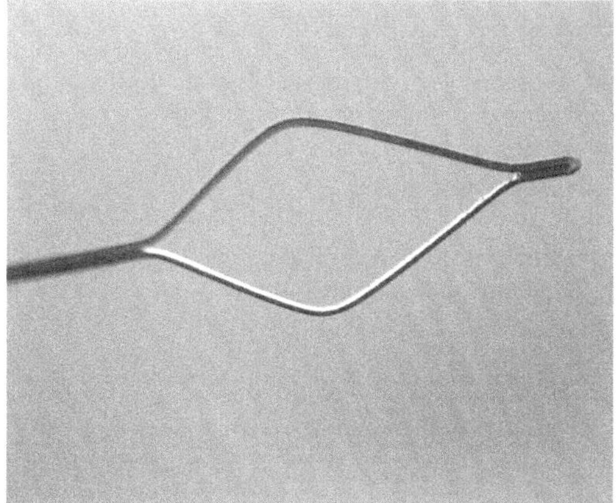

Fig. 38. Marker in form of a rhombus (*Courtesy of* PolyDiagnost; with permission.) originally made to mark regions under endoscopic control before surgery of the mamma. These devices might also be helpful to identify regions inside the salivary glands. Normally, however, the transillumination effect is sufficient for this task.

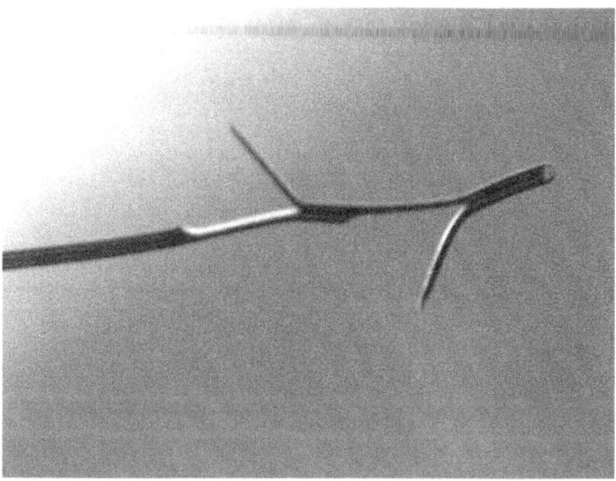

Fig. 39. Another marker, in form of a hook. (*Courtesy of* PolyDiagnost; with permission.)

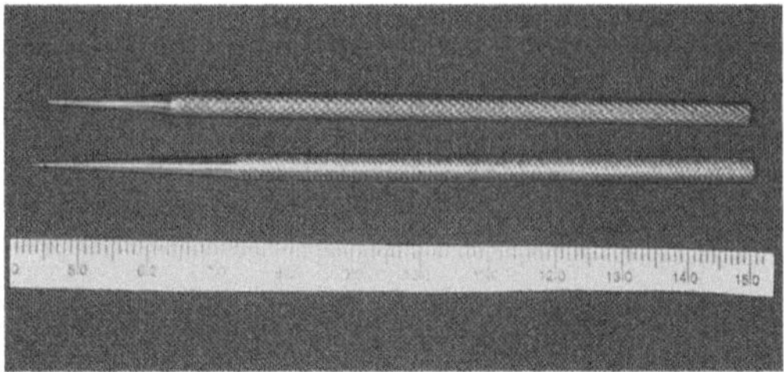

Fig. 40. Two different types of conical dilators used for identification and dilatation of the papillae of the ducts. The lower one with the sharp tip is only suitable for initial identification and dilatation as its use is associated with the danger of damage to the mucosal lining of the duct. The upper one with the blunt tip can be used for effective dilatation without this danger.

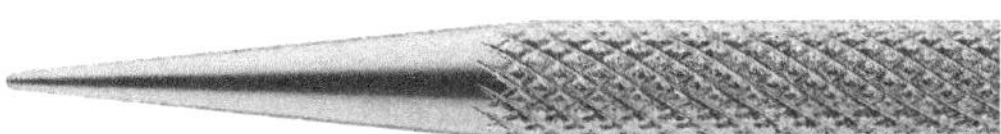

Fig. 41. Enlargement of the blunt tip of a conical dilator (described previously). (*Courtesy of* Karl Storz, Tuttlingen, Germany; with permission.)

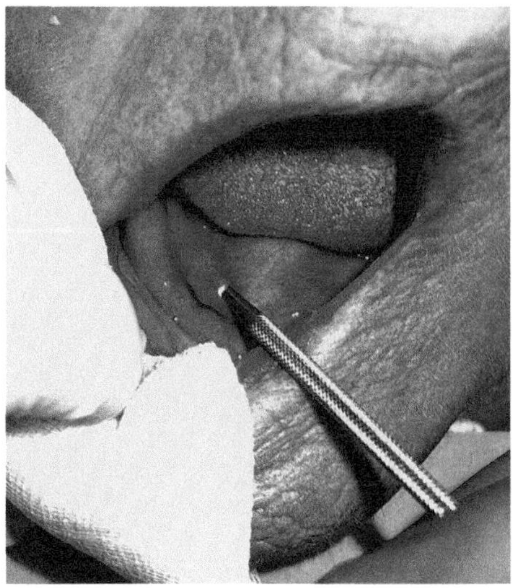

Fig. 42. Dilatation of the papilla of the right Wharton's duct with a conical instrument. (*Courtesy of* Geisthoff UW. Techniques for multimodal salivary gland stone therapy. Operative Tech Otolaryngol 2007;18:332–40; with permission.)

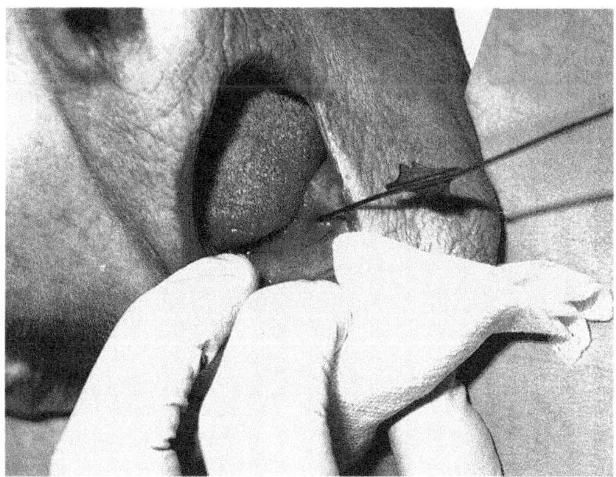

Fig. 43. Introduction of a blunt probe gives information about the patency, diameter, and direction of the duct.

Forceps

Mainly, two different types of forceps are manufactured: grasping forceps with a serrated surface on the jaws and biopsy cup forceps with sharp cutting edges (**Figs. 21** and **22**). The latter can also be used for stone fragmentation and removal. Both can be used for the careful dilatation of strictures by opening the jaws. Typical diameters are 0.78 and 1.0 mm. Although different handles are provided, experience shows that handles that allow a good visualization of the rotation of the instrument tip are advantageous.

Baskets

Baskets are classified by the number and form of their wires and tips and whether or not they have a separate outer sheath (**Fig. 23**). A basket without an outer sheath can

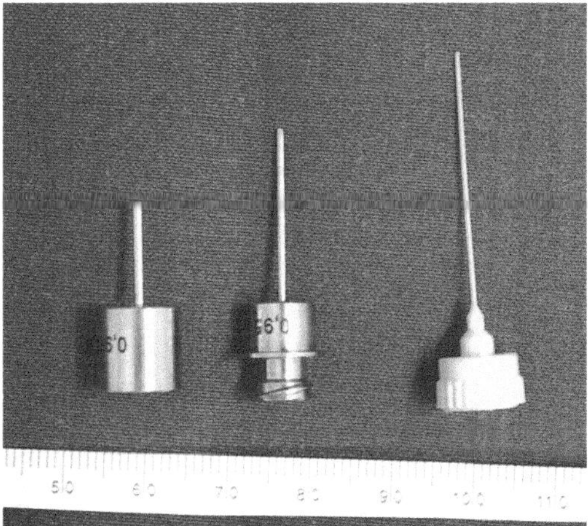

Fig. 44. Components of the Solex (Soft Lumen Expander) system (PolyDiagnost). This system can effectively be used to identify and dilate the papillae of the ducts. The inner parts can be removed while the outer part (*left*) can remain in place and act as a port for multiple removals and reintroductions of an endoscope. The system is available in different sizes.

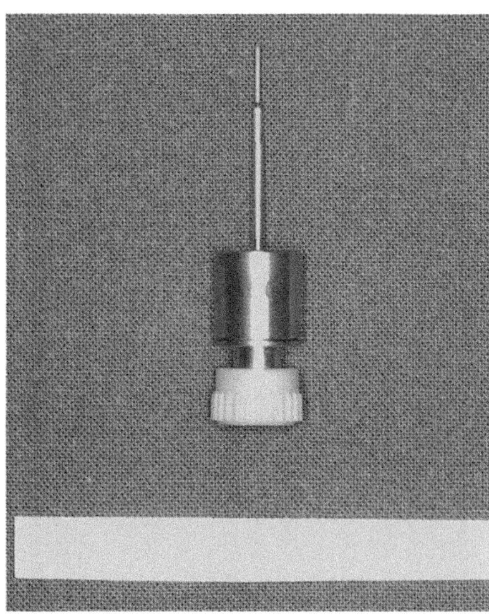

Fig. 45. The Solex system ready for use (PolyDiagnost). A danger of the system is that the tip of the plastic obturator might be sheered off when retracting it. This can be avoided when knowing about this danger and using it carefully.

be used in a fine working channel and is reusable. These models are often weaker than other ones (PolyDiagnost). To the author's knowledge, only one manufacturer provides reusable baskets with separate outer sheaths (outer diameter: 1 mm, Spiggle & Theis). Different handles are provided; however, a visualization of the rotation is less important than for forceps (**Fig. 24**). Baskets with a high number of wires (more than 4) are especially useful for small stones. Strong wires (eg, made from nitinol, Cook Medical) expand the duct. By doing this, the stone sometimes enters this large artificial "cavity" almost by itself. Strong wires can be useful to surpass stenotic duct areas

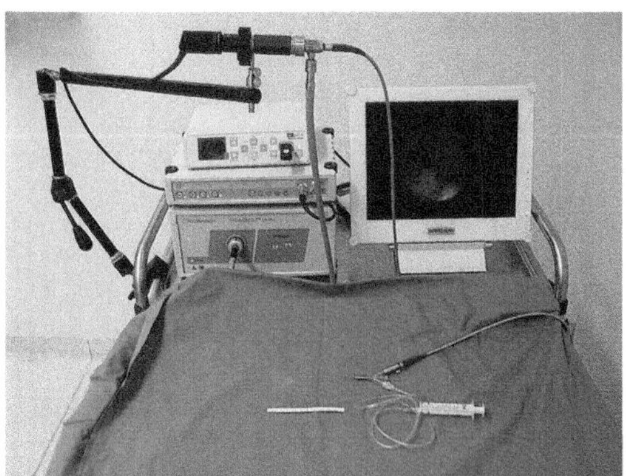

Fig. 46. Basic setup for sialendoscopy with an endoscope, irrigation, endoscopic camera system, light source, and video documentation system. In this case, the use of a camera system without zoom objective is possible. One of the oculars for the modular semirigid endoscope is available with an integrated zoom (PolyDiagnost).

when pulling out a captured stone. Alternatively, baskets with weak wires are less probable to cause a blockage as they often break when strong forces have to be applied. The well established distributors for sialendoscopy are Gyrus ACMI, Karl Storz, PolyDiagnost, and Spiggle & Theis; all sell different baskets. Additionally, there are producers for urologic and gastroenterologic procedures. Cook Medical offers a variety of different and high-quality urology baskets, including some with special features (eg, a separate channel provided for the insertion of a laser fiber to fragment the captured stone) (**Fig. 25**). To the author's knowledge, however, this expensive system has not yet been used for salivary stones.

Graspers

Graspers are a mixture of forceps and baskets (**Fig. 26**). Previously, they were also distributed by Gyrus ACMI and Karl Storz. To the author's knowledge, however, only Almikro still sells them.

Laser Fibers

A large variety of laser fiber diameters and connectors are available from multiple manufacturers. For intracorporeal laser lithotrips, only bare fibers are used (**Fig. 27**). The fibers are fragile and, therefore, should not be angularly bent. An off-label option for rigid or semirigid endoscopes with small working channels is to strip the bare fiber out of its plastic coating to allow the introduction of the smaller-diameter denuded fiber. One risk with this maneuver is that the bare fiber can break and jam within the working channel and destroy the endoscope.

An additional possibility for the transmission of laser light has been described by the working group around Nahlieli.[16] A metal hollow waveguide can be used to transmit the light of an erbium:yttrium-aluminum—garnet laser. The system is more rigid than regular fibers, however, and has a relatively large outer diameter (1 mm).

Drills

Microburrs have diameters of 0.38 to 0.4 mm (**Fig. 28**). They can be used for stone fragmentation and dilatation of filiform or complete stenoses. An electrically powered motor system and a shifter system (PolyDiagnost) can be especially helpful for hard stones (**Figs. 29** and **30**). The treatment of stenoses or soft stones can be done by manually twizzle-rotating the burrs. Two distributors are Karl Storz and PolyDiagnost. The working channels of some endoscopes are too long for use with these burrs.

Balloons

Low-pressure latex and high-pressure balloons are made (Karl Storz; Balton, Warsaw, Poland; and Sialo Technolgy). The former have only limited efficacy, mainly for thin membrane-like strictures (**Fig. 31**). They have a high risk of rupturing. The latter require a special syringe system for inflation. Some of them can be used through the working channels of endoscopes (**Fig. 32**). Similar to baskets, however, a large variety of high-quality balloons are offered for endovascular treatment. Some of these balloons have small cutting blades (Flextome Cutting Balloon Dilatation Device or Peripheral Cutting Balloon Device, Boston Scientific, Natick, Massachusetts). Some of these balloons are useable on salivary pathologies. Additionally, nearly all endovascular balloons allow the use of a guide wire. For sialendoscopy the combination of endoscopy, guide wire, and an external imaging technique may be used to apply the Seldinger technique.[17]

Stents/Drains

The use of stents is controversial.[12,18,19] One possible use is in the prevention of restenosis after the dilatation of ductal strictures. Soft polyurethane stents of different forms and sizes help to individualize case treatments (Sialo Technology) (**Fig. 33**). An alternate to using the insertion device provided with the stents is to slide them over the endoscope and place them using endoscopic control (**Fig. 34**). The soft consistency might be beneficial to prevent scarring but can make insertion difficult. Also, the soft device may be compressed by scar tissue in some cases. Therefore, the author also uses custom-made drains made from more rigid intravenous cannulas (**Figs. 35** and **36**). It is important to have a phalange at one end of the stent; this prevents the stent from sliding into the duct and creating a foreign-body problem. This happened one time in the author's experience and the drain inside Stensen's duct had to be identified and drawn out under sonographic control. Stents and drains usually are removed by 1 month after insertion.

Cytology Brushes and Markers

These two devices were developed for endoscopy in the mammary glands but may also be used in salivary ducts. Cytology brushes are an option when a tumor is suspected in an area that is not easily accessible by a biopsy forceps (**Fig. 37**). Markers are used to mark suspected regions before operations (**Figs. 38** and **39**). In sialendoscopy, however, the transillumination effect is an established alternative to locate a target region for external approaches.

Instruments Used to Facilitate the Introduction of Endoscopes

The insertion of the endoscopes is an essential and sometimes difficult part of a sialoscopy. Conical dilatators often play a crucial role in the identification and dilatation of the duct papillae (**Figs. 40–42**). Introducing a blunt probe gives information about the patency, diameter, and direction of the duct (**Fig. 43**). A sophisticated tool to identify, dilate, and keep the papilla open is the Soft Lumen Expander (Solex by PolyDiagnost) (**Figs. 44** and **45**).

Further Equipment

An endoscopic camera system, a light source, and a monitor are necessary (**Fig. 46**). A recording unit can also be advantageous. A strong light source is recommended due to the length of the optical fibers. It should be possible, however, to modify light intensities to assure appropriate light levels for different endoscopes and to prevent heat formation. Therefore, it is recommended to use camera and recording systems with high light sensitivities. The resolution of most video systems is sufficient as resolution is limited more by the number of endoscope pixels. A sialendoscope with an integrated zoom ocular is made (PolyDiagnost). Otherwise, the camera systems used should have optical zoom options. Most of the systems incorporate these features.

SUMMARY

A large variety of different endoscopes, instruments, and ancillaries equipment are commercially available from various companies. It is important to select the specific equipment suitable to the problem of an individual case. Compatibility of endoscopes and instruments should be considered.

REFERENCES

1. Zenk J, Hosemann WG, Iro H. Diameters of the main excretory ducts of the adult human submandibular and parotid gland: a histologic study. Oral Surg Oral Med Oral Pathol Oral Radiol Endod 1998;85(5):576–80.
2. Katz P. [New therapy for sialolithiasis]. Inf Dent 1991;73(43):3975–9 [in French].
3. Katz P. Endoscopie des glandes salivaires [Endoscopy of the salivary glands]. Ann Radiol 1991;34(1–2):110–3.
4. Gundlach P, Scherer H, Hopf J, et al. [Endoscopic-controlled laser lithotripsy of salivary calculi. In vitro studies and initial clinical use]. HNO 1990;38(7):247–50 [in German].
5. Konigsberger R, Feyh J, Goetz A, et al. [Endoscopic controlled laser lithotripsy in the treatment of sialolithiasis]. Laryngorhinootologie 1990;69(6):322–3 [in German].
6. Sterenborg H, van den Akker HP, van der Meulen C. Laserlithotripsy of salivary stones: a comparison between the pulsed dye laser and Ho: YAG laser. Lasers Med Sci 1990;5:357–62.
7. Marchal F, Dulguerov P, Becker M, et al. Specificity of parotid sialendoscopy. Laryngoscope 2001;111(2):264–71.
8. Nahlieli O, Baruchin AM. Endoscopic technique for the diagnosis and treatment of obstructive salivary gland diseases. J Oral Maxillofac Surg 1999;57(12):1394–401.
9. Pajkos A, Vickery K, Cossart Y. Is biofilm accumulation on endosope tubing a contributor to the failure of cleaning and decontamination? J Hosp Infect 2004;58:224–9.
10. Geisthoff UW, Lehnert BK, Verse T. Ultrasound-guided mechanical intraductal stone fragmentation and removal for sialolithiasis: a new technique. Surg Endosc 2006;20(4):690–4.
11. Nahlieli O, London D, Zagury A, et al. Combined approach to impacted parotid stones. J Oral Maxillofac Surg 2002;60(12):1418–23.
12. Nahlieli O, Iro H, McGurk M, et al. Minimal invasive methods and procedures for the treatment of salivary gland sialolithiasis. In: Nahlieli O, Iro H, McGurk M, et al, editors. Modern management preserving the salivary glands. Herzeliya (Israel): Isradon; 2007. p. 136–76.
13. Marchal F. A combined endoscopic and external approach for extraction of large stones with preservation of parotid and submandibular glands. Laryngoscope 2007;117(2):373–7.
14. McGurk M, MacBean A, Fan KF, et al. Conservative management of salivary stones and benign parotid tumours: a description of the surgical techniques involved. Ann R Australas Coll Dent Surg 2004;17:41–4.
15. Geisthoff UW. [Sialendoscopy]. HNO 2008;56(2):105–7 [in German].
16. Raif J, Vardi M, Nahlieli O, et al. An Er:YAG laser endoscopic fiber delivery system for lithotripsy of salivary stones. Lasers Surg Med 2006;38(6):580–7.
17. Seldinger SI. Catheter replacement of the needle in percutaneous arteriography; a new technique. Acta Radiol Diagn (Stockh) 1953;39(5):368–76.
18. Iro H, Zenk J, Koch M, et al. The Erlangen salivary gland project - part 1: sialendoscopy in obstructive diseases of the major salivary glands. Tuttlingen (Germany): Endo-Press; 2008.
19. Baurmash HD. Discussion: endoscopic technique for the diagnosis and treatment of obstructive salivary gland diseases. J Oral Maxillofac Surg 1999;57:1401–2.

20. Arzoz E, Santiago A, Garatea J, et al. Removal of a stone in Stensen's duct with endoscopic laser lithotripsy: a case report. J Oral Maxillofac Surg 1994;52: 1329–30.
21. Gundlach P, Hopf J, Linnarz M. Introduction of a new diagnostic procedure: salivary duct endoscopy (sialendoscopy) clinical evaluation of sialendoscopy, sialography, and X-ray imaging. Endosc Surg Allied Technol 1994;2(6):294–6.
22. Nahlieli O, Neder A, Baruchin AM. Salivary gland endoscopy: a new technique for diagnosis and treatment of sialolithiasis. J Oral Maxillofac Surg 1994;52(12): 1240–2.
23. Zenk J, Benzel W, Iro H. New modalities in the management of human sialolithiasis. Minim Invasive Ther Allied Technol 1994;3:275–84.
24. Iro H, Zenk J, Benzel W. Laser lithotripsy of salivary duct stones. Adv Otorhinolaryngol 1995;49:148–52.
25. Ito H, Baba S. Pulsed dye laser lithotripsy of submandibular gland salivary calculus. J Laryngol Otol 1996;110(10):942–6.
26. Iro H, Zenk J, Waldfahrer F, et al. [Current status of minimally invasive treatment methods in sialolithiasis]. HNO 1996;44(2):78–84 [in German].
27. Arzoz E, Santiago A, Esnal F, et al. Endoscopic intracorporeal lithotripsy for sialolithiasis. J Oral Maxillofac Surg 1996;54(7):847–50.
28. Yuasa K, Nakhyama E, Ban S, et al. Submandibular gland duct endoscopy. Diagnostic value for salivary duct disorders in comparison to conventional radiography, sialography, and ultrasonography. Oral Surg Oral Med Oral Pathol Oral Radiol Endod 1997;84(5):578–81.
29. Nahlieli O, Baruchin AM. Sialoendoscopy: three years' experience as a diagnostic and treatment modality. J Oral Maxillofac Surg 1997;55(9):912–8.
30. Hopf JUG, Hopf M, Gundlach P, et al. Miniature endoscopes in otorhinolaryngologic applications. Minim Invasive Ther Allied Technol 1998;7(3):209–18.
31. Marchal F, Becker M, Vavrina J, et al. Diagnostic et traitement des sialolithiases [Diagnosis and treatment of salivary gland stones]. Schweizerische Ärztezeitung 1998;79(22):1023–8.
32. Kerr PD, Krahn H, Brodovsky D. Endoscopic laser lithotripsy of a proximal parotid duct calculus. J Otolaryngol 2001;30(2):129–30.
33. Chu DW, Chow TL, Lim BH, et al. Endoscopic management of submandibular sialolithiasis. Surg Endosc 2003;17(6):876–9.
34. Zenk J, Koch M, Bozzato A, et al. Sialoscopy—initial experiences with a new endoscope. Br J Oral Maxillofac Surg 2004;42(4):293–8.
35. Geisthoff UW. Techniques for multimodal salivary gland stone therapy. Operat Tech Otolaryngol Head Neck Surg 2007;18:332–40.

Basic Sialendoscopy Techniques

Urban W. Geisthoff, Priv.-Doz. Dr. med.[a,b,*]

KEYWORDS

• Sialendoscopy • Sialolithiasis • Minimally invasive techniques
• Salivary strictures • Salivary gland stones

Sialendoscopy, begun in 1988,[1–4] is now an established procedure for the diagnosis of salivary disease[5–7] and is a method to control minimally invasive interventions to treat salivary obstructions.[6–8] In this article a discussion of indications and the different aspects of basic sialendoscopy technique are presented.

INDICATIONS

Diagnostic indications include suspicion of obstructive salivary disease (diagnostic endoscopy). Therapeutic indications include the following: treatment of salivary stones (including fragmentation, removal, and stone localization for external approaches); dilatation of strictures and localization of strictures for external approaches; management of chronic sialadenitis by irrigation; and management of recurrent juvenile sialadenitis.

Diagnostic Sialendoscopy

Careful patient history is the first step in ascertaining presence of obstructive salivary disease. Typically, gland swelling is associated with food intake. Inspection and palpation is sometimes helpful; however, ultrasonography is the most important diagnostic procedure. Applying a sialagogue during sonography can help to detect the cause and region of obstruction.[8] In most cases, treatment can be planned with the information obtained by history and sonography. In some cases additional information may be necessary. The most relevant aspects regarding planning of treatment, to which plain sonography is of limited use, are the following:

1. The distinction between a nonechogenic stone and a stricture (qualitative assessment): In the case of a suspected stricture a nonechogenic stone should be excluded using other methods (eg, sialendoscopy).

Urban Geisthoff consulted with Spiggle & Theis, Overath, Germany, and Gyrus ACMI, Tuttlingen, Germany, for the development of instruments without any financial benefit thus far.
[a] University of the Saarland, Medical Faculty, Kirrberger Street, D-66421 Homburg/Saar, Germany
[b] Department of Otorhinolaryngology, Holweide Hospital, Hospitals of the City of Cologne, Cologne, Germany
* HNO, KHS Holweide, Neufelder Street 32, D-51067 Koeln, Germany.
E-mail address: http://www.geisthoff.de

Otolaryngol Clin N Am 42 (2009) 1029–1052
doi:10.1016/j.otc.2009.08.004 oto.theclinics.com
0030-6665/09/$ – see front matter

2. The quantitative assessment of the obstruction using sonography: It is often difficult to measure the three-dimensional size of a stone or to assess the length and number of stenotic areas.
3. The state of the distal duct system in the event that an intraductal approach is planned: It may be useful to assess the duct and its diameter distal of the obstruction to ensure that the duct is wide and straight enough for the instruments, to which plain sonography is poorly suited. These considerations are also important in determining whether the fragments produced by extracorporeal shock wave lithotripsy are easily washed out by the saliva from the duct system. For sonographically controlled procedures it is also important to know if there are kinks and branchings that might complicate approaching the obstruction.[9]

Both sialendoscopy and sialography (sialogram) can be used to ascertain the three aspects listed previously. Sialography gives a better overview of the whole duct system and can give information about areas not reachable by sialendoscopy (eg, behind extreme kinks and strictures).[5] Disadvantages are radiation exposure and false-positive stone detections because of air bubbles. Sialendoscopy allows visualizing the pathology directly. Both, sialendoscopy and fluoroscopy can also be used to control therapeutic interventions so that it is possible to switch from diagnostics to treatment within the same session.[8,10]

Therapeutic Sialendoscopy

Apart from using the endoscope for the dilatation of strictures within the duct system, sialendoscopy is not a treatment itself but rather a method of visual control for therapeutic procedures.[5]

Fragmentation and extraction of stones

Sialolithiasis is the most frequent reason for salivary duct obstruction. The aim of treatment is to completely remove the stone. Various approaches exist and endoscopic techniques are only one part of the whole spectrum of possibilities (**Table 1**).[5–8] It can be advantageous to combine different approaches (multimodal therapy).[5–8]

The information obtained during diagnosis determines the choice of treatment. The most important parameters are the patient history of complaints and complications; the position, size, and number of stones; the diameter of the duct between the stone and the papilla; and the surgeon's experience with the particular techniques.[8]

For the most part, the smallest stones can be removed conservatively. For this, patients are asked to use sialagogues (eg, chewing gum, cherry pits, and so forth) and to massage their glands regularly. This approach is often very helpful as an auxiliary fragment clearing measure for use after other treatment types. If stones are recalcitrant, other treatment options are discussed. **Figs. 1** and **2** list other therapeutic techniques to be used depending on the location of stones.[6]

For basic sialendoscopy several parameters should be considered. The normal parotid and submandibular ducts have diameters of about 1.5 mm with bottlenecks up to 0.5 mm at the papillae.[11] The mean diameters of the observed stones may have some variability ranging from about 3 to 8 mm, depending on individual experience.[12,13] It has been suggested that a stone's maximum diameter should not be larger than 150% of the anterior ducts and that the absolute diameters should not exceed 3 to 5 mm for Stensen duct and 4 to 7 mm for Wharton duct if it is to be removed without fragmentation.[12,14] It is sometimes possible, however, to remove stones with even larger maximum diameters if their form is streamlined (eg, if they are highly ellipsoid). The chances for removal are reduced if the stone is not mobile

Table 1
Overview of the spectrum of therapeutic options for obstructive salivary disease

Method	Approach
Gland extirpation (not for distal stones)	External
Slitting of the duct	Transoral

Intraductal therapy
Tasks
  Stone removal
  Stone fragmentation
  Duct dilatation
Devices
  Basket, grasper, forceps, suction, balloon, stent, drill, laser
Methods of control
  Blind/tactile
  Endoscopic
  Ultrasound
  Fluoroscopic
	Transoral

Extracorporeal shock wave lithotripsy	External
Minimal incision and combined approaches from the outside for parotid stones	External

Adapted from: Geisthoff UW. Techniques for multimodal salivary gland stone therapy. Operat Tech Otolaryngol 2007;18:332–40; with permission.

because of adherence to the duct, or if it is located in a diverticulum. In the latter cases there is an increased risk of the basket instrument jamming in the duct.[10]

An advanced application for sialendoscopy for salivary stones includes the localization of the stone by skin transillumination as an aid to external approach.[7,15–17]

Dilatation of stenoses and strictures Relatively few data exist regarding the treatment of salivary duct strictures.[18–21] It is generally agreed that long strictures have a worse prognosis than short stenoses. Multiple technical options exist to dilate a duct (see **Table 1**). Endoscopically controlled procedures are especially helpful for short, membrane-like stenoses or where stenoses begin at duct branchings. The latter ones can be very difficult to treat with fluoroscopically or sonographically controlled procedures; filiform-like openings might not be identified by these methods. Disadvantages of the endoscopically controlled balloon dilatation are that the diameter of the duct created by the inflated balloon can only be assessed after deflation and that it may also be difficult to determine the position of the tip of the balloon. It can be helpful to combine endoscopy with one of the other imaging techniques (multimodal therapy).[8] A useful technique for difficult stenosis or stricture cases is the placement of a guidewire using endoscopic control. The guidewire is then left in place while the endoscope is removed. Lastly, a balloon or hollow conical dilatator (**Fig. 3**A) is placed over the guidewire and the dilatation procedure is continued under sonographic or fluoroscopic control.[22]

Management of chronic sialadenitis Sialendoscopy has been used successfully to treat adult chronic sialadenitis.[7,23] The mechanism is probably clearance of mucous plugs and dilatation of the duct by irrigation and might be the same as for chronic juvenile parotitis. A less invasive procedure may be performed by just irrigating the duct with a catheter without endoscopy.[24]

Management of recurrent juvenile sialadenitis Recurrent juvenile parotitis can be treated successfully as with adult chronic sialadenitis using sialendoscopy.[25–27]

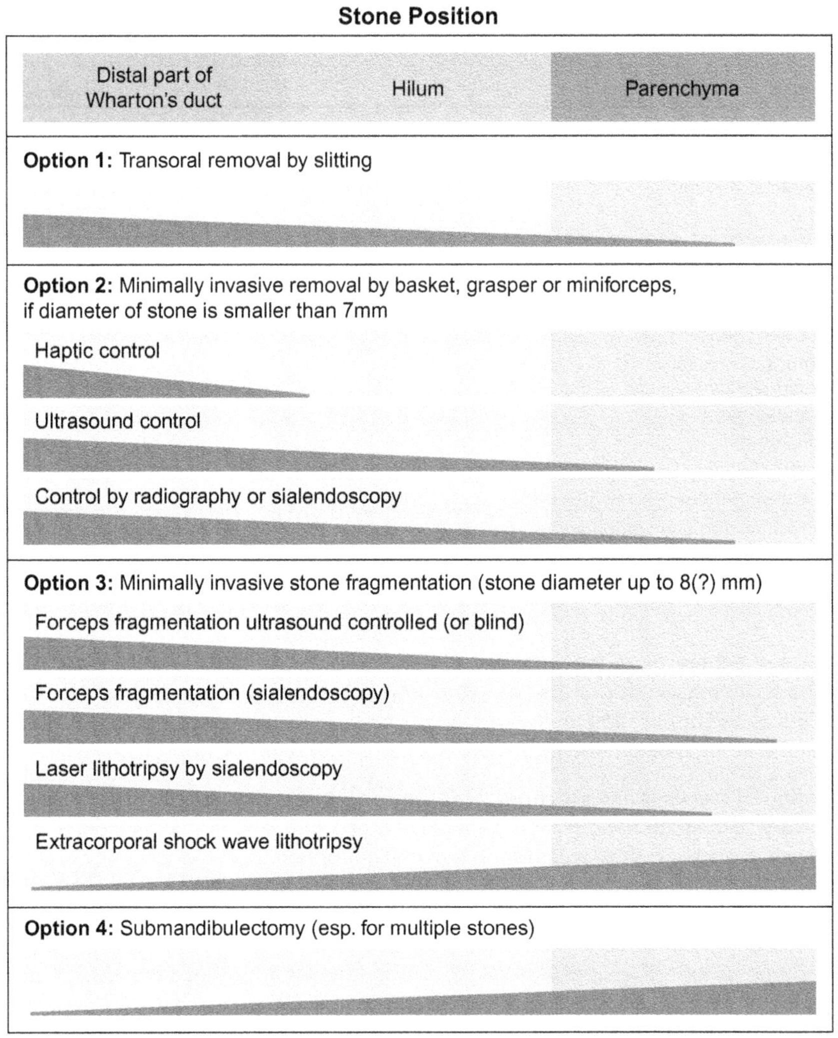

Stone Position

Distal part of Wharton's duct	Hilum	Parenchyma

Option 1: Transoral removal by slitting

Option 2: Minimally invasive removal by basket, grasper or miniforceps, if diameter of stone is smaller than 7mm

Haptic control

Ultrasound control

Control by radiography or sialendoscopy

Option 3: Minimally invasive stone fragmentation (stone diameter up to 8(?) mm)

Forceps fragmentation ultrasound controlled (or blind)

Forceps fragmentation (sialendoscopy)

Laser lithotripsy by sialendoscopy

Extracorporal shock wave lithotripsy

Option 4: Submandibulectomy (esp. for multiple stones)

Fig. 1. Selection of therapeutic options for submandibular stones dependent on their localization. Option 1: The success rate of slitting the distal duct is about 100%.[36] Localization of posterior stones should be possible haptically or by diaphanoscopy for option 1.[17,36] Option 2: Tactilely controlled procedures have a good chance of success if the stone inside the distal duct can be palpated with one hand while the other hand steers the instrument to capture the stone. Ultrasound-guided techniques are more difficult when branchings of the duct system have to be navigated (this also applies to option 3). In contrast, endoscopically and radiographically controlled interventions allow for better control inside the duct system. Option 3 (see also option 2): Endoscopic forceps fragmentation often can be performed further proximally inside the duct system than laser lithotripsy because it was found that stones can be pushed forcefully posterior by laser energy. If the stone is far posterior in a smaller duct it might occlude the duct and lead to abscesses. Extracorporeal shock wave lithotripsy can be very difficult when the stone is near the floor of mouth because the reflections of saliva can resemble those of stones on the ultrasound imaging screen.

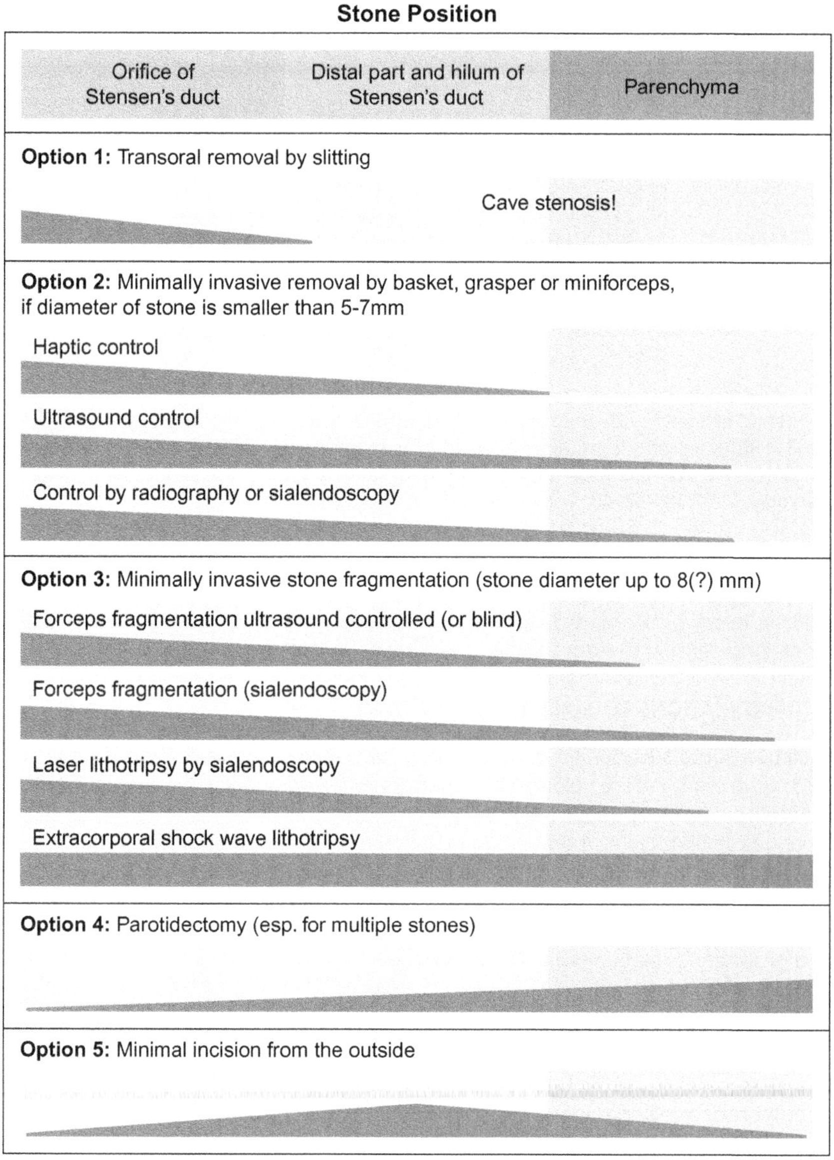

Stone Position

Orifice of Stensen's duct	Distal part and hilum of Stensen's duct	Parenchyma

Option 1: Transoral removal by slitting

Cave stenosis!

Option 2: Minimally invasive removal by basket, grasper or miniforceps, if diameter of stone is smaller than 5-7mm

Haptic control

Ultrasound control

Control by radiography or sialendoscopy

Option 3: Minimally invasive stone fragmentation (stone diameter up to 8(?) mm)

Forceps fragmentation ultrasound controlled (or blind)

Forceps fragmentation (sialendoscopy)

Laser lithotripsy by sialendoscopy

Extracorporal shock wave lithotripsy

Option 4: Parotidectomy (esp. for multiple stones)

Option 5: Minimal incision from the outside

Fig. 2. Selection of therapeutic options for parotid stones dependant on their localization (see also legend for **Fig. 1**). Option 1: In contrast to the submandibular duct system, slitting of Stensen duct should be used only in selected cases for very distal stones because there is a high risk of postoperative stricture.[6] Option 3: Extracorporeal shock wave lithotripsy for parotid stones has a higher success rate than for submandibular stones. Identification of the stones is usually much easier. Option 5: A minimal incision from the outside is easier when the stone is near the surface and inside one of the larger duct segments.

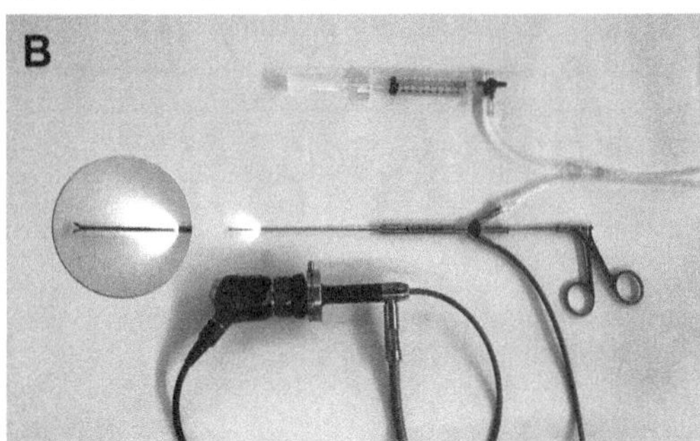

Fig. 3. (*A*) Hollow conical dilatator to be placed over a guidewire. (*Courtesy of* Karl Storz, Tuttlingen, Germany; with permission.) (*B*) Typical set-up for sialendoscopy: the sialendoscope is connected to a light source, a video unit by a camera, and an irrigation system. (*From* Geisthoff UW. Techniques for multimodal salivary gland stone therapy. Operat Tech Otolaryngol 2007;18:332–40; with permission of Elsevier.)

Sialography may also be useful (Dr P Katz, personal communication, 2007). The latter normally does not require general anesthesia as is often necessary for sialendoscopy. It is associated with radiation exposure, however, and iodinated contrast material remains long-term in the duct system as a basis for this treatment.

CONTRAINDICATIONS TO SIALENDOSCOPY

Sometimes acute sialadenitis is named as an absolute contraindication[7] because the swollen duct wall is more vulnerable to perforation. Additionally, the endoscopic view is hampered by mucopurulent debris. Uncommonly, conservative treatment including intravenous antibiotics and oral antiphlogistics did not show sufficient effect to avoid a sonographically proved imminent abscess. In these uncommon cases, diagnostic sialendoscopy was then carefully performed to confirm that a sonographically controlled ductal procedure on the stone was possible and curative.[9] Acute sialadenitis is probably a relative contraindication.

SIDE EFFECTS

Reported side effects and complications include the following[12,14,28]:

- Temporary swelling caused by irrigation (2–3 hours, 100%)
- Wire-basket blockages (6%)
- Canal wall perforations (0.3%–6%)
- Recurrence of symptoms (1%–6%)
- Temporal lingual nerve paresthesia (0.5%)
- Ranula (1%)
- Postoperative infection (2%)
- Ductal strictures (0.3%–3.5%)

GENERAL PRINCIPLES FOR SIALENDOSCOPIC PROCEDURES

Choice of the Appropriate Endoscope

For interventional endoscopies it is often advantageous to start with a fine-caliber diagnostic endoscope. It is less invasive because only a slight dilatation of the papilla is needed and only rarely a papillotomy. Trauma to the duct walls is minimal so that no iatrogenic lesions interfere with the assessment. The narrow diameter and greater flexibility make the procedure easier and allow for the inspection of parts that are not accessible with a larger interventional scope. Important information is gained, such as if a stricture is of short length and more easily treatable with the interventional scope. Another example is that it is often possible to pass by stones with the diagnostic scope by passing between the concretion and the duct wall and measuring the length of the stone and the proximal duct condition. This is important for therapeutic decisions, such as whether a basket can be opened behind the stone.

Preparation of the Optical System and Orientation of the Endoscope

A typical set-up for sialendoscopy includes the connection of the endoscope to a camera system with a monitor, a light source, and an irrigation system (**Fig. 3**B). It is important to know the exact orientation of the endoscope with respect to the picture on the monitor before starting the procedure. For this reason the scope should be passed over a test region with lettering and the orientation can be corrected by repositioning the camera. At the same time acuity, zoom, and white balance can be adjusted. The surgeon should know about the orientation of the working channel relative to the scope's objective lens. In selected cases it can be advantageous to rotate the position of the scope within one's hands to a new "zero position" and correct the camera position respectively. This avoids viewing the target upside down on the monitor screen. At the same time it allows defining the position of the instrument leaving the working channel in any desired position relative to the optical axis. This can be of help, for example, when grabbing a stone with a forceps, surpassing a stone with a basket, or entering a stenotic duct with a balloon. Especially with larger instruments the instrument and not the optical axis of the endoscope is centered within the duct system. Foreseeing, choosing, and calculating the direction of this shift can be very helpful.

Anesthesia for Sialendoscopy

Dilatation of the papilla and diagnostic endoscopy are not very painful and often no anesthesia is necessary. The situation is vice versa for interventional sialendoscopy. In most cases an anesthetic irrigation of the duct system is sufficient by using an intravenous cannula or using the rinsing or working channels of an endoscope; xylometazolin 2% or bupivacaine 3% are used to flush the duct system. Additional local anesthesia injections or even regional blockage of nerves are sometimes necessary. Indications for general anesthesia are limited to more complicated problems and also to many children. Some authors recommend initially starting all sialendoscopy procedures under general anesthesia.

Operative Time

The average time needed for sialendoscopy is about 60 minutes,[14] 57 ± 39 minutes for an interventional sialendoscopy for single sialoliths, and 89 ± 42 minutes for multiple sialoliths.[12] It is comparable with the classic gland resection. It has a lower risk of side effects, however, and preserves the gland.

Introducing the Endoscope

The first step is identification of the papilla. This can sometimes be difficult and time consuming. The use of magnifying loupes or a microscope can be helpful. One way to enhance the visibility of the papilla is to massage the gland with one hand, which pushes saliva to open the papilla and make it visible. Simultaneously, it is possible

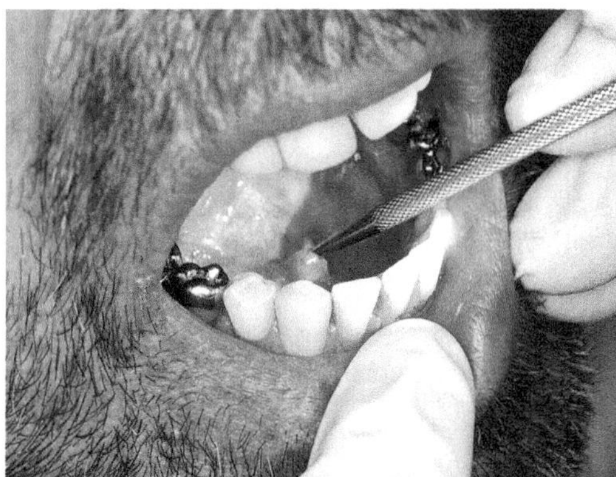

Fig. 4. Introduction of a conical dilatator into the papilla of Wharton duct at the anterior tip of the sublingual fold.

to introduce a conical dilatator into the opening with the other hand (**Fig. 4**). This technique can be enhanced by using sialagogues (eg, ascorbic acid, lemon juice). It has recently been suggested to swab the region of the papilla with methylene blue, which might further facilitate the procedure.[29] The papilla of Stensen duct can be found opposite to the second upper molar (**Fig. 5**). Wharton duct enters the oral cavity at the anterior tip of the sublingual fold (see **Fig. 4**). Sometimes it is difficult to differentiate the Wharton duct papilla from the papillae of the minor sublingual ducts; sometimes it is covered by a mucosal fold. Because the anterior floor of mouth mucosa is quite loose it can be stabilized by grabbing it posterior-superior to the punctum with a toothed forceps. The natural papilla diameters are about 0.5 mm.[30] Most cases need a papilla dilatation done with a conical dilatator. Two different types of dilatators are available: one "dilator" with a sharp tip and the other "bougie" with a blunter tip (**Figs. 6** and **7**). The pointed one is good for entering a visibly very small papilla and starting dilatation until the blunt one fits. Forceful dilatation with the dilatators should be avoided because it can perforate the duct and create a false passage. The dilatators can also be used to identify a papilla tactilely by moving over the region of its

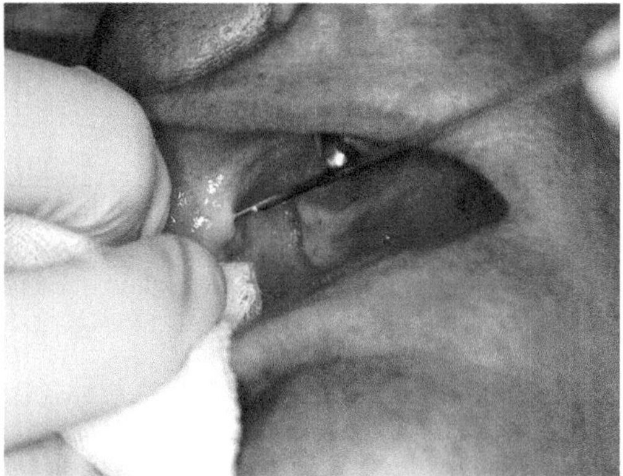

Fig. 5. Introduction of a forceps followed by an endoscope into Stensen duct. The papilla can be found in the region opposite to the second upper molar.

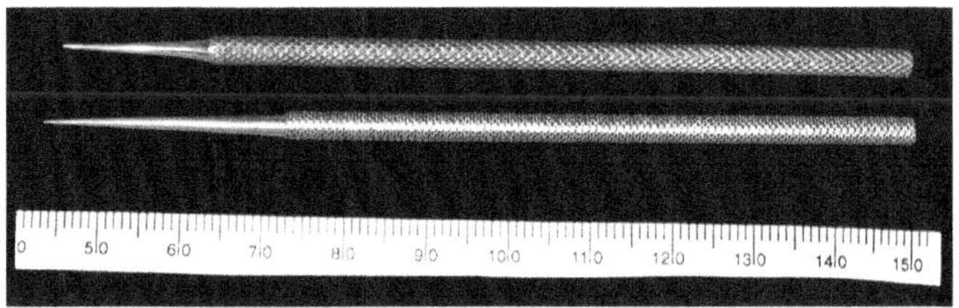

Fig. 6. Two different types of dilatators exist: one with a sharp tip (*bottom*) and one with a blunter tip (*top*).

expected position and "dropping" into it. A caution when identifying Wharton papilla is that a minor sublingual duct can be cannulated and a false lumen created. When in doubt a blunt probe should be introduced to check for the length, patency, and direction of the duct (**Fig. 8**).

A further way to dilate the duct is by using the Solex system (soft lumen expander; Polydiagnost, Pfaffenhofen, Germany) (**Fig. 9**). After removing the inner obturators a port remains that allows the introduction of the endoscope (**Fig. 10**). This system is especially helpful in cases in which multiple introductions of the scope might be necessary or if the diameter of the papilla shrinks very quickly after dilatation.

Sometimes it is not possible to identify the Wharton duct papilla by using dilatators, especially if there is a stricture in the distal duct. In this case, a surgical exploration cutdown can be used to identify the submandibular duct, open it, and introduce the endoscope. Often a small papillotomy is sufficient whereby the mucosa is opened slightly dorsal to the expected position of the papilla under local anesthesia (**Fig. 11**). If it is not possible to identify the duct, the incision is extended dorsally. The medial border of the sublingual gland is identified and this gland is retracted laterally. In the surgical plane beneath the sublingual gland both the duct and the lingual nerve can be identified. The duct is opened lengthwise and the endoscope introduced. The endoscope can also be introduced into a ductomy even further posteriorly (eg, after stone extraction to check for further stones).

Introduction of large therapeutic endoscopes into ducts is sometimes difficult because their outer diameter is often similar to the maximum diameter of the duct.[30] When it is not possible to gently introduce the scope it can be very helpful to apply the Seldinger technique.[22,31] An instrument (eg, guidewire, closed basket, or miniforceps) is inserted into the working channel of the endoscope (small guidewires can even fit through larger irrigation channels). The instrument is then introduced into the duct followed by the endoscope, which is slid over the instrument and into the duct (**Fig. 12**).

Irrigation

Irrigation is crucial for vision during sialendoscopy. Without irrigation the duct collapses. Additionally, irrigation helps to remove debris, such as fibrin or small stone fragments. Isotonic saline is the fluid of choice. Some surgeons recommend the use of an IV bag connected by intravenous tubing to the irrigation port of the endoscope

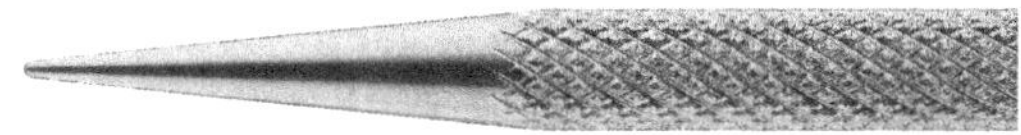

Fig. 7. Detail of a dilatator with a blunted tip. (*Courtesy of* Karl Storz, Tuttlingen, Germany; with permission.)

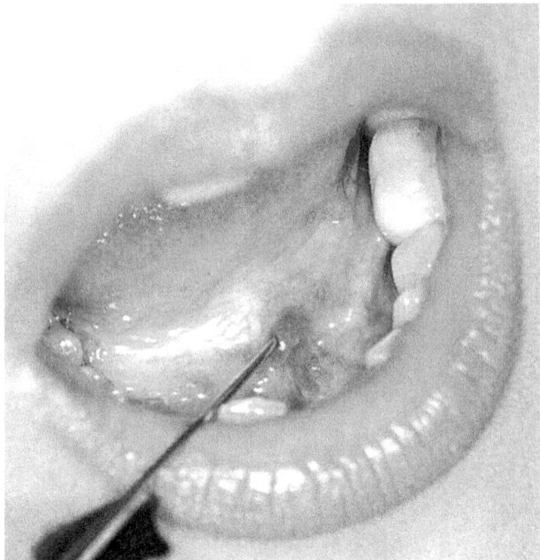

Fig. 8. Introduction of a blunt probe into Wharton duct. By checking for length, patency, and direction one can simultaneously make sure that a duct of part of the sublingual gland has not been cannulated.

because this provides continuous pressure. Others use larger syringes (50–100 mL) for continuous or smaller ones (10–20 mL) for intermittent irrigation. Air bubbles should be flushed out of the tubing and the endoscope because they hamper vision (**Fig. 13**). To avoid new bubbles the tips of the syringes should be held downward during irrigation. When using a therapeutic endoscope it can be advantageous to irrigate by way of the large working channel first and switch to the smaller irrigation channel when starting the intervention.

Surpassing Kinks

The endoscopes have a view angle of 70 to 120 degrees limited to the front. It is sometimes difficult to identify the secondary and tertiary branches connecting to the main duct system at an angle. Entering these side-branches might not be possible. Passing

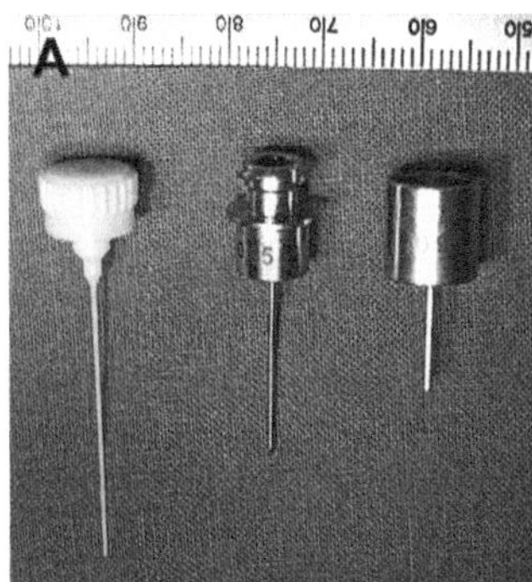

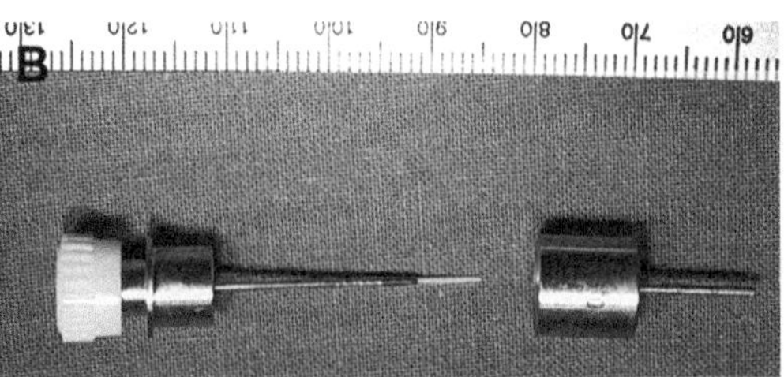

Fig. 9. (*A, B*) Port system for microendoscopes that can be used to dilate the papillae of ducts (Solex soft lumen expander, Polydiagnost, Pfaffenhofen, Germany). The inner part can be removed after successful introduction and dilatation; the outer part can remain as a port.

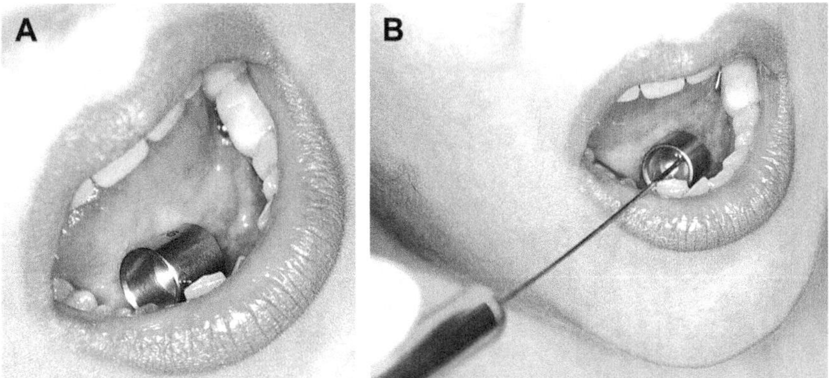

Fig. 10. (*A, B*) Solex inside the papilla of Wharton duct after removal of the inner part. The port allows easy introduction of an endoscope.

through kinks within the main duct can also be difficult (video 1, "Kink in the main part of Wharton's duct"; video 2, "Normal left Stensen's duct"; and video 3, "Guidewire technique to surpass a stenotic area of the left Stensen's duct" available at: http://www.oto.theclinics.com). Both rigid classic and the more flexible nitinol endoscopes have advantages that may be used to surmount the problem. The latter ones can be bent to follow a kink. The tip of the classic rigid endoscope is often easier to steer and more force can be applied to the tissue. This can be used to straighten a kink. This maneuver can be enhanced by using the Seldinger technique. In this method, the kink is first passed through by an (optionally prebent) instrument previously inserted into the working channel of the endoscope. Afterward, the endoscope follows by sliding over the instrument. In some cases it might be helpful to manipulate the gland from the outside during endoscopy to try to straighten the kink. This is often a very difficult procedure. Even slight manipulations on the outside can lead to massive internal movements interfering with endoscopic vision by duct wall contact.

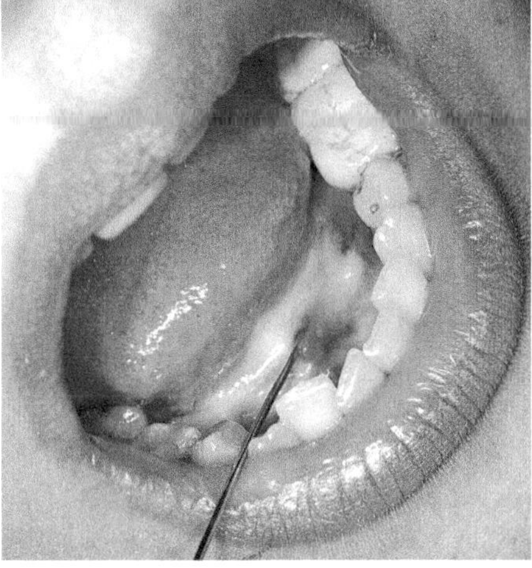

Fig. 11. Small papillotomy of Wharton duct to allow the introduction of a larger endoscope.

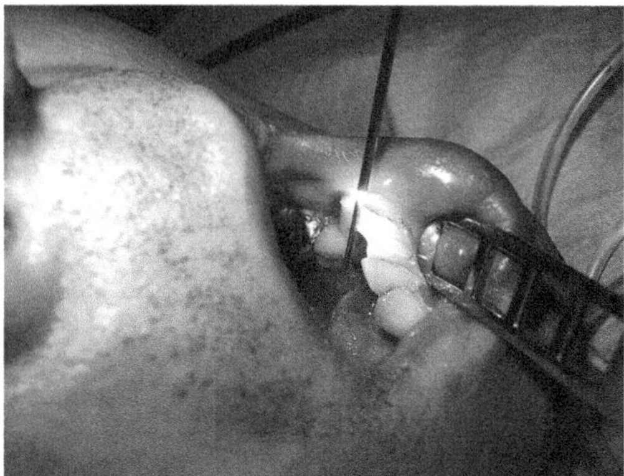

Fig. 12. Application of the Seldinger technique to introduce a larger endoscope into Wharton duct. First an instrument (in this case closed miniforceps) is introduced into the duct and then the endoscope is slid over it to follow into the duct.

Surpassing Stenoses and Strictures

Even after successful dilatation of strictures it can be difficult to pass through the pathologic area of the duct. Again, one good option is the use of the Seldinger technique (see video 3, "Normal left Stensen's duct" available at: http://www.oto.theclinics.com). The main advantage is that the endoscope always stays centered within the confines of the duct. This helps to avoid perforations of the duct. The endoscopes themselves, however, should be used only very carefully to dilate strictures because their front end has sharp right angle edges. Other methods should be used beforehand (see later).

DIAGNOSTIC ENDOSCOPY

Diagnostic endoscopy is usually a technically straightforward procedure. In some ways it resembles rigid bronchoscopy. Ear-nose-throat physicians are often able to

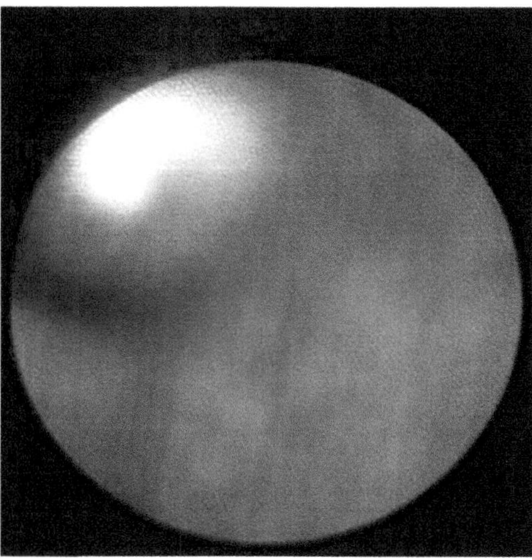

Fig. 13. Air bubble inside Wharton duct hampering vision.

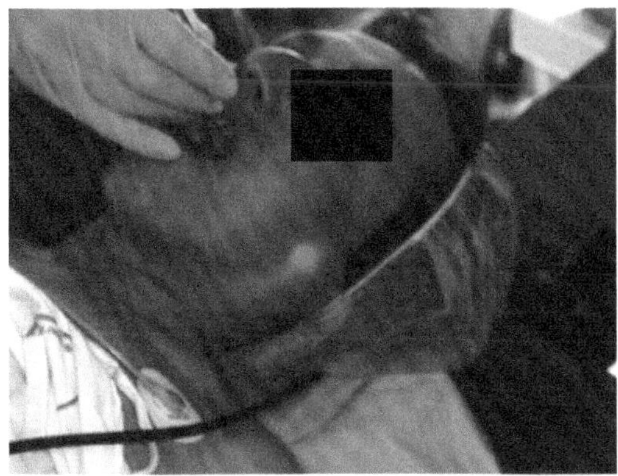

Fig. 14. The transillumination effect allows one to determine the position of the tip of the endoscope from the outside.

familiarize themselves with it quite quickly. The principle is to arrive at the pathology by following the duct system. The position of the tip of the endoscope can be determined by palpation, centimeter calibrations, or from the outside by the transillumination effect (**Fig. 14**). To track the endoscope even more precise guidance can be achieved by simultaneously using ultrasound (**Fig. 15**). If the reason or location of the obstruction is not known, the ductal system is inspected systematically distal to proximal (see video 2). Sometimes mucous and mucous strands are attached to stones and are seen on approaching the stone, before the actual stone is seen (see video 1; **Fig. 16**). Irrigation alone is sometimes not sufficient for mucous removal. In this case, suction applied by using small syringes (2–5 mL) applied directly without any tubing to the irrigation channel, or preferably to the working channel, can be very helpful (**Fig. 17**). Irrigation channels, because of their small diameters, can get blocked by this procedure and extracorporeal flushing of the channel clears the channel.

THERAPEUTIC ENDOSCOPY

Experience helps to successfully individualize treatment for each particular duct problem, although general techniques form the basis for therapy.

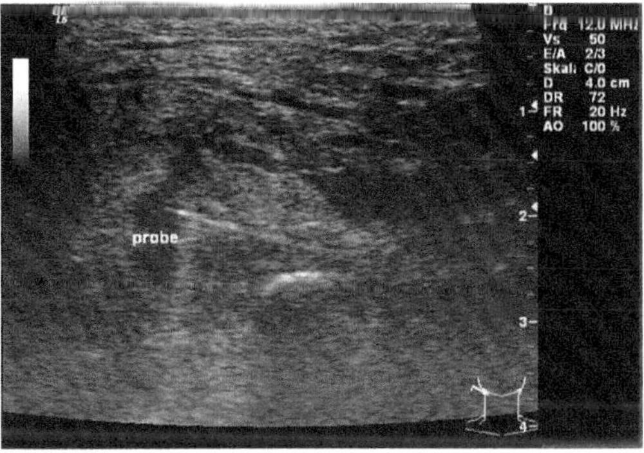

Fig. 15. Ultrasound image of the right parotid gland with an endoscope (*probe*) inside. The simultaneous use of ultrasound allows a precise intraoperative guidance of the endoscope.

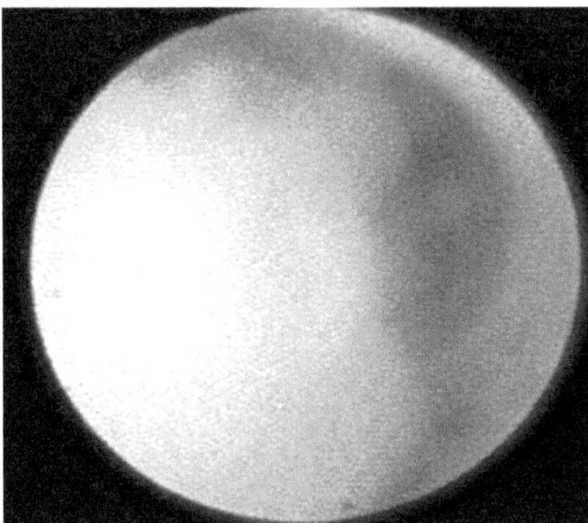

Fig. 16. Mucous strand attached to a stone inside Wharton duct (see also video 1, which shows mucous strands attached to a stone indicating its position).

Stones

Together with stenoses and strictures, stones are the main cause of obstructive salivary disease. Forceps, baskets, graspers, suctions, and balloons can be used to remove stones with an endoscopic control. Fragmentation is possible by using forceps, drills, and different laser systems (see **Table 1**).

It is of primary importance to note the relationship between the diameters of the stone and the duct. It begins the decision-making process as to what is realistically possible using any one or a combination of techniques, for example when deciding if stone removal without prior fragmentation technique should be attempted or if extracorporeal lithotripsy should be used.

Suction

Suction applied through the irrigation or working channel of the endoscope only can be used to remove dust-like stone fragments. It is important to be very close to the stone dust when starting suction because both the collapsing duct walls and the stone

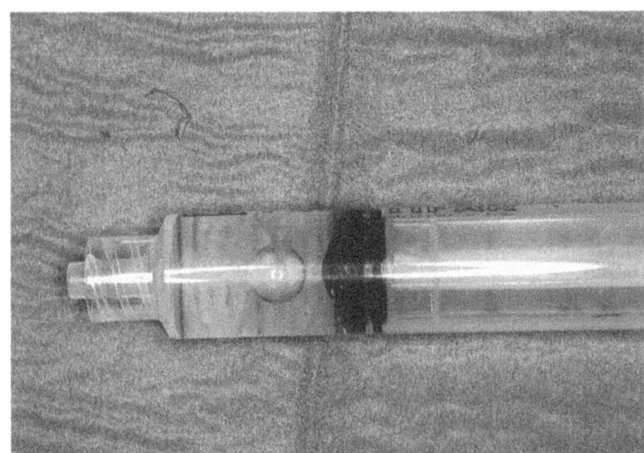

Fig. 17. Mucous plug (*outside the syringe*) and thick saliva (*inside*), which was inside a blocked Wharton duct. It was removed by suction with the syringe using the working channel of an endoscope.

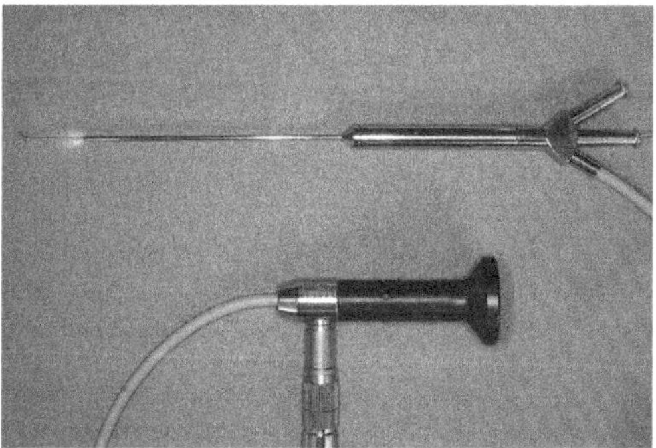

Fig. 18. Example of a compact semirigid endoscope (Spiggle & Theis, Overath, Germany) with a working channel of 1 mm, which allows the introduction of quite stable forceps as shown. The existence of the irrigation channel (0.2-mm diameter) can be noted by the second Luer-lock tube at the back part of the endoscope. The endoscope has a large outer diameter of 1.7 mm and often Seldinger technique has to be applied for insertion (see previously).

in front of the optical system totally interrupt vision. The value of this technique is limited.

Balloons

Above all, small (2–3 mm), round, mobile stones and multiple small fragments can be removed using balloons.[14] The balloon is inflated just behind the stones and slowly pulled out with the stones just in front of the balloon. The application of this technique is limited to the smallest stones.

Forceps: fragmentation and removal

The maximum diameter of certain sialendoscopic working channels is 1.02 mm (**Fig. 18**). The maximum forceps diameter is 1 mm (**Fig. 19**). The usual length of the jaw is about 3 mm. Consequently, the forces that these instruments can apply are

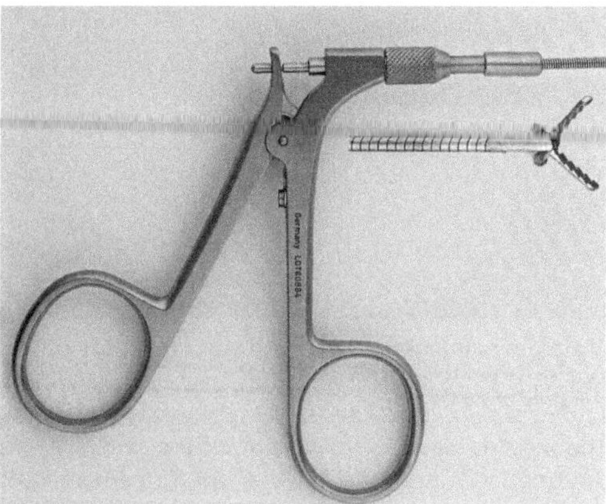

Fig. 19. Grasping forceps with serrated surface on the prongs and with a handle, which allows one to determine the orientation of the prongs quite easily (forceps handle). (*Courtesy of* Spiggle & Theis, Overath, Germany; with permission.)

very low and they are only suitable to crush small or soft stones. One advantage of this instrument is that it can be used for the extraction of the fragments. Large stones can be grasped. A change in the diameter of the duct, however, can prevent the extraction of the complete stone (**Fig. 20**, video 4, "Endoscopically controlled fragmentation of stones" forceps part, available at: http://www.oto.theclinics.com). When trying to surmount a stenosis soft stones can break. A positive feature of the forceps is that the instrument does not jam in the duct (versus a basket). The endoscopic forceps can break with the broken parts in loose contact with the main instrument or retrievable with another forceps from the duct; back-up instruments are important.

Baskets

A large variety of baskets exist. The main reason for this is that they were primarily designed for urologic and gastroenterologic purposes. A drawback to always consider is that baskets might get jammed in the duct with larger stones or fragments (see indications). Often stones can be released again after capturing them with baskets when jamming is imminent. Some types of baskets break quite easily and the jamming can be resolved. The more durable versions have the advantage that high forces can be applied to extract the fragments. Often it is possible to dislodge the stone and move it to a position where slitting of the papilla or the duct is possible (**Fig. 21**). Extended incision of Stensen duct should be avoided, however, because of the risk of severe duct stenosis.[6]

Technically, it is advantageous to open the basket behind the stone or at least in the region of the maximum diameter of the stone. By turning, pushing, and pulling

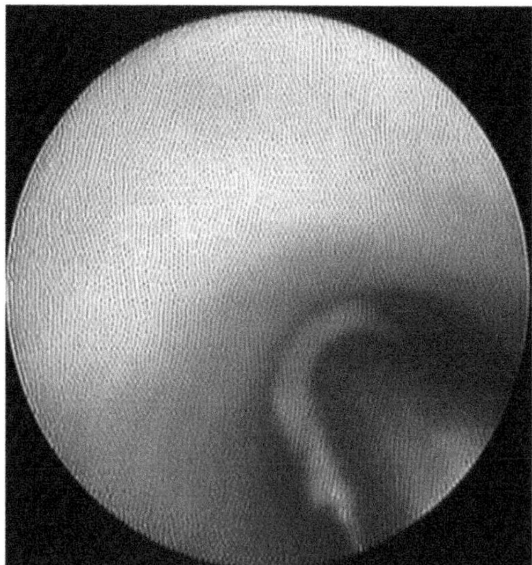

Fig. 20. Endoscopically controlled grasping and fragmentation of a stone in the hilum region of Wharton duct. A slitting in local anesthesia was not possible in this case because of a strong gag reflex. The picture illustrates some typical aspects of the forceps technique: the advancement of the forceps leads to a deviation of the optical axis of the scope toward the duct walls, and the relatively large diameter of the forceps occupies a significant part of the visible lumen of the duct and the stone. The forceps technique is often performed by a mixture of visual and tactile control. (*From* Geisthoff UW. Techniques for multimodal salivary gland stone therapy. Operat Tech Otolaryngol 2007;18:332–40; with permission of Elsevier.)

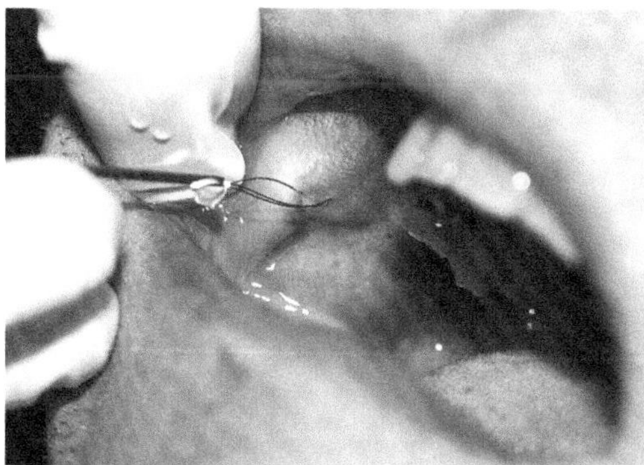

Fig. 21. Dislocation of a stone of the right Stensen duct to a position near the papilla. The basket is blocked at this position; it was possible to free the stone and the basket by a small papillotomy. (*From* Geisthoff UW. Techniques for multimodal salivary gland stone therapy. Operat Tech Otolaryngol 2007;18:332–40; with permission of Elsevier.)

movements on the basket the stone is engaged by the basket. Closure and extraction are the final steps (**Fig. 22**, video 5, "Endoscopically controlled basket removal of a stone in the hilum region of Stensen's duct," available at: http://www.oto.theclinics.com).

Graspers

Graspers are a combination of baskets and forceps (**Fig. 23**). They can be used to grasp even large stones. No space behind the stone is required. The forces applied are quite weak because of the small size and construction principle and fragmentation of stones is not possible. There is no relevant risk of blockage. Usually, there is good control of the procedure.

Drills

Drilling can be used to produce holes in stones. This is quite time consuming, but results in a stone that looks like Swiss cheese with scaffolding remaining, similar to the use of a holmium:yttrium-aluminum-garnet (Ho:YAG) laser (see later; video 6, available at: http://www.oto.theclinics.com). It is often impossible to destroy this scaffold by further drilling. The holes, however, can be used to apply forceps for fragmentation or for extraction (see video 4; **Fig. 24**).

Lasers

Various lasers have been used for intracorporeal lithotripsy, among them the XeCl-excimer, flash-lamp pulsed dye, the Ho:YAG, and the erbium:YAG laser. One important advantage of most lasers is that the fibers have small diameters (sometimes only 200 μm). Because the fibers are flexible they can also be used in flexible endoscopes. These properties allow applying high-watt intensities for fragmentation to stones even in the periphery of the duct system or behind stenotic areas. Disadvantages of lasers are their high costs, tissue damage including perforations of the duct, and the development of abscesses requiring gland removal.[2]

In contrast to other lasers mentioned, the beam of the erbium:YAG laser is not transmitted through a fiber but through a hollow guide with an outer diameter of 1 mm. This is a disadvantage. The fragments produced, however, are smaller than for most other laser types and can be removed easily by irrigation.[32]

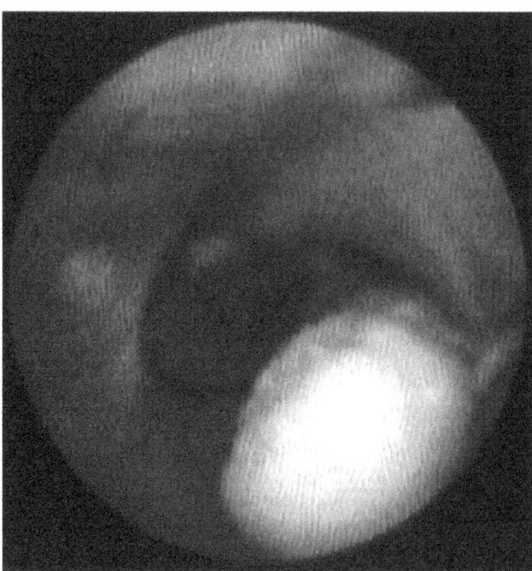

Fig. 22. Endoscopically controlled entrapping of a stone in the hilum region of Stensen duct using a basket without a separate outer sheath (ie, the basket opens directly in front of the endoscope). (*From* Geisthoff UW. Techniques for multimodal salivary gland stone therapy. Operat Tech Otolaryngol 2007;18:332–40; with permission of Elsevier.)

Usually, a Ho:YAG laser is used because the color absorption in stones is good and most hospitals also use it in urologic procedures. Technically, the laser fiber is directed toward the stone until the pilot beam is visible on its surface; then the working laser is started (see video 4, available at: http://www.oto.theclinics.com; **Figs. 25–27**). Vision is often reduced by floating fragments, interrupting the case until irrigation, baskets, or forceps are used to remove the fragments. The procedure is time consuming mainly because of the frequent "fragment" interruptions, but also to avoid tissue damage.

Treatment of Strictures

Endoscopically controlled treatment of stenoses and strictures includes the use of balloons, forceps, drills, and stents (see **Table 1**).

Drills

Manually rotated drills can initially be used to open filiform narrowings so that other instruments can later be used. The drill avoids the drawback of lasers, which can shrink surrounding tissue as they vaporize or coagulate the target.

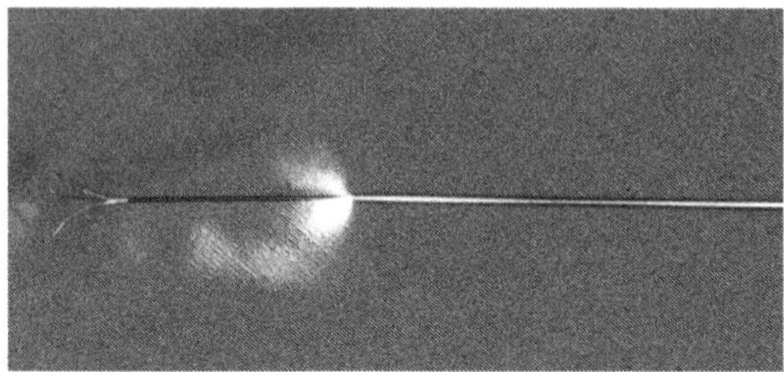

Fig. 23. A grasper inside the working channel of a compact semirigid sialendoscope.

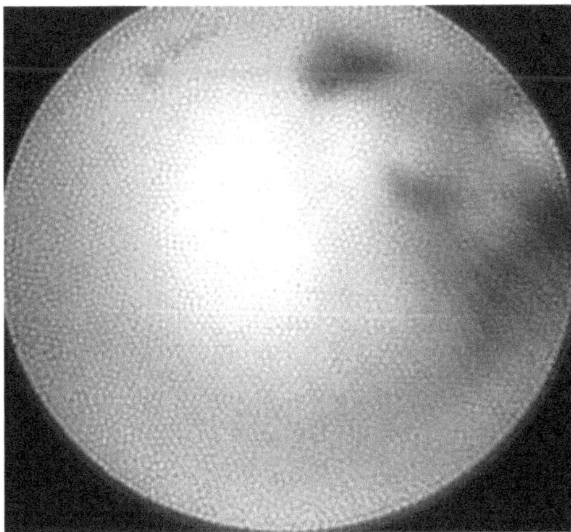

Fig. 24. Endoscopically controlled fragmentation of a stone inside the parotid gland with a drill. The stone nearly occludes the duct. In the upper part of the picture a bore hole already produced by the drill (visible on the right side of the picture) can be seen. (*From* Geisthoff UW. Techniques for multimodal salivary gland stone therapy. Operative Tech Otolaryngol 2007;18:332–40; with permission of Elsevier.)

Balloons

There are only a few balloons that fit within the working channels of sialendoscopes. The others are placed within the duct and then the endoscope follows. Alternatively, either sonography or fluoroscopy can be used to visualize the inflated balloon. The balloon is pushed into the narrowing and inflated. At that moment, optical control is lost because the inflated balloon prevents vision (video 7, "Balloon dilatation of

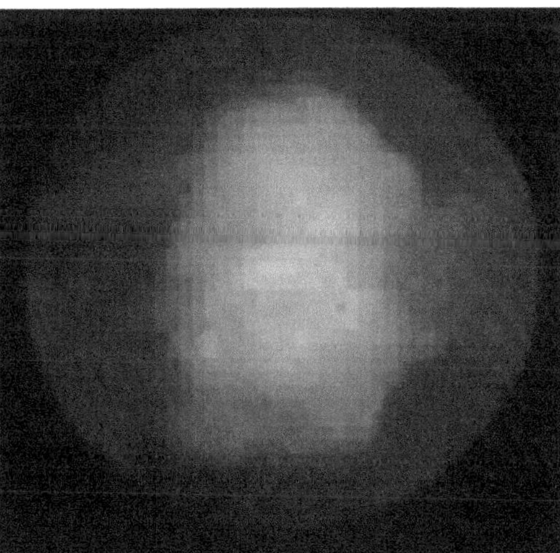

Fig. 25. Endoscopically controlled fragmentation of a stone inside Stensen duct using a flash lamp pulsed dye laser. The fiber is directed toward the stone. (*From* Geisthoff UW. Techniques for multimodal salivary gland stone therapy. Operat Tech Otolaryngol 2007;18:332–40; with permission of Elsevier.)

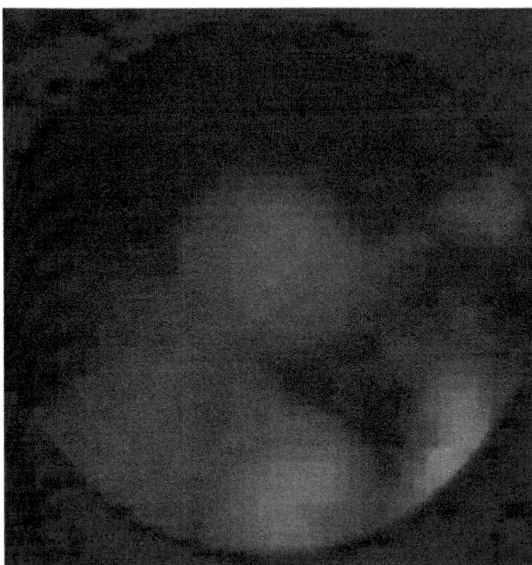

Fig. 26. The stone from **Fig. 25** has been broken up to multiple small fragments. (*From* Geisthoff UW. Techniques for multimodal salivary gland stone therapy. Operat Tech Otolaryngol 2007;18:332–40; with permission of Elsevier.)

a stenosis inside the parotid gland," available at: http://www.oto.theclinics.com). It might be necessary to repetitively inflate and deflate the balloon several times with increasing pressure until the stricture is opened sufficiently. In the case of a stricture serial advancement of the balloon may be necessary to open the entire extent of the

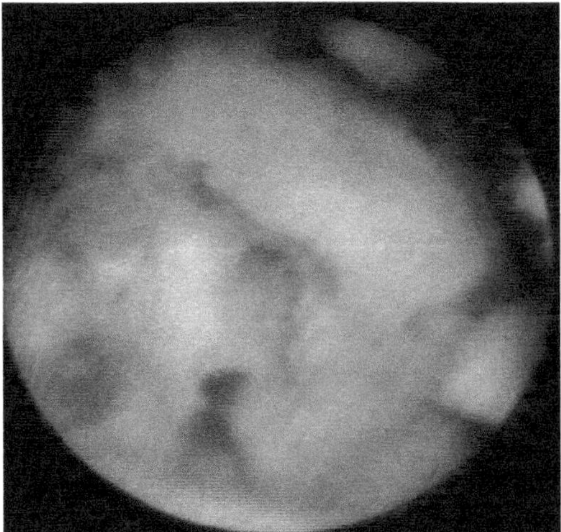

Fig. 27. The effect of the Ho:YAG laser is different from the flash lamp pulsed dye laser. The latter leads to a disruption of the stone into multiple fragments, whereas the former resembles the effect of a drill. The stone shown in the picture is situated within the hilum region of a submandibular gland. It has been treated with a Ho:YAG laser and a large scaffold with multiple holes remains. Part of this scaffold was broken down and removed with forceps.

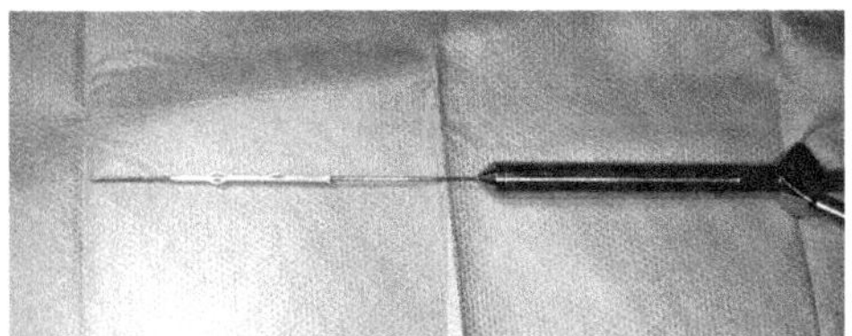

Fig. 28. Drain (Sialotechnology, Ashkelon, Israel) mounted on an endoscope (Spiggle & Theis, Overath, Germany) ready for placement under endoscopic view.

narrowed duct. Low- and high-pressure balloons exist. The former should be handled with care because they might rupture prematurely (video 8, "Removal of ruptured balloon inside the parotid gland," available at: http://www.oto.theclinics.com).

Forceps

Forceps that fit through the working channels of endoscopes are quite delicate. They can be used, however, for careful dilatations of membranous strictures. In contrast to balloons, the opening process can be well controlled and the instruments are reusable. Manufacturers advise against this use of their forceps because they are made to withstand closing but not opening forces (video 9, "Forceps dilatation of a stenosis inside the parotid gland," available at: http://www.oto.theclinics.com).

Stents and drains

The opinions about the use and terminology of stents and drains are divergent.[7,33,34] Their use has been shown to be beneficial in a number of cases. Although some minor membrane-like stenoses do well without stents, they are probably helpful in preventing recurrence. To place a stent using an endoscope it is slipped over the endoscope. After passing the stenotic area, the endoscope is retracted (**Figs. 28–30**, video 10, "Endoscopically controlled placement of a stent," available at: http://www.oto.theclinics.com). The drain should be kept in place for up to 1 month.

Chronic Sialadenitis and Recurrent Juvenile Sialadenitis

Sialendoscopy is performed as a treatment option both for chronic sialadenitis and recurrent juvenile sialadenitis.[26,27,35] By irrigation with saline the duct systems are dilated and cleared of mucous substances and debris. Up to 60 mL of saline are used for each gland even in children.[26] Additional instillation of cortisone (eg, 100 mg

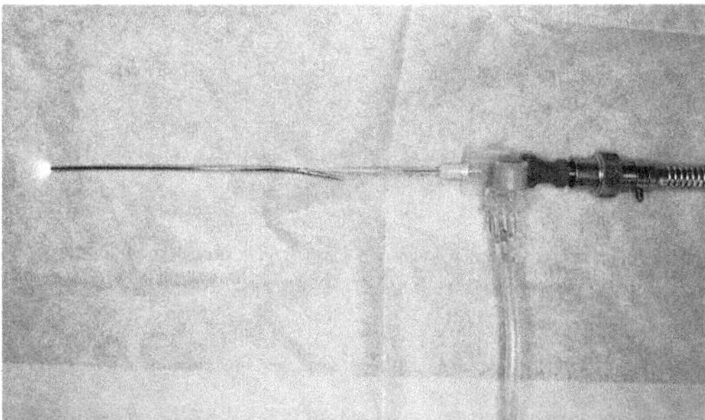

Fig. 29. Custom-made drain mounted on the optic system of a modular endoscope (Karl Storz, Tuttlingen, Germany). The drain was made from an IV-cannula; a second IV-cannula is used to allow irrigation.

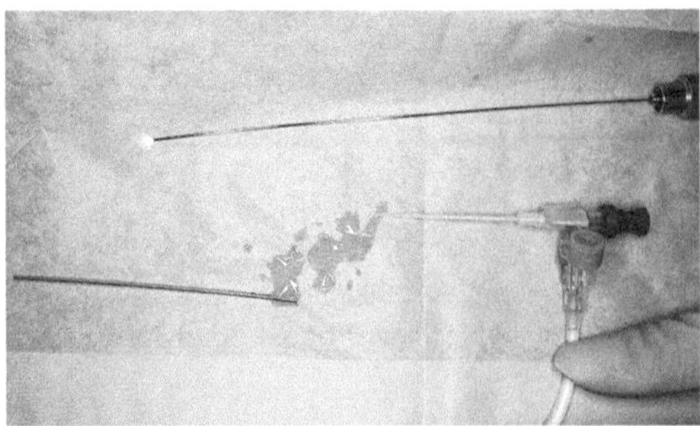

Fig. 30. Components of the system for endoscopically controlled deployment for drains as shown in Fig. 29. An IV-cannula as a drain and a second one for irrigation are mounted on the optic system of a modular endoscope (Karl Storz, Tuttlingen, Germany).

hydrocortisone), the use of balloons, and perioperative antibiosis might be helpful. Otherwise, the procedure resembles diagnostic endoscopy. Procedures for children are usually performed under general anesthesia, whereas local anesthesia is sufficient for adults. In some adult cases the temporary insertion of a stent may be considered.[35]

SUMMARY

Diagnostic sialendoscopy is an important technique to help the physician understand salivary duct pathology. For effective treatment of the obstructed duct, multiple techniques using combinations of different approaches may be used. Interventional procedures using the sialendoscopic technique are a significant part of the broad spectrum of minimally invasive procedures for the treatment of obstructive salivary disease.

APPENDIX: SUPPLEMENTARY MATERIAL

Supplementary material can be found in the online version at doi:10.1016/j.otc.2009.08.004.

REFERENCES

1. Katz P. [New therapy for sialolithiasis]. Inf Dent 1991;73(43):3975–9 [in French].
2. Gundlach P, Scherer H, Hopf J, et al. [Endoscopic-controlled laser lithotripsy of salivary calculi: in vitro studies and initial clinical use]. HNO 1990;38(7):247–50 [in German].
3. Konigsberger R, Feyh J, Goetz A, et al. [Endoscopic controlled laser lithotripsy in the treatment of sialolithiasis]. Laryngorhinootologie 1990;69(6):322–3 [in German].
4. Sterenborg H, van den Akker HP, van der Meulen C. Laserlithotripsy of salivary stones: a comparison between the pulsed dye laser and Ho:YAG laser. Laser Med Sci 1990;5:357–62.
5. Geisthoff UW. [Sialendoscopy]. HNO 2008;56(2):105–7 [in German].
6. McGurk M, Nahlieli O, Iro H, et al. Modern management of sialolithiasis: a consensus document. In: Nahlieli O, Iro H, McGurk M, et al, editors. Modern management preserving the salivary glands. Herzeliya (Israel): Isradon; 2007. p. 177–84.
7. Nahlieli O, Iro H, McGurk M, et al. Minimal invasive methods and procedures for the treatment of salivary gland sialolithiasis. In: Nahlieli O, Iro H, McGurk M, et al,

editors. Modern management preserving the salivary glands. Herzeliya (Israel): Isradon; 2007. p. 136–76.
8. Geisthoff UW. Techniques for multimodal salivary gland stone therapy. Operat Tech Otolaryngol 2007;18:332–40.
9. Geisthoff UW, Lehnert BK, Verse T. Ultrasound-guided mechanical intraductal stone fragmentation and removal for sialolithiasis: a new technique. Surg Endosc 2006;20(4):690–4.
10. Brown JE, Drage NA, Escudier MP, et al. Minimally invasive radiologically guided intervention for the treatment of salivary calculi. Cardiovasc Intervent Radiol 2002; 25(5):352–5.
11. Zenk J, Hosemann WG, Iro H. Diameters of the main excretory ducts of the adult human submandibular and parotid gland: a histologic study. Oral Surg Oral Med Oral Pathol Oral Radiol Endod 1998;85(5):576–80.
12. Marchal F, Dulguerov P, Becker M, et al. Specificity of parotid sialendoscopy. Laryngoscope 2001;111(2):264–71.
13. Zenk J, Iro H. [Sialolithiasis and its treatment]. Laryngol Rhinol Otol 2001;80(S1): S115–36 [in German].
14. Nahlieli O, Shacham R, Bar T, et al. Endoscopic mechanical retrieval of sialoliths. Oral Surg Oral Med Oral Pathol Oral Radiol Endod 2003;95(4): 396–402.
15. McGurk M, MacBean A, Fan KF, et al. Conservative management of salivary stones and benign parotid tumours: a description of the surgical techniques involved. Ann R Australas Coll Dent Surg 2004;17:41–4.
16. Nahlieli O, London D, Zagury A, et al. Combined approach to impacted parotid stones. J Oral Maxillofac Surg 2002;60(12):1418–23.
17. Marchal F. A combined endoscopic and external approach for extraction of large stones with preservation of parotid and submandibular glands. Laryngoscope 2007;117(2):373–7.
18. Koch M, Iro H, Zenk J. Role of sialoscopy in the treatment of Stensen's duct strictures. Ann Otol Rhinol Laryngol 2008;117(4):271–8.
19. Nahlieli O, Shacham R, Yoffe B, et al. Diagnosis and treatment of strictures and kinks in salivary gland ducts. J Oral Maxillofac Surg 2001;59(5):484–90.
20. Ngu RK, Brown JE, Whaites EJ, et al. Salivary duct strictures: nature and incidence in benign salivary obstruction. Dentomaxillofac Radiol 2007;36(2):63–7.
21. Salerno S, Lo CA, Comparetto A, et al. Sialodochoplasty in the treatment of salivary-duct stricture in chronic sialoadenitis: technique and results. Radiol Med 2007;112(1):138–44.
22. Seldinger SI. Catheter replacement of the needle in percutaneous arteriography: a new technique. Acta Radiol 1953;39(5):368–76.
23. Ziegler CM, Steveling H, Seubert M, et al. Endoscopy: a minimally invasive procedure for diagnosis and treatment of diseases of the salivary glands: six years of practical experience. Br J Oral Maxillofac Surg 2004;42(1):1–7.
24. Antoniades D, Harrison JD, Epivatianos A, et al. Treatment of chronic sialadenitis by intraductal penicillin or saline. J Oral Maxillofac Surg 2004;62(4):431–4.
25. Shacham R, Droma EB, London D, et al. Long-term experience with endoscopic diagnosis and treatment of juvenile recurrent parotitis. J Oral Maxillofac Surg 2009;67(1):162–7.
26. Nahlieli O, Shacham R, Shlesinger M, et al. Juvenile recurrent parotitis: a new method of diagnosis and treatment. Pediatrics 2004;114(1):9–12.
27. Quenin S, Plouin-Gaudon I, Marchal F, et al. Juvenile recurrent parotitis: sialendoscopic approach. Arch Otolaryngol Head Neck Surg 2008;134(7):715–9.

28. Koch M, Zenk J, Iro H. [Diagnostic and interventional sialoscopy in obstructive diseases of the salivary glands]. HNO 2008;56(2):139–44 [in German].
29. Luers JC, Vent J, Beutner D. Methylene blue for easy and safe detection of salivary duct papilla in sialendoscopy. Otolaryngol Head Neck Surg 2008;139(3): 466–7.
30. Zenk J, Zikarsky B, Hosemann WG, et al. [The diameter of the Stensen and Wharton ducts: significance for diagnosis and therapy]. HNO 1998;46(12):980–5 [in German].
31. Chossegros C, Guyot L, Richard O, et al. A technical improvement in sialendoscopy to enter the salivary ducts. Laryngoscope 2006;116(5):842–4.
32. Raif J, Vardi M, Nahlieli O, et al. An Er:YAG laser endoscopic fiber delivery system for lithotripsy of salivary stones. Lasers Surg Med 2006;38(6):580–7.
33. Iro H, Zenk J, Koch M, et al. The Erlangen salivary gland project. Part 1: sialendoscopy in obstructive diseases of the major salivary glands. Tuttlingen (Germany): Endo-Press; 2008.
34. Baurmash HD. Discussion: endoscopic technique for the diagnosis and treatment of obstructive salivary gland diseases. J Oral Maxillofac Surg 1999;57: 1401–2.
35. Nahlieli O, Bar T, Shacham R, et al. Management of chronic recurrent parotitis: current therapy. J Oral Maxillofac Surg 2004;62:1150–5.
36. Zenk J, Constantinidis J, Al Kadah B, et al. Transoral removal of submandibular stones. Arch Otolaryngol Head Neck Surg 2001;127(4):432–6.

Advanced Sialoendoscopy Techniques, Rare Findings, and Complications

Oded Nahlieli, DMD[a,b,*]

KEYWORDS

- Sialoendoscopy • Sialolithiasis
- Extracorporeal shock wave lithotripsy • Salivary
- Complications

Obstructive sialadenitis, with or without sialolithiasis, represents the most common inflammatory disorder of the major salivary glands.[1] Sialolithiasis is one of the major causes of sialadenitis. Calculi in the salivary glands can be found in 1.2% of the general population.[2] Other common salivary gland pathologies (besides tumors) are sialadenitis, strictures, and kinks. The diagnosis and treatment of this problem has been traditionally hampered by limitations of the standard imaging techniques. Satisfactory management depends on the surgeon's ability to reach a precise anatomic diagnosis and, in the case of sialoliths, to most accurately locate the obstruction.

Traditionally, sialoliths in the submandibular or parotid ducts and glands were divided into two groups[3,4]: stones that can be removed by the intraoral sialolithotomy approach, located usually in the anterior part of the duct; and stones that cannot be removed by the intraoral approach necessitating extirpation of the entire gland (sialadenectomy). Another pathology that required gland removal was concurrent or recurrent sialadenitis.

WHY MINIMALLY INVASIVE PROCEDURES FOR THE TREATMENT OF SIALOLITHIASIS?

The morbidity following traditional surgery for parotid and submandibular sialadenectomy includes a number of complications. Neurologic damage following superficial parotidectomy is of primary concern, because between 16% and 38% cases suffer

---

Dr Nahlieli is a consultant for Sialotechnology, Ashkelon, Israel.

[a] Department of Oral and Maxillofacial Surgery, Barzilai Medical Center, Ashkelon 78306, Israel

[b] Faculty of Medicine, Ben Gurion University of the Negev, Beer Sheva, Israel

[*] Department of Oral and Maxillofacial Surgery, Barzilai Medical Center, Ashkelon 78306, Israel.

E-mail address: nahlieli@yahoo.com

Otolaryngol Clin N Am 42 (2009) 1053–1072

doi:10.1016/j.otc.2009.08.007 oto.theclinics.com

0030-6665/09/$ – see front matter

temporary nerve weakness and 9% suffer permanent damage.[5,6] During submandibular gland removal there is a 7% risk of permanent marginal mandibular nerve damage and a 3% risk of damage to the lingual nerve.[7] Frey syndrome, facial scarring, greater auricular nerve numbness, sialocoeles, and salivary fistula also contribute to the morbidity of the traditional procedure.[8]

During the past decade, rapid developments in medical technology, such as optical miniaturization, lithotripsy equipment, microinstruments, and the influence from other surgical specialties, pushed development of new methods of analogous noninvasive and minimally invasive treatment.[9] Although it is possible to successfully treat salivary stones with traditional techniques, the use of the new methods was applied to advanced ductal cases. Because of the innovations, a surgeon became able to solve more complicated cases without major surgery and to perform the cases with less morbidity assuming the return of the gland to function.

The endoscopic system armamentarium requires an endoscope with at least 6000 pixels, a focal depth of 2 to 15 mm, and at least a 70° wide field of view. The diameter of one endoscope system (Modular Salivascope; PolyDiagnost, Pfaffenhofen, Germany) is 0.5 mm and uses four different disposable sleeves: 0.9, 1.1, 1.6, and 2 mm (**Fig. 1**A–C). The 0.9-mm sleeve has an irrigation channel and port for the telescope and is designed only for diagnostic purposes. The 1.1-mm system has three channels for the telescope, irrigation, and a special channel for surgical instruments. The 1.6- and 2-mm have the same number of channels but can accommodate large-size instruments to the working channel. The optical part, the telescope, is autoclavable.[10–12] Other endoscope models offered for advanced cases are Polydiagnost Salivascope flex, Type PD ZS 2001 1.1 mm (PolyDiagnost, Pfaffenhofen, Germany); Sialoview MDI 1.1 mm (Millennium, Islandia, New York); and Erlangen model (Karl Storz, Tuttlingen, Germany).

The endoscopic systems used in the author's study were the Modular Salivascope (PolyDiagnost, Pfaffenhofen, Germany); Polydiagnost Salivascope flex, Type PD ZS 2001 1.1 mm (PolyDiagnost, Pfaffenhofen, Germany); and the Sialoview MDI 1.1 mm (Millennium, Islandia, New York). The instruments used in his studies were microbaskets, miniforceps, minibiopsy forceps, high-pressure balloons, and microdrills for dilatation; brushes for cytology; and microneedles for injection (PolyDiagnost, Pfaffenhofen, Germany; and Sialotechnology, Ashkelon, Israel).

Recently, a miniature extracorporeal shock wave lithotriptor (ESWL) (Sialotechnology, Ashkelon, Israel) (**Fig. 1**D, E) was developed to assist in sialolithiasis management. It has a miniature generator and applicator, focal point depth of 15 × 15 × 25 mm, large focus zone at 50% of 35 mm, and a penetration depth of 120 mm. The size of the generator is 52 cm height × 42 cm length (20 kg weight) and the working head is reduced to fit the dimensions of the head and neck region. The usual technique delivers 1000 to 1500 shock waves per session. The miniature lithotripter can use an ultrasonic aiming system, or can be directed to the stone using endoscopic identification with the transillumination effect and also clinical findings.

This article assesses the value of and strategies for using the multitude of newly developed instruments and combinations of use, such as lithotripsy-sialoendoscopy methods, for advanced salivary gland sialolithiasis cases.

ADVANCED TECHNIQUES FOR ADVANCED CASES

When to Use Combined ESWL and Endoscopic Techniques?

In the past 2 years, 94 patients (43 males and 51 females, aged from 6–87 years) have been enrolled into the combined treatment. Sixty had pathology of the submandibular gland and 34 had pathology of the parotid gland.[10]

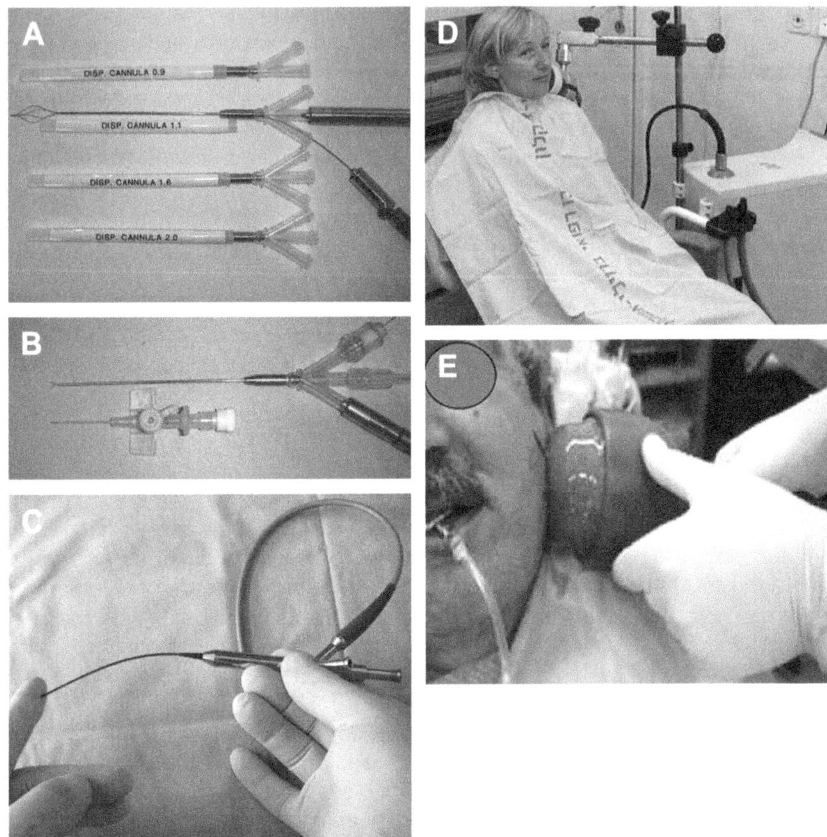

Fig. 1. (*A*) The modular salivascope with a telescope inside, disposable sleeves, and a miniature basket. (*B*) A 1.1-mm modular salivascope with integrated grasping forceps. (*C*) A 1.1-mm salivascope. (*D*) The miniature external lithotripter. (*E*) An intraoperative view; identification of parotid stone with the help of the sialoendoscope and adaptation of the lithotripter applicator.

Inclusion criteria for submandibular gland cases were (1) small (<5 mm) stone in secondary ducts or intraparenchymal stone (14 patients were selected); (2) small (<5 mm) fixed stone in the main duct in the hilus region (20 patients were selected); and (3) medium to large (>5 mm) hilar stone attached to the surrounding tissue, immobile or difficult to palpate (26 patients were selected).

Inclusion criteria for parotid gland cases were (1) small (<5 mm) stone in the main or secondary duct proximal from the middle part of the duct (eight patients were selected); (2) small (<5 mm) stone in secondary ducts or intraparenchymal stone (11 patients were selected); and (3) medium to large (>5 mm) hilar stone attached to the surrounding tissue, immobile or difficult to palpate (15 patients were selected). Exclusion criteria (same for both locations) were small (<5 mm) mobile stones in the main duct and medium to large (>5 mm) hilar mobile palpable stone.

Surgical Approach

Ultrasound and endoscopy assisted in location of the stone.[3,4,10,13] The endoscope was then used to instill the salivary gland with lidocaine 2%. Lidocaine helps to numb the entire gland and the subsequent isotonic saline inflation is needed to protect the salivary parenchyma. In all patients, external lithotripsy was first applied at low energy levels up to 130 atm with 1000 to 1500 shockwaves for each session. Three sessions of ESWL per patient are usually administered with 1-month interval between each session.

Following lithotripsy, an assessment is made to determine the outcome using plain radiograph, sialogram, ultrasound, CT, or sialoendoscopy. Thereafter, a purely endoscopic procedure or endoscopy-assisted open approach is chosen to finish treatment of the stones. Three types of treatment might be performed: (1) lithotripsy; (2) lithotripsy plus intraductal endoscopic approach (pure endoscopy); and (3) lithotripsy plus endoscopic-assisted extraductal open approach (stretching procedure for submandibular stones[4] or extraoral approach for parotid stones).[3] The second and third methods are used in cases when a salivary stone is not eliminated by lithotripsy alone.

CASE PRESENTATIONS

Lithotripsy (Sole Treatment)

A 45-year-old woman failed attempt in removal of a right submandibular stone using sialoendoscopy. The patient had suffered from multiple swellings of the right submandibular gland for 5 years. Panorex (Morita, Tokyo, Japan) radiograph demonstrated a 5-mm stone in the hilum region, which was difficult to palpate and which was attached to the surrounding tissues. Endoscopic exploration could not demonstrate the stone in the ductal system so the diagnosis of an intraparenchymal stone in the hilum region was made (**Fig. 2**A).

ESWL with the miniature lithotripter was applied with low energy levels up to 130 atm. A total of 1000 shockwaves per session was administrated for three sessions with a month interval between. Following the third session, the stone was still clinically palpable and the patient was to be scheduled for an endoscopic-assisted extraductal approach. Just before the endoscopic procedure, however, a sialogram was performed and surprisingly it demonstrated exfoliation of the stone, which was very easily removed by massage of the gland (see **Fig. 2**B, C). Endoscopic exploration following the removal of the stone showed dilated ducts but no additional stones or strictures were noted. In follow-up for over 16 months the gland remained asymptomatic and secretion of clear saliva could be noticed from the gland orifice.

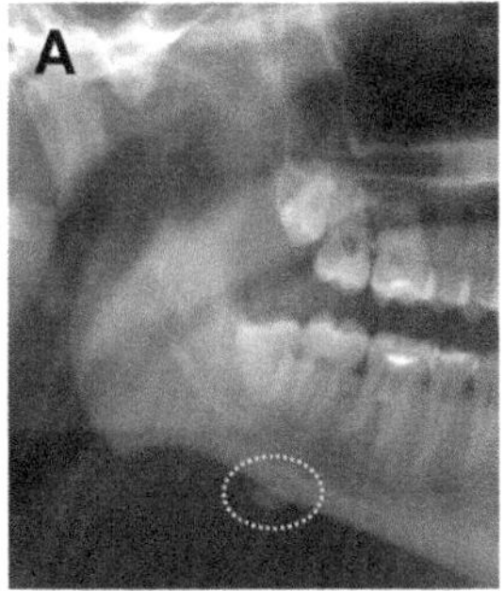

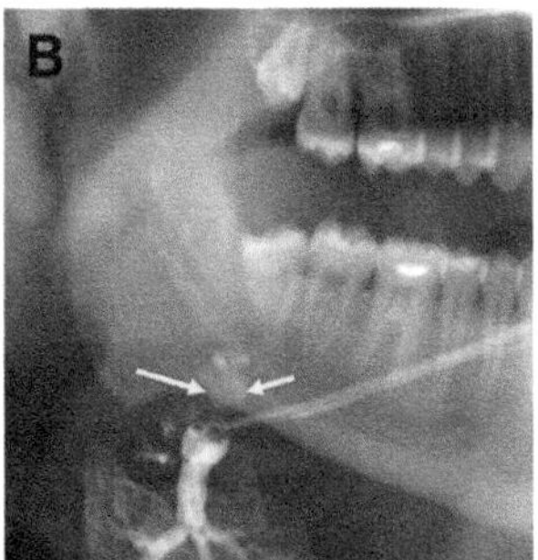

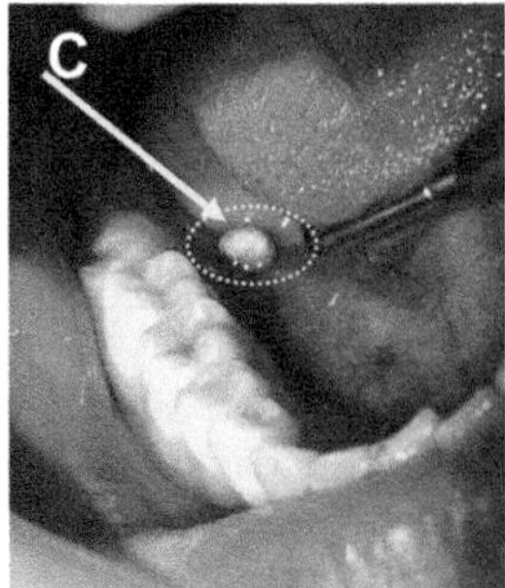

Fig. 2. (*A*) Panorex view demonstrating (*circle*) deep submandibular stone. (*B*) Sialogram of the same patient after the external lithotripsy procedures; note the stone location (*arrows*). (*C*) Intraoral view of the patient after the lithotripsy procedure with the stone exfoliated from the gland (*arrow, circle*).

Lithotripsy Plus Intraductal Endoscopic Approach (Purely Endoscopy)

A 62-year-old man had a sialolith of the left parotid gland. Clinical examination revealed swelling of the left parotid gland with purulent secretion from the left Stensen duct (**Fig. 3**A). Facial CT demonstrated a 4-mm stone located in the right parotid hilum (**Fig. 3**B). Endoscopic diagnostic exploration of the gland revealed the same 4-mm stone located in secondary duct without any possibility to reach the stone endoscopically.

ESWL with the miniature lithotripter was applied with low energy levels up to 130 atm. A total of 1000 shockwaves per session was administered for three sessions with a month interval between. Following the third session the stone was located

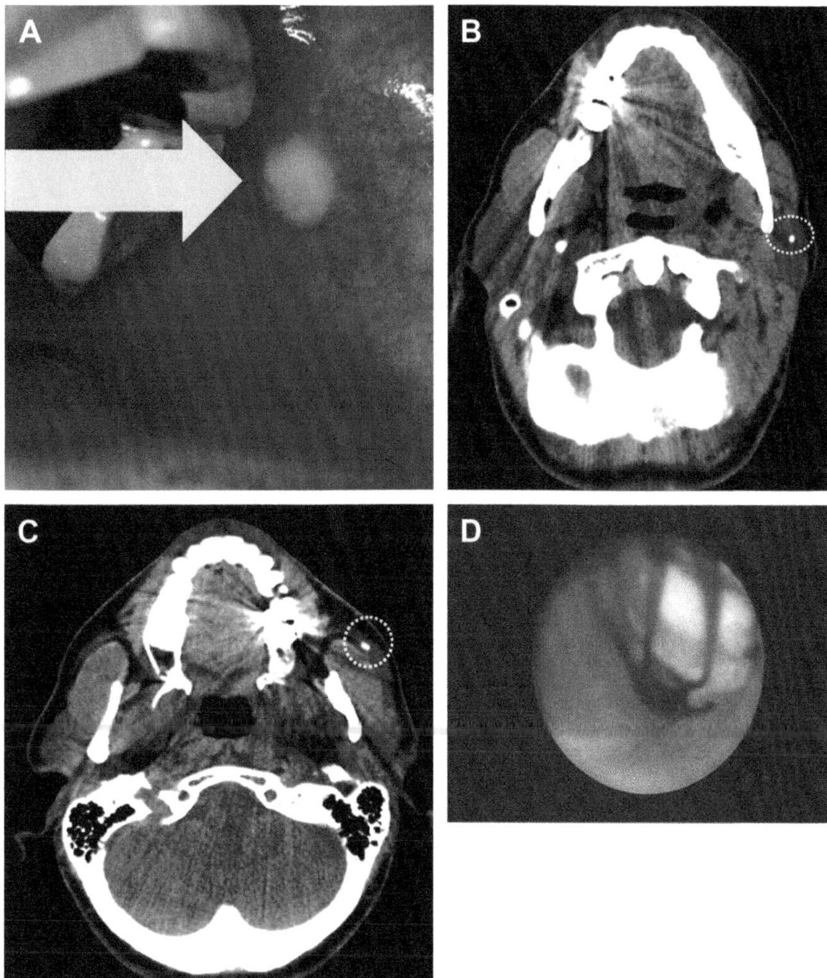

Fig. 3. (*A*) Purulent secretion from the Stensen duct orifice. (*B*) CT scan of the same patient with stone located in the parotid hilum region (*circle*). (*C*) CT scan after the third lithotripsy session; note the new location of the stone in the anterior third of the Stensen duct (*circle*). (*D*) Intraoperative sialoendoscopic view of the same patient during the retrieving procedure of the stone.

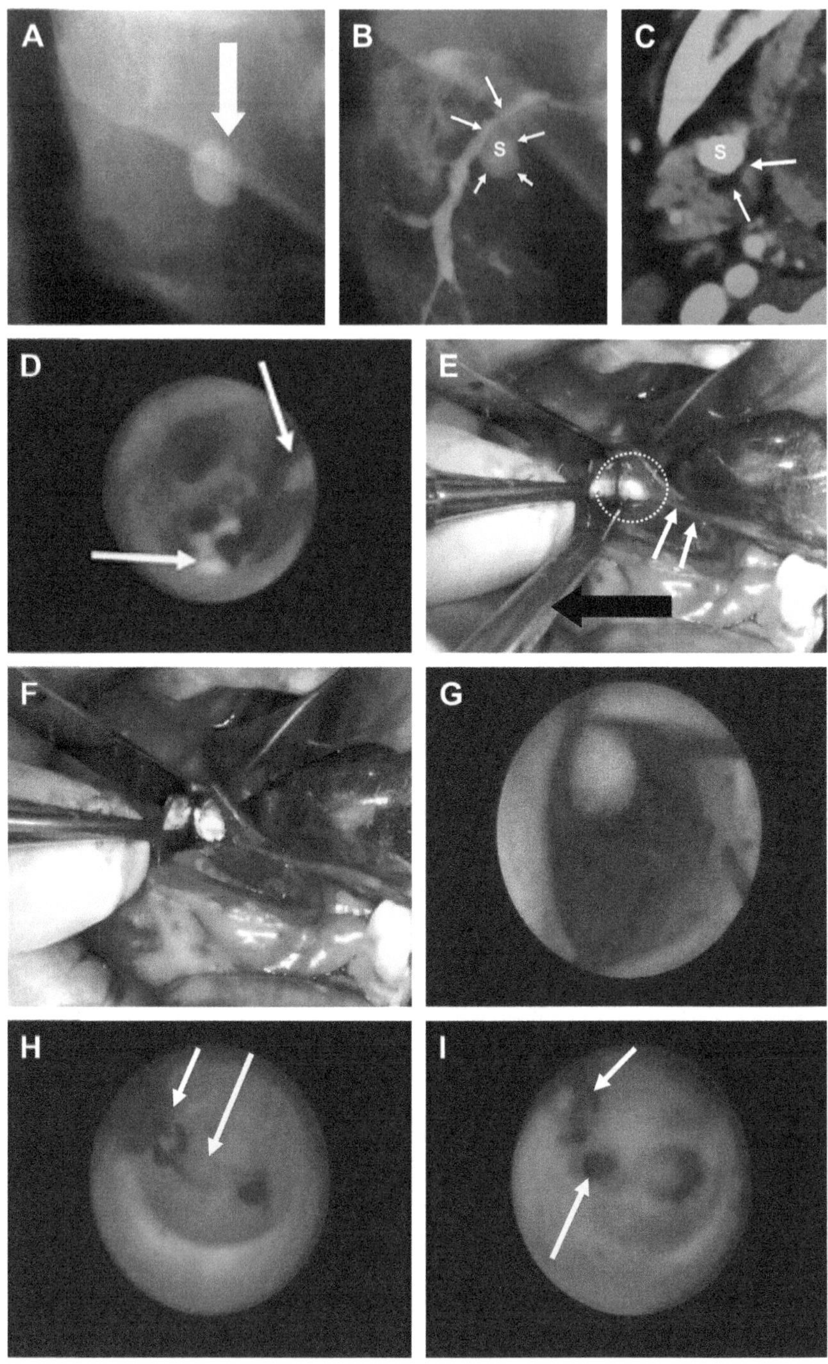
A
B
S
C
S
D
E
F
G
H
I

with CT scan in the anterior third of the Stensen duct (**Fig. 3**C). Endoscopic removal of the stone was carried out under local anesthesia using a four-wire basket (**Fig. 3**D). Sialodrain (Sialotechnology, Ashkelon, Israel) was introduced into the duct for 1 month. During a 12-month follow-up, the gland was asymptomatic and secretion of clear saliva could be noticed from the duct orifice.

Lithotripsy Plus Endoscopic-Assisted Extraductal Open Approach (Submandibular Stretching Procedure)

A 45-year-old man presented a deep left submandibular stone. The patient suffered from multiple episodes of swelling. Clinical evaluation revealed a very deep stone located inside the gland and fixed to the surrounding inflamed tissues. Imaging including Panorex, sialogram, and CT scan demonstrated a round 7-mm stone extraductally compressing the Wharton duct (**Fig. 4**A–C). Endoscopic exploration of the Wharton duct revealed the stone to be posterior to the hilar region in one of the secondary branches of the duct. Only the upper part of the stone could be observed (the tip of an iceberg); the main part of the stone was located inside the salivary parenchyma (**Fig. 4**D).

Three sessions of ESWL were administrated with 1000 shock waves per session at low energy levels up to 130 atm. After the third session, the stone was better palpated and seemed to be mobile. Under local anesthesia, a diagnostic endoscopy demonstrated the stone within the main duct but because of the narrow diameter of the duct it was not possible to use the intraductal approach. Endoscopic assistant technique (stretching technique) was indicated and the stone was removed (**Fig. 4**E, F). Sialoendoscopic exploration following the sialolithtomy revealed a small sialolith in the secondary duct and a stricture posterior to the stone. The stone was retrieved with the aid of a microbasket and the stricture dilated with a microdrill and a high-pressure balloon (**Fig. 4**G–I). Sialodrain was inserted for 1 month. Follow-up 8 months later revealed an asymptomatic gland with a clear salivary secretion.

Fig. 4. (*A*) Lateral radiograph view of deep submandibular stone (*arrow*). (*B*) Sialogram of the same patient demonstrating the location of the stone extraductally (*white arrows* and S show the stone, *yellow arrows* direct to the duct). (*C*) CT scan axial view; note the location of the stone in the gland (*arrows* and S) and the position of part of it into the duct. (*D*) An endoscopic view of the same stone. Note on the right the miniforceps (*white arrow*). Yellow arrow directs to the edge of the stone locating mainly in the parenchyma. (*E*) Intraoperative view of the extraductal stretching procedure. The stone (*circle*) inside the duct in the hilum region before the incision (*black arrow*, scalpel). Note the narrowness of the duct (*white arrows*) preventing intraductal removal. (*F*) Intraoperative view immediately after the incision. The stone located outside the duct before its removal. (*G*) Endoscopic view of the same patient after the stone removal. Retrieval of small additional stone from the secondary duct with four-wire basket. (*H*) Stricture obstructing secondary duct (*yellow arrow*) and small miniature drill directed to open it (*white arrow*). (*I*) Immediately following the drill procedure (*white arrow*, drill); the lumen of the duct is opened (*yellow arrow*). (*J*) CT demonstrating two stones in the left parotid gland. The first is in the hilus (*yellow circle*) and the second is in the middle part of the Stensen duct (*white circle*). (*K*) An intraoperative view. The black arrow directs to the biopsy marker and the yellow circle demonstrates the methylene blue around the stone location. (*L*) Removal of the hilar stone by rhytidectomy approach. (*M*) Removal of the second stone. Identification of the stone is done by the salivascope (*yellow arrows*) by the previous stone location. The white arrow directs to the transillumination effect demonstrated at the location of the stone. (*N*) Postoperative view of the same patient 1 week following the rhytidectomy approach.

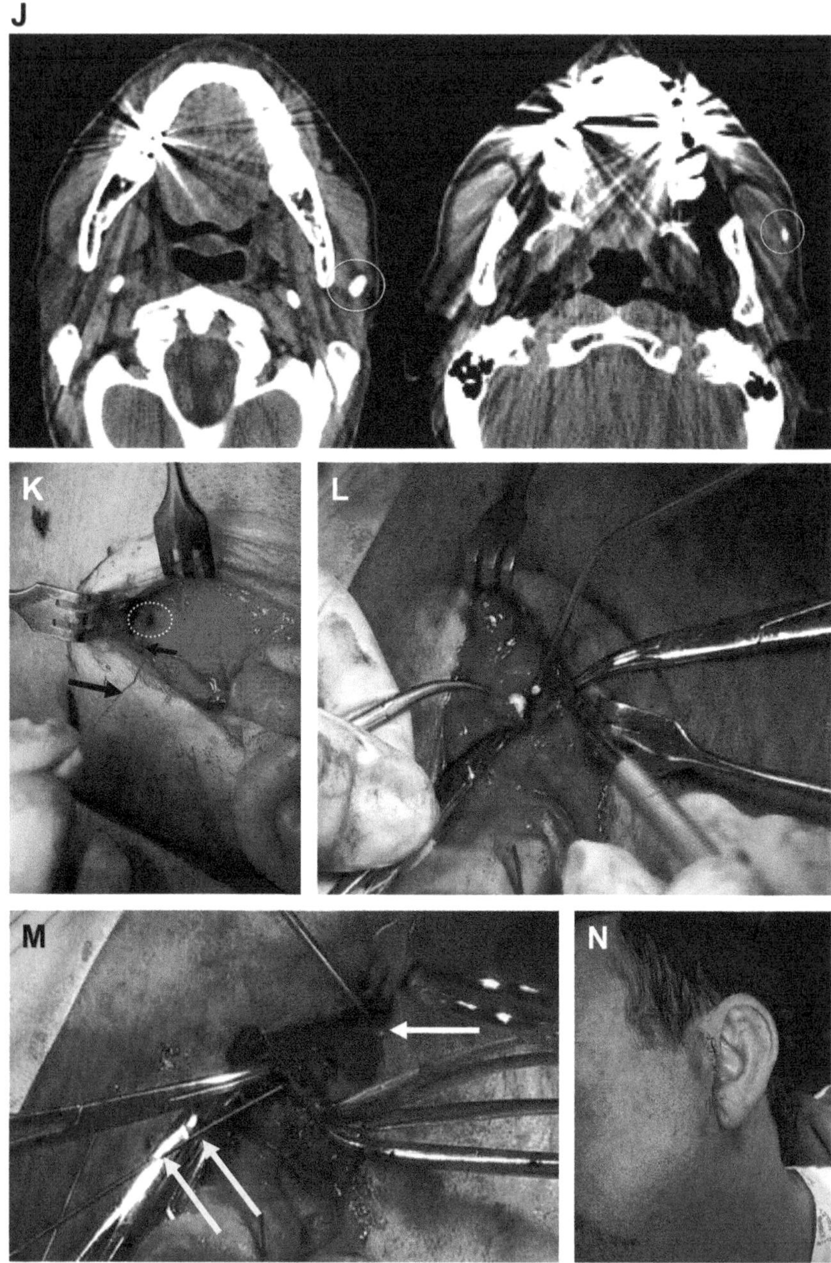

Fig. 4. (*continued*)

Lithotripsy Plus Endoscopic-Assisted Extraoral Approach

A 52-year-old man had a long-standing swelling of his left parotid gland. The patient suffered from multiple episodes of swelling and was hospitalized three times for IV antibiotic treatment and drainage.

CT demonstrated two stones (**Figs.** 4J–N) in the left parotid gland, the first stone located in the hilar region and the second stone located anterior to this region. The duct was totally obstructed in the anterior part to the second stone. Two attempts for endoscopic stone removal were unsuccessfully performed at another clinic.

On physical examination, a hard swelling of the left parotid region was noticed from the retroauricular region to the middle cheek area. Intraoral examination revealed complete obstruction of the Stensen duct, located a few millimeters posterior to the orifice. The patient was scheduled for superficial parotidectomy at another hospital.

Three sessions of ESWL were administrated with miniature lithotripter. Following the third session of lithotripsy there was a remarked reduction of the swelling in the parotid region. The patient was scheduled for sialolithotomy by external open parotid approach.

Under general anesthesia, the hilar stone was located with the aid of ultrasound and was marked with biopsy marker and injection of methylene blue into the stone location (**Fig.** 4K). By way of a rhytidectomy approach the first stone in the hilar region was explored and removed with the aid of a small dental excavator (**Fig.** 4L). Following the removal of this stone, a Salivascope flex, 1.1 mm, was inserted from the previous stone location to locate the anterior stone. The second stone was located and removed with the aid of the endoscope using the transillumination effect (**Fig.** 4M).

The next step was to create a new ductal opening to the gland. An 18-gauge veinline was inserted from the location of the second stone toward the mouth into the original location of the Stensen duct.

Parotid duct drain (Sialotechnology, Ashkelon, Israel) was inserted from the mouth with the aid of the veinline toward the location of the hilar region. The drain was fixed with 3/0 Vicryl sutures to the cheek mucosa and the incisions of the stones' regions were sutured thoroughly with 4/0 Vicryl sutures. The rhytidectomy flap was sutured with 5/0 nylon (**Fig.** 4N). Pressure dressing was applied for 24 hours. After 4 weeks, the parotid duct drain was removed. Follow-up 3 months later revealed an asymptomatic and normally functioning gland. The cosmetic result was satisfactory.

Lithotripsy Plus Endoscopic-Assisted Extraductal Open Approach for Giant Stones

A 68-year-old woman had constant swelling of her right submandibular gland. On physical examination, a large, hard swelling was detected, fixed to the surrounding tissues. Lateral radiographs demonstrated exceptionally significant stone occupying the location of the submandibular gland (**Fig.** 5A).

ESWL with the miniature lithotripter was applied for three sessions. After the last session the stone was palpated easily and was mobile. Under general anesthesia, by the extraductal stretching approach, the stone was exposed and easily extracted from the gland (**Fig.** 5B); two sialodrains were introduced into the stone location (**Fig.** 5C). The patient's postoperative course was uneventful and 1 year later the gland was completely asymptomatic with clear saliva observed from the new orifices.

From experience during 2 years of extensive use of these techniques, this combination seems to be successful and safe. Total elimination of the stone by lithotripsy alone was achieved in 32% (N = 30) of the cases; in 29% (N = 27) of lithotripsy cases, intraductal endoscopic assistance was needed. In 39% (N = 37) the removal of a stone was achieved with the help of endoscopic-assisted extraductal open approach.

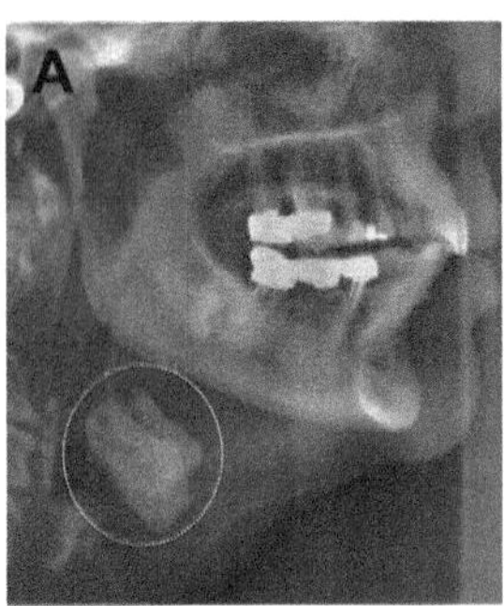

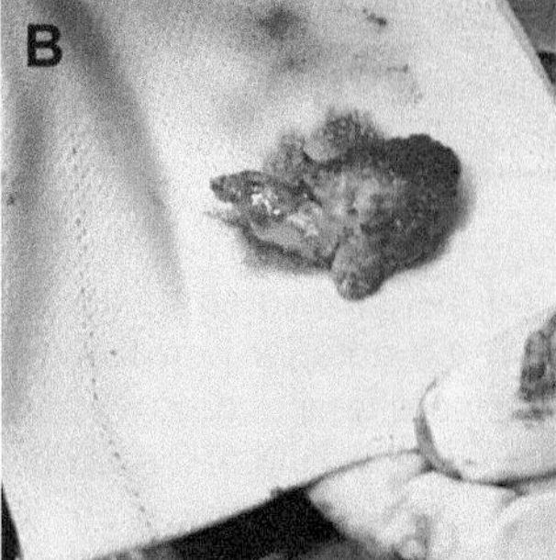

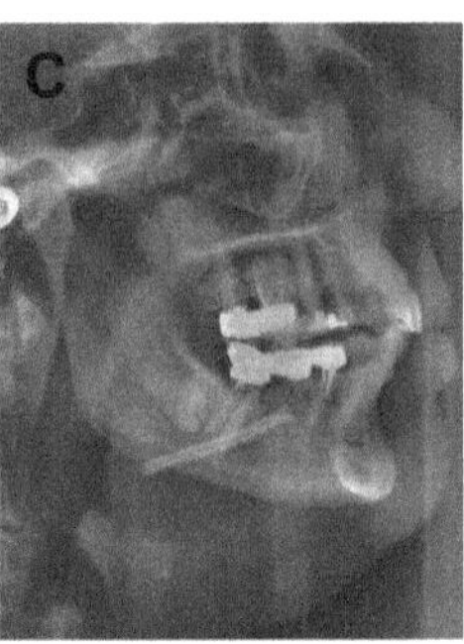

Fig. 5. (*A*) Lateral radiograph with huge stone occupying the location of the right submandibular gland (*circle*). (*B*) The stone after the extraction. (*C*) Lateral radiograph after the extraction of the stone with two sialodrains located in the space following the stone removal.

Six-month follow-up revealed an absence of symptoms in all cases when lithotripsy or lithotripsy plus intraductal endoscopic approach were performed. In cases when endoscopy-assisted extraductal approach was used, 35 (95%) out of 37 patients remained nonsymptomatic. Postoperative follow-up was carried out from 6 to 24 months.

RARE FINDINGS IN SIALOENDOSCOPY

During 15 years of sialoendoscopic experience the author has encountered several rare conditions that were responsible for ductal obstruction of the salivary glands.[2,3,10,12–19] The list of the conditions from more to less frequent follows:

1. Extraductal stones
2. Nonsalivary stones, calcifications of foreign bodies
3. Stones in the submandibular or sublingual gland
4. Obstruction caused by salivary tissue
5. Foreign bodies
6. Tumors that mimic sialadenitis and stones

Although rare, these findings have the potential to cause severe morbidity and delay in the correct diagnosis.

Extraductal stones present a delicate problem. The ability to extract stones solely by endoscopic technique is based on the presence of the stone in the ductal lumen. The existence of a stone partially or completely inside the parenchyma presents a dilemma requiring the use of other techniques. These types of stones can be diagnosed mainly by sialoendoscopic exploration. The correct diagnosis can also be made by conventional sialogram and MRI sialogram, and less accurately by ultrasound and CT (**Fig. 6**A, B).

Division of these stones is by their location: (1) completely embedded in the parenchyma (no possibility to observe it by the ductal system); (2) partially embedded in the parenchyma (only a small part of the stone is inside the ductal lumen) (**Fig. 6**C); and (3) the main part of the stone is in the duct (the lesser part is in the parenchyma).

In groups 1 and 2 the direction of the procedures should be toward ESWL extraductal open approaches. In group 3, the treatment depends on the stone diameter: if the stone is smaller than 5 mm the treatment is endoscopic removal; in cases with stones larger than 5 mm the preferred treatment is extraductal open extraction.

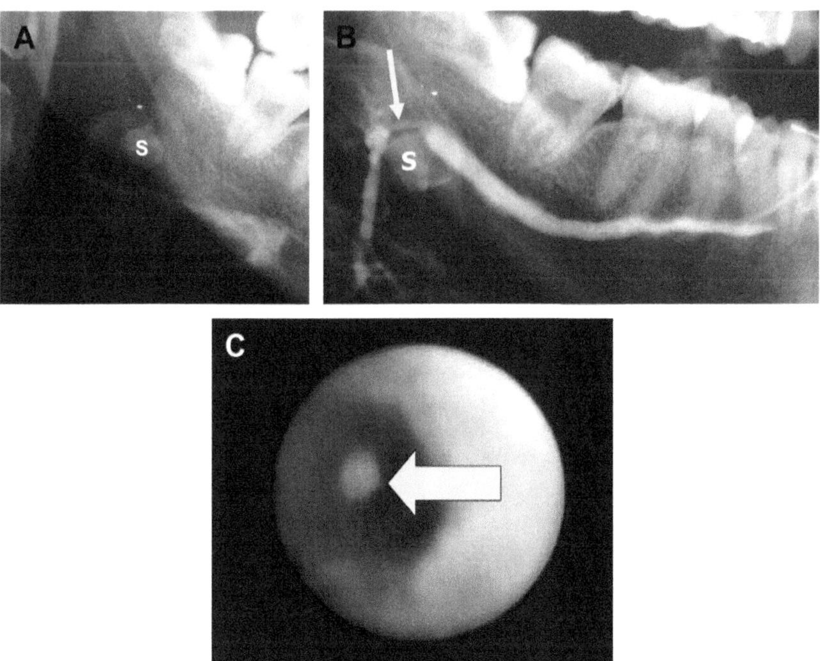

Fig. 6. (*A*) Panorex radiograph of 27-year-old patient referred with swelling of the right submandibular gland. Stone is demonstrated in this imaging in the location of the gland (S). (*B*) Sialogram of the same patient; note the extraductal nature of the stone (S) compressing the main duct (*arrow*). (*C*) Endoscopy demonstrating partially embedded stone in the parenchyma (*arrow*); only a small part of the stone is inside the ductal lumen (tip of iceberg).

In the case of nonsalivary stones and calcifications of foreign bodies, radiopaque lesions in the salivary region are blamed as salivary stones.[20–22] There are a number of calcifications that are not stones.[23,24] The most common calcifications are tonsiliths, phlebolith calcifications in blood vessels, lymph nodes, and foreign bodies including vascular clips following carotid endarethrectomy surgery (**Fig. 7**A). Combinations of stones and other calcifications is even more rare, but possible (**Fig. 7**B).

Stones in the sublingual glands present very challenging findings. The relationship between the submandibular gland and the sublingual gland is still unclear but in many instances there is direct connection between the two ductal systems, which sometimes makes the diagnosis regarding the origin and the location of the stone problematic (**Fig. 8**). The correct diagnosis of these rare findings is a combination of methods, such as sialogram, sialoendoscopy, CT, ultrasound Doppler, and MRI.

Obstruction caused by salivary tissue itself is perhaps the most novel type of rare finding. During sialoendoscopic treatment the author encountered new phenomenon that was not familiar: a few cases with obstruction caused by enlargement of part of the salivary tissue. This phenomenon is more likely to occur in the parotid gland because of the hypertrophy of the accessory lobe (**Fig. 9**), but cases of sublingual enlargement that caused Wharton duct occlusion also were observed. Diagnosis is performed mainly by pure sialogram, and CT or MRI sialogram. There is no other imaging modality that can help in these cases, including endoscopy, because the obstruction results from the surrounding tissue that is not in the duct. The treatment

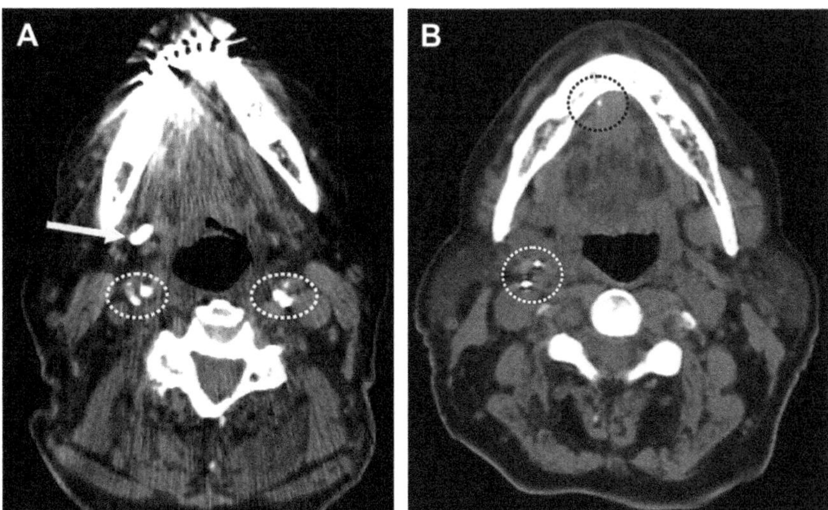

Fig. 7. (*A*) *Yellow arrow* demonstrates stone in the right submandibular gland, the bilateral *yellow circles* surround calcifications in the carotid region. (*B*) A 71-year-old patient presented with intermittent swelling of the right submandibular gland. Axial CT demonstrates a small stone near the Wharton duct orifice (*black circle*). Two vascular clips are shown following endarterectomy (*white circle*) performed 6 years ago.

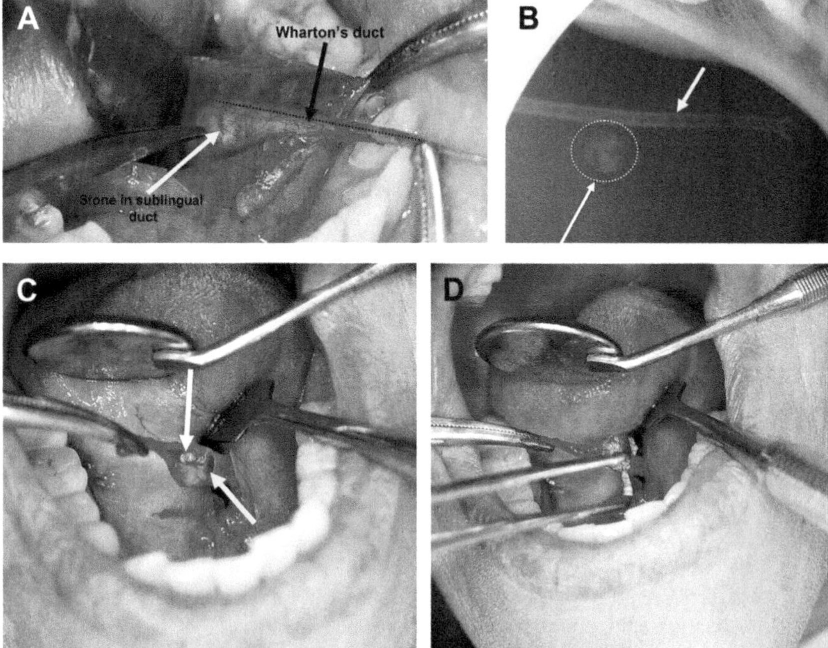

Fig. 8. (*A*) An intraoperative view of patient with a stone located in the sublingual duct. The lachrymal probe is inside the Wharton duct (*black line*). (*B*) Intraoperative occlusal radiograph of the same patient. Radiopaque drain introduced into the Wharton duct (*yellow arrow*); the stone in the sublingual duct (*white circle, white arrow*). (*C*) White arrow directs to the stone, the yellow arrow directs to the Wharton duct. (*D*) The removal of the stone.

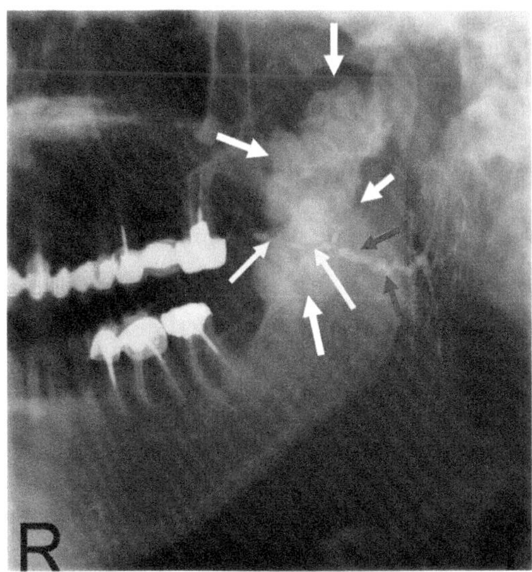

Fig. 9. Obstruction of parotid gland because of a huge enlargement of the accessory lobe. In the sialogram the accessory lobe is marked with *white arrows*. The obstructed anterior duct is marked with *yellow arrows*. The dilated posterior duct is marked with *red arrows*.

of choice is to locate the exact location of the pathology and to use a sialoballoon to dilate the obstruction; if possible, a sialodrain can be inserted.

Foreign bodies are a rare, but possible, pathology that can be blamed for obstructing the ductal system of the salivary glands. During the endoscopic procedure, the author encountered 15 patients with obstruction symptoms in which the endoscopic exploration revealed a foreign body inside the ductal system. Nine of them appeared inside the submandibular and six in the parotid gland. Seven of them were associated with stone formation and seven patients were children. In six patients the foreign bodies were hair shafts (**Fig. 10**A). In the other nine cases the particles were identified as a fragment of a tea leaf (**Fig. 10**B, C), fish bone, and toothbrush fibers. This foreign body phenomenon demonstrates the ability of particles from the oral region to gain access into the gland ducts by an unknown scenario. The only method to diagnose this rare condition is by way of the sialoendoscopic approach.

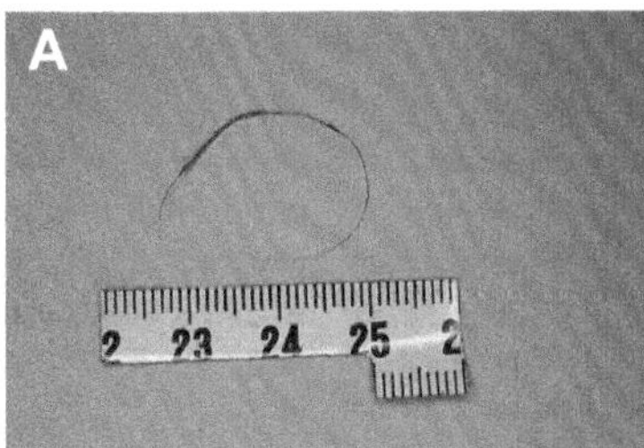

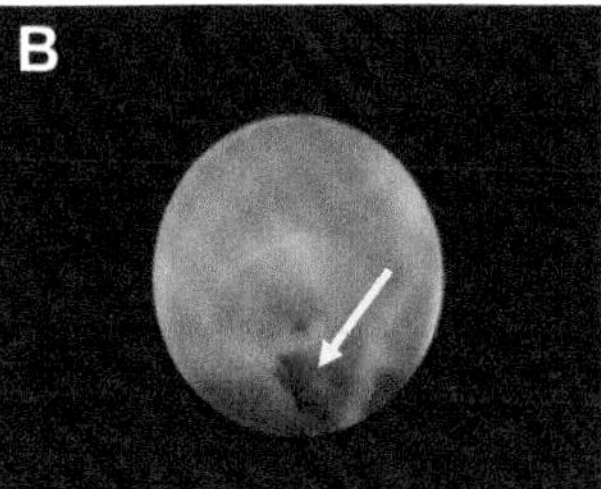

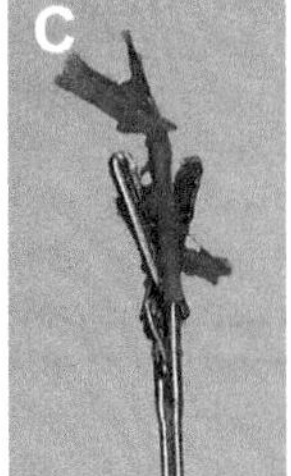

Fig. 10. (*A*) Hair follicle removed from the Stensen duct; note the formation of stone around the follicle. (*B*) A sialoendoscopic view of the submandibular hilum. Note a planet fragment located in the middle of the hilum (*arrow*). (*C*) Removal of the fragment with miniforceps; the particle was examined and proved to be a leaf of tea.

Tumors mimicking sialadenitis and stones are the most serious rarities, which can affect the prognosis of a patient and could delay an adequate treatment. Deep tumors that pressure the gland and obstruct the main duct can cause such a stone mimicry. Experiences faced by the author include Hodgkin lymphoma mimicking submandibular sialdenitis, carotid body tumor mimicking parotid chronic sialadenitis (**Fig. 11**A), juvenile parotid lymphangioma and hemangioma mimicking juvenile recurrent parotitis (**Fig. 11**B), tuberculosis mimicking submandibular stones and sialadenitis, and submandibular cyst obstructing the ductal system.

Complications

Several main types of complications follow sialoendoscopic procedures, including strictures; excessive swelling; perforations (false rout); ranula; and lingual nerve paresthesia. Strictures are the main complication pathology following sialoendoscopic procedures.[25–28] Postoperative strictures are well-known complications in ductal surgery in other organs, such as in urology bile duct and nasolachrimal endoscopic surgery. The risk for such a complication remains after each operative endoscopic surgery. In the author's experience, the risk for this complication is 2.5%. In a review of 1589 cases, 39 patients suffered from postoperative strictures, 30 underwent successful dilation, and 9 underwent sialadenectomy.

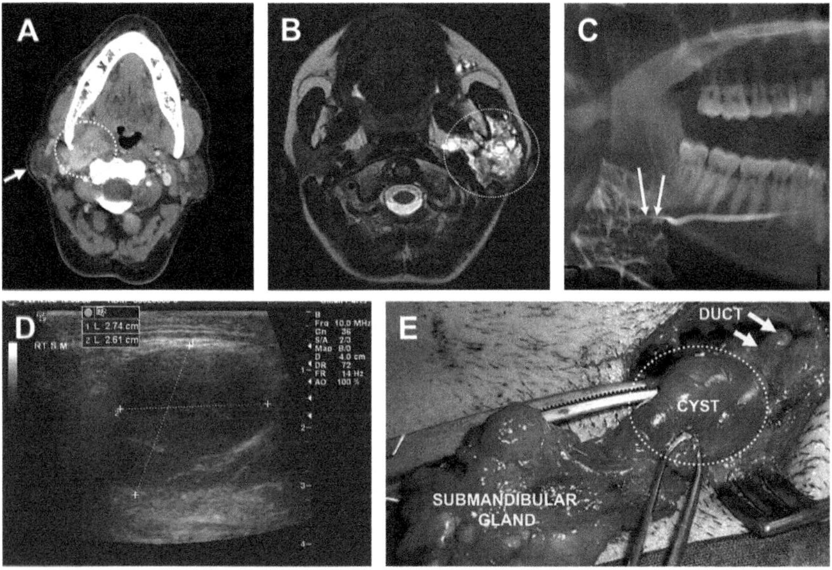

Fig. 11. (*A*) CT of 66-year-old woman with carotid body tumor (*yellow circle*) causing compression of the right parotid gland (*white arrow*) and intermittent swelling of the gland mimicking chronic recurrent parotitis. (*B*) MRI of 10-year-old child with juvenile parotid lymphangioma (*circle*) mimicking juvenile recurrent parotitis. (*C*) Sialogram of 32-year-old patient suffering from intermittent swelling of the right submandibular gland for 1-year period. *Yellow arrows* indicate the obstruction region. (*D*) Ultrasound of the same patient demonstrates organized hypoechoic lesion with sharp borders and homogenous content in the right submandibular gland. (*E*) Intraoperative view during the sialadenectomy procedure; note the cyst compressing the submandibular duct (*arrow*) causing obstruction of the gland.

The strictures can be identified by continued swelling of the gland following stone extraction without any evidence of an additional stone or stone particle intraductally. The absence of saliva or reduced salivary secretion from the orifice of the affected gland is also characteristic. Most postoperative strictures are near the orifice region. Usually, prevention of strictures can be achieved by the insertion of sialodrain following every surgical endoscopic procedure with intraglandular irrigation with hydrocortisone, 100 mg, which prevents most postoperative stricture formation. The treatment of stricture in the orifice area could be performed with a dilator and irrigation of the duct with hydrocortisone, 100 mg. Treatment of strictures in other parts of the ductal system is the same as for primary strictures (ie, mainly by high-pressure sialoballoon, miniforceps, and miniature drills) (**Fig. 12**A, B).

Perforation (false passage) of the duct can happen in two main locations: orifice of the duct, caused by separation of the ductal wall from the oral mucosa; and intraductally, during sialoendoscopic mechanical procedures, such as stone removal and stricture dilation. The identification of this pathology is made mainly by the endoscopic picture, which does not show the ductal lumen structures. Another sign is excessive swelling in the region of the perforation caused by leakage of the irrigation solution into the surrounding tissue. Careful observation of the ductal anatomy and irrigation when the practitioner identifies the lumen part of the duct helps prevent this complication. The complication is best treated by identification of the exact location of the perforation and insertion of sialodrain if possible (**Fig. 13**).

Excessive swelling following sialoendoscopy is usually caused by obstruction of the main duct, perforation of the duct, or excessive irrigation. It can be prevented or treated by insertion of a drain, administering of intravenous steroids, and gentle massage of the affected gland and hydration.

Ranula formation is a well-known outcome following surgical procedures in the floor of the mouth.[29,30] Formation of ranula can occur in patients following submandibular sialoendoscopy. From the author's last review on 1589 cases, 1152 glands underwent submandibular or sublingual sialoendoscopic surgery; 29 (2.5%) of them developed ranula; 27 of them underwent successful marsupialization; and 2 underwent sublingual sialadenectomy.

The formation of ranula is proportional to the extensivity of the procedure. Patients who underwent endoscopic-assisted intervention, such as the stretching procedure, were more prone to this complication. Some patients suffering from ranula have multiple pathologies in their secretary system of both the submandibular and the sublingual ductal system. The formation of ranula is the expression of these multiple pathologies.

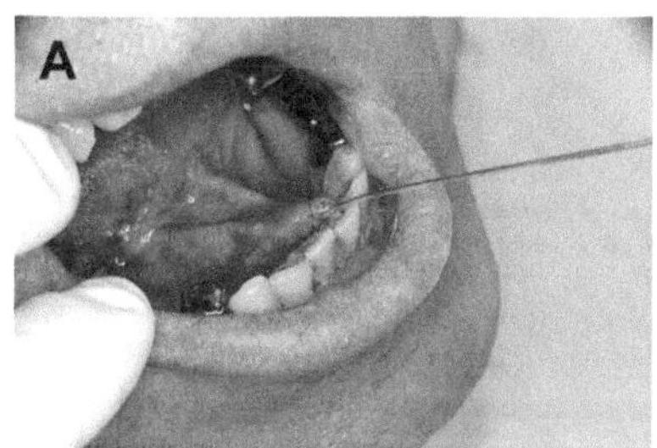

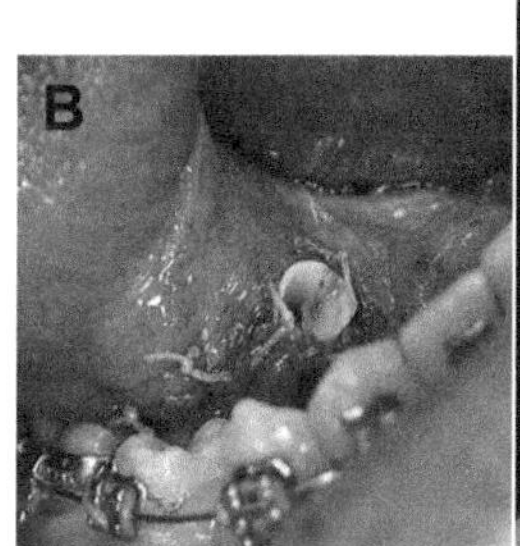

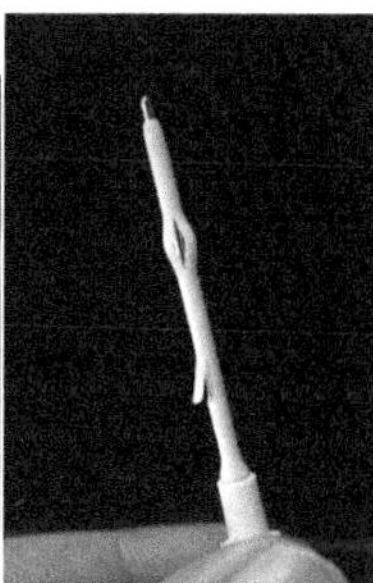

Fig. 12. (*A*) Dilation procedure of the Wharton duct with high-pressure balloon. (*B*) Sialodrain is inserted into the Wharton duct following the dilation procedure.

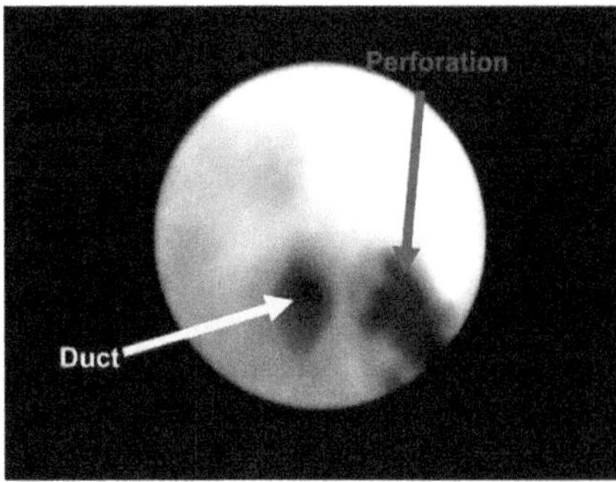

Fig. 13. Intraoperative view demonstrates perforation during sialoendoscopy of the parotid duct.

Ranula is usually identified by swelling, mostly blue, in the floor of the mouth. The treatment is very simple: unroofing or marsupialization and insertion of iodoform gauze with suturing with 4/0 Vicryl sutures for 2 weeks. In 93% of cases this procedure solves the problem (**Fig. 14**). In a few cases, a second attempt at marsupialization might be needed. In 7% (two) of the patients with postoperative ranula an intraoral sublingual sialadenectomy is the solution.

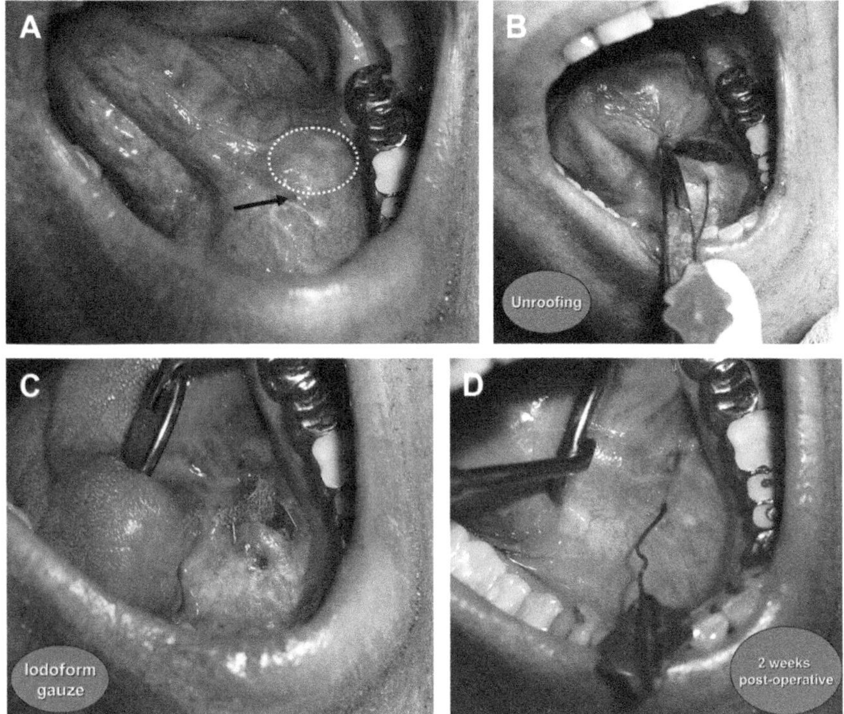

Fig. 14. (*A*) Ranula following sialoendoscopy of the left submandibular gland (*white circle*). *Black arrow* indicates the new duct opening. (*B*) Unroofing (marsupialization) procedure; lachrymal probe is inserted into the Wharton duct. (*C*) Iodoform gauze is packed into the cavity. (*D*) The postoperative view 2 weeks following the procedure.

Lingual nerve paresthesia and anesthesia is a rare complication of sialoendoscopy of the submandibular gland. It can happen mainly in the endoscopic-assisted procedure, stretching technique. During a purely endoscopic procedure, it can happen only because of perforation of the duct. In the author's experience, only five (0.4%) patients suffered from temporary lingual nerve paresthesia. Knowledge of the lingual nerve anatomy and the relation between the nerve and the duct is paramount to preventing the complication (**Fig. 15**). If the lesion occurs, steroid treatment should be administered.

DISCUSSION

Until recently, low success rate and very expensive equipment were the main obstacles preventing surgeons from using the described techniques for advanced problems. The rapid development in miniaturization of equipment, the reduction in equipment price, and the combination with other minimally invasive techniques give the lithotripsy technique a place in the armamentarium of the treatment of sialolithiasis.

The combination of lithotripter and sialoendoscope can be very effective. The endoscopic removal of residual stones after the lithotripsy procedures is easier and less complicated. The shock waves disconnect the stone from the ductal wall and reduce the volume of the stone. Disconnection of the stone from the surrounding ductal tissue seems to be the major positive effect of the lithotripsy procedure.

This combined lithotripsy-endoscopy approach might help to overcome the various sizes, locations, and most of the obstruction pathologies because it involves multiple techniques and technologies: pure endoscopy, endoscopic assistance technique, and external lithotripsy can be combined in a treatment of the same patient. The implementation of these three methods relies on the advantages of each method and can lead to effective treatment of most of the obstructive and inflammatory salivary conditions.

The treatment philosophy of the lithotripsy procedure has been changed from its original usage as a solo technique to its implementation as an adjuvant technique. As an adjuvant, the author adapted the miniature lithotripter and the low energy levels to detach the stone from ductal tissues without breaking it into fragments. Disconnecting the outer cortex of the stone during or after lithotripsy and the positive effect on

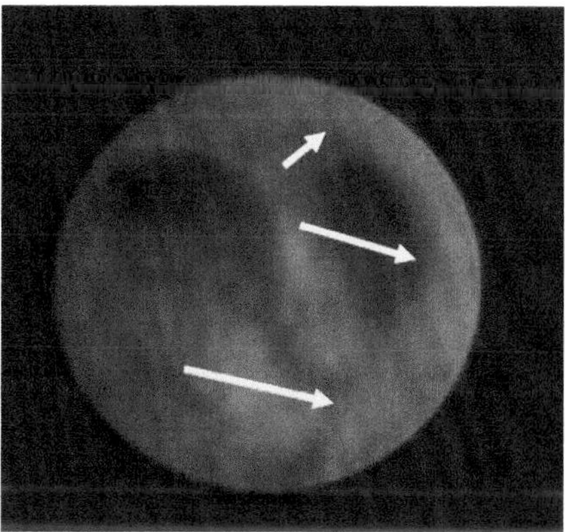

Fig. 15. Intraoperative view during sialoendoscopy. The yellow arrows indicate the prominence of the lingual nerve location, near the hilum of the submandibular gland.

scar tissue provides a possibility for saliva leakage to the oral cavity by going around the stone.

Regaining normal gland function after lithotripsy in cases with medium to large stones is a welcome addition to positive results for the patient. Additional research is needed to evaluate this phenomenon; however, some speculations are possible. One can speculate that revascularization angiogenesis might occur in the affected salivary gland similar to the effect of cardiac shock wave therapy. This might be a suitable explanation, assuming that one used the same energy levels that were used in the cardiac shock wave research and treatment. External shock wave therapy has generated great interest in cardiology since the first report of enhanced neovascularization by shock wave application at the tendon-bone junction in a dog model.[31] It was then found that in patients with chronic refractory angina external shock wave therapy was safe and well tolerated. It improved symptoms, exercise capacity, and myocardial perfusion.[32] Some hints were allowed in favor of formation of new capillary networks.[33] If indeed this is also the case for salivary glands, the newly proposed treatment might add significantly to the therapeutic capacities in cases of sialolithiasis with gland atrophy.

ESWL is an old technique with the main advantage of being noninvasive. The first report on the use of shock waves to fragment sialoliths appeared in 1986.[34] The problems at that time seemed caused by the large-sized lithotripsy machine with a very broad focus that caused damage of dental fillings and periostial irritation. Development of smaller machines with a more finely focused wave beam led to further improvement of the method that reached a success rate 50% to 60% for stone removal and up to 100% for alleviation of symptoms.[35,36] It was not previously used for treatment as an adjuvant technique with low-level energy of salivary gland diseases and the innovation demonstrates that it might be used in this field with significant success. Additional research is needed to assess whether this novel technique reduces the incidence of significant complications.

Major complications are infrequent and in general can be salvaged by standard salivary gland surgery.[28] The rare findings and complications encountered during extensive experience and described in this article help the practitioner to use diagnostic and treatment techniques safely.

SUMMARY

Lithotripsy combined with intraductal or extraductal endoscopic-assisted treatment for sialolithiasis is a highly effective surgical method for removal of salivary stones, especially for deep parenchymal and advanced sialolithiasis cases. This method helps to avoid resections of salivary glands and represents a further development of minimally invasive surgical technique. Rare findings and complications during endoscopic procedures are also discussed.

REFERENCES

1. Mandel L, Witek EL. Chronic parotitis diagnosis and treatment. J Am Dent Assoc 2001;132:1707–11.
2. Rauch S, Gorlin RJ. Diseases of the salivary glands. In: Gorlin RJ, Goldman HM, editors. Oral pathology. St Louis (MO): Mosby; 1970. p. 962–1060.
3. Nahlieli O, London D, Zagury A, et al. Combined approach to impacted parotid stones. J Oral Maxillofac Surg 2002;60:1418–23.

4. Nahlieli O, Shacham R, Zagury A, et al. The ductal stretching technique: endoscopic assisted technique for submandibular stones. Laryngoscope 2007;117(6):1031–5.
5. Mra Z, Komisar A, Blaugrund SM. Functional facial nerve weakness after surgery for benign parotid tumours: a multivariate statistical analysis. Head Neck 1993;15:147–52.
6. Owen ER, Banerjee AK, Kissin M, et al. Complications of parotid surgery: the need for selectivity. Br J Surg 1989;76:1034–5.
7. Milton SM, Thomas BM, Bickerton RC. Morbidity study of submandibular gland excision. Ann R Coll Surg Engl 1986;68:148–50.
8. Lari N, Chossegros C, Thiery G, et al. Sialendoscopy of the salivary glands. Rev Stomatol Chir Maxillofac 2008;109(3):167–71, Epub 2008 Jun 3.
9. Nahlieli O, Nakar LH, Nazarian Y, et al. Sialoendoscopy: a new approach to salivary gland obstructive pathology. J Am Dent Assoc 2006;137(10):1394–400.
10. Nahlieli O, Shacham R, Zagury A. Combined external lithotripsy and endoscopic techniques for advanced sialolithiasis cases. J Oral Maxillofac Surg 2009, in press.
11. Wagner N, von Buchwald C, Hoved-Hals-Kirurgisk Selskab Dansk. Sialoendoscopy: endoscopy of the larger salivary glands. The Danish society for head and neck surgery. Ugeskr Laeger 2007;169(12):1107 [in Danish].
12. Shacham R, Droma EB, London D, et al. Long-term experience with endoscopic diagnosis and treatment of juvenile recurrent parotitis. J Oral Maxillofac Surg 2009;67(1):162–7.
13. Nahlieli O, Nazarian Y. Sialadenitis following radioiodine therapy: a new diagnostic and treatment modality. Oral Dis 2006;12(5):476–9.
14. Nahlieli O, Shacham R, Shlesinger M, et al. Juvenile recurrent parotitis: a new method of diagnosis and treatment. Pediatrics 2004;114(1):9–12.
15. Nahlieli O, Shacham R, Yoffe B, et al. Diagnosis and treatment of strictures and kinks in salivary gland ducts. J Oral Maxillofac Surg 2001;59(5):484–90.
16. Nahlieli O, Eliav E, Hasson O, et al. Pediatric sialolithiasis. Oral Surg Oral Med Oral Pathol Oral Radiol Endod 2000;90(6):709–12.
17. Nahlieli O, Baruchin AM. Long-term experience with endoscopic diagnosis and treatment of salivary gland inflammatory diseases. Laryngoscope 2000;110(6):988–93.
18. Nahlieli O, Baruchin AM. Endoscopic technique for the diagnosis and treatment of obstructive salivary gland diseases. J Oral Maxillofac Surg 1999;57(12):1394–401 [discussion: 1401–2].
19. Nahlieli O, Baruchin AM. Sialoendoscopy: three years' experience as a diagnostic and treatment modality. J Oral Maxillofac Surg 1997;55(9):912–8 [discussion: 919–20].
20. Hosal AS, Fan C, Barnes L, et al. Salivary duct carcinoma. Otolaryngol Head Neck Surg 2003;129(6):720–5.
21. Kurabayashi T, Ida M, Yoshino N, et al. Differential diagnosis of tumours of the minor salivary glands of the palate by computed tomography. Dentomaxillofac Radiol 1997;26(1):16–21.
22. Kodaka T, Debari K, Sano T, et al. Scanning electron microscopy and energy-dispersive X-ray microanalysis studies of several human calculi containing calcium phosphate crystals. Scanning Microsc 1994;8(2):241–56.
23. Savica V, Calò LA, Monardo P, et al. Salivary phosphorus and phosphate content of beverages: implications for the treatment of uremic hyperphosphatemia. J Ren Nutr 2009;19(1):69–72.

24. Savica V, Calò L, Santoro D, et al. Salivary phosphate secretion in chronic kidney disease. J Ren Nutr 2008;18(1):87–90.
25. Marchal F, Chossegros C, Faure F, et al. Salivary stones and stenosis: a comprehensive classification. Rev Stomatol Chir Maxillofac 2008;109(4):233–6, Epub 2008 Sep 5.
26. Quenin S, Plouin-Gaudon I, Marchal F, et al. Juvenile recurrent parotitis: sialendoscopic approach. Arch Otolaryngol Head Neck Surg 2008;134(7):715–9.
27. Nahlieli O, Bar T, Shacham R, et al. Management of chronic recurrent parotitis: current therapy. J Oral Maxillofac Surg 2004;62(9):1150–5.
28. Walvekar RR, Razfar A, Carrau RL, et al. Sialendoscopy and associated complications: a preliminary experience. Laryngoscope 2008;118(5):776–9.
29. Nahlieli O, Droma EB, Eliav E, et al. Salivary gland injury subsequent to implant surgery. Int J Oral Maxillofac Implants 2008;23(3):556–60.
30. Mandel L. Plunging ranula following placement of mandibular implants: case report. J Oral Maxillofac Surg 2008;66(8):1743–7.
31. Caspari GH, Erbel R. Revascularization with extracorporeal shock wave therapy: first clinical results. Circulation 1999;100(Suppl 18):84–9.
32. Gutersohn A, Caspari G, Marlinghaus E. Autoangiogenesis induced by cardiac shock wave therapy (CSWT) increases myocardial perfusion in endstage CAD patients. CH Z Kardiol 2004;93(Suppl 3).
33. Fukumoto Y, Ito A, Uwatoku T, et al. Extracorporeal cardiac shock wave therapy ameliorates myocardial ischemia in patients with severe coronary artery disease. Coron Artery Dis 2006;17(1):63–70.
34. Marmary Y. A novel and non-invasive method for the removal of salivary gland stones. Int J Oral Maxillofac Surg 1986;15:585–7.
35. Iro H, Benzel W, Zenk J, et al. Minimally invasive treatment of sialolithiasis using extracorporeal shock waves. HNO 1993;41:311–6.
36. Zenk J, Bozzato A, Winter M, et al. Extracorporeal shock wave lithotripsy of submandibular stones: evaluation after 10 years. Ann Otol Rhinol Laryngol 2004;113(5):378–83.

Alternatives for the Treatment of Salivary Duct Obstruction

Mark McGurk, MD, FRCS, FDSRCS, DLO[a,*],
Jackie Brown, BDS, MSc, FDSRCPS, DDRRCR[b]

KEYWORDS

- Salivary obstruction • Salivary calculi • Duct strictures
- Sialendoscopy • Interventional sialography
- Balloon ductoplasty • Stone extraction
- Gland preserving surgery

SALIVARY DUCT OBSTRUCTION ALTERNATIVE TREATMENT OVERVIEW

This article considers the radiologically and endoscopically guided management of benign salivary duct obstruction. Salivary stones and strictures account for most benign duct obstructions.[1] Traditional management has fallen between the conservative approach (gland massage and review) and surgical lithectomy or sialadenectomy. Alternative treatments for these common causes of salivary obstruction have been sought to offer resolution of symptoms without extensive surgery or coexistence with long-term symptoms. Among these minimally invasive techniques, the per-ductal interventions, such as interventional sialography and sialendoscopy, have become firmly established, offering a solution that may be performed as a simple outpatient procedure under local anesthesia in selected cases.

SALIVARY DUCT STRICTURES

Problems and Aims of Treatment

Strictures, most common in the parotid duct, can take several forms: approximately 66% of cases involve a single point lesion; around 33% are multiple point obstructions along the duct (known as sialadochitis) or a continuous band of fibrous tissue forming a diffuse stricture that may extend over a length of several millimeters. The

[a] Department of Maxillofacial Surgery, Floor 23, Tower Wing, King's College London Dental Institute at Guy's, King's College and St Thomas' Hospitals, Guy's Hospital, Great Maze Pond, London SE19RT, UK
[b] Department of Dentomaxillofacial Radiology, Floor 23, Tower Wing, King's College London Dental Institute at Guy's, King's College and St Thomas' Hospitals, Guy's Hospital, Great Maze Pond, London SE19RT, UK
* Corresponding author.
E-mail address: mark.mcgurk@kcl.ac.uk (M. McGurk).

Otolaryngol Clin N Am 42 (2009) 1073–1085
doi:10.1016/j.otc.2009.08.011 oto.theclinics.com
0030-6665/09/$ – see front matter

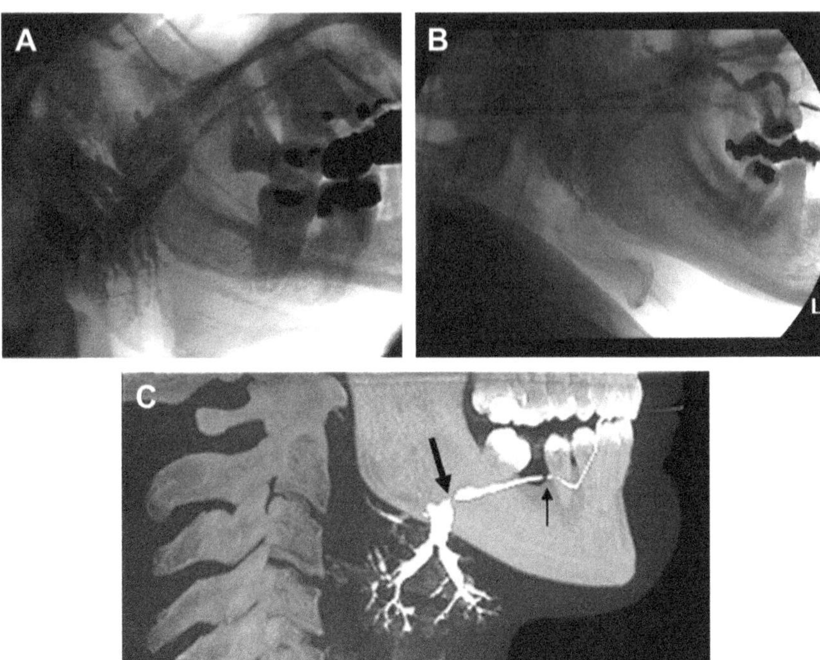

Fig. 1. Parotid sialograms showing (*A*) a diffuse stenosis within the proximal portion of the main extraglandular duct, (*B*) multiple point strictures within the main parotid duct. (*C*) A cone beam computed tomographic sialogram of the submandibular gland showing a small stone in the distal duct (*small arrow*) and a point stricture in the genu region of the proximal duct (*large arrow*).

morphology, number, and position of these strictures is best demonstrated by sialography. This imaging forms the basis for interventional treatment planning (**Fig. 1**).

Sialography demonstrates that the common sites of parotid strictures are at the entry to the hilum of the parotid gland and the point where the duct curves over the anterior border of the masseter muscle to enter the oral cavity.

Endoscopic evidence suggests that evolving strictures, which probably equate to sialadochitis (**Fig. 1**B), commence as fibrous rings in the duct wall, giving it a similar appearance to the lumen of the trachea. Endoscopic examination of duct stenosis demonstrates a condensation of scar tissue within the duct wall giving it a pale, opaque, and avascular appearance (**Fig. 2**).

The clinical manifestation of obstruction is the mealtime syndrome (prandial swelling); but the clinical picture of salivary strictures is different from that of obstruction by a stone. Swelling of the gland does not always occur in relation to food intake; frequently, it is worse on waking, and the symptoms may develop over several days. Sometimes the swelling is released with a sudden gush of saliva. The scarred duct has a tendency to backfill and stagnant saliva has a tendency to gel, so that the ducts are seen to be filled with thick mucous plugs on endoscopic examination (**Fig. 3**). Thus, the probable cause of acute obstruction is a plug washed forward and impacted into a stricture. With time and massage, the plug eventually squeezes through the stricture, followed by a surge of saliva. To minimize the risk of acute obstruction, a constant flow of saliva should be maintained by regular use of sialagogues (chewing gum), supported by regular

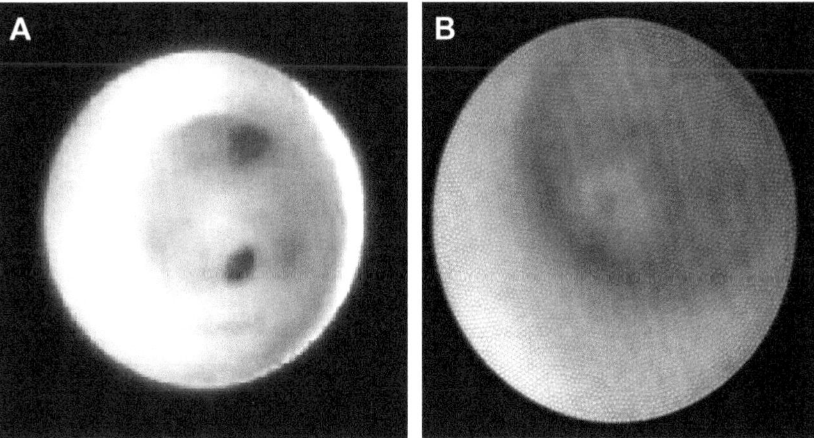

Fig. 2. (*A*) Endoscopic image showing early avascular change within the duct wall and stenosis reducing lumen diameter. (*B*) Endoscopic image showing occlusion of the duct by pale scar tissue.

gland massage. The aim of treatment, however, is to relieve stenosis and thus allow free outflow of saliva, preventing the formation of mucous plugs and allowing any that do form to be expelled readily.

Management of Salivary Strictures

Acute obstructive symptoms can be managed by stricture dilation, which can take several forms. Modest strictures can be dilated by endoscopic irrigation. Point strictures can be released by cutting the fibrous band with a hand drill through an endoscope (PolyDiagnost GmbH, Pfaffenhofen, Germany), after which the lumen springs open. Established strictures (both point and diffuse) can be stretched by intraluminal

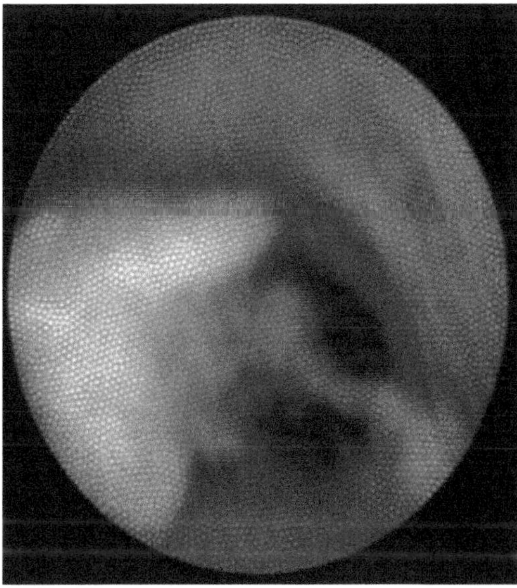

Fig. 3. Mucous plugs within the duct lumen.

balloon dilatation. Salivary balloon ductoplasty was first described in 1992 as a potential technique for the nonoperative elimination of benign salivary duct strictures.[2] It has since become the most widely reported technique; several case reports and small case series agree on the benefits of this technique for relieving salivary duct stenosis without the problems of surgical intervention, particularly in the parotid gland where these are most common.[3–6] This minimally invasive technique may be undertaken under radiological or endoscopic guidance and under local anesthesia. Radiological guidance requires a preoperative sialogram to localize the stricture, followed by insertion of the angioplasty balloon, using the fluoroscopic image to guide the balloon into the stricture before inflating it. A balloon slightly wider than the normal duct lumen is advised. A balloon with high inflation pressure or, alternatively, a cutting balloon, is advocated to release these dense fibrous strictures. Cutting balloons are a new technology and are constructed as conventional angioplasty balloon catheters, but with small microtome blades mounted along the length of the balloon itself. These blades are deployed as the balloon inflates, and are forced out into the vessel or duct wall to make minimal, superficial incisions across the surface of the band of stenotic tissue (**Fig. 4**). The cutting balloon is a 2-cm long, 3.5F, 90-cm overall catheter, with typical inflation diameter of 2.5 mm. These balloons have been used in vascular and nonvascular interventional radiology as a more conservative and controlled way of incising through circumferential occlusions, and they have been found to reduce damage to vessel walls, yet achieve more precise relief from stenosis.[7,8]

The technique is essentially the same when used with an endoscope, except that the balloon is positioned under direct vision, passed down the duct beside the endoscope, and forced forward through the stenosis. A postoperative sialogram is recommended to confirm successful elimination of the stricture (**Fig. 5**).

Technique for radiologically guided balloon sialoplasty

The number and location of strictures is identified on a preoperative sialogram. Digital subtraction sialography is helpful in eliminating large dense superimposed objects, such as teeth and restorations.[5] Local anesthesia may be obtained by infiltration along the anterior parotid duct and by per-ductal instillation of local anesthetic solution, such as 2% lidocaine. With radiographic contrast in situ in the duct and under fluoroscopic guidance, a 2-cm long angioplasty balloon, slightly wider than the desired duct diameter, is inserted over a hydrophilic guidewire that is passed along the main excretory duct. A parotid duct may be dilated with a balloon between 2.5 and 4 mm in diameter (when inflated), dependent on the degree of preexisting adjacent dilatation. The balloon catheter should ideally be on a reasonably rigid shaft to allow it to be pushed through tight proximal strictures, and it should reach pressures of at least 10 to 15

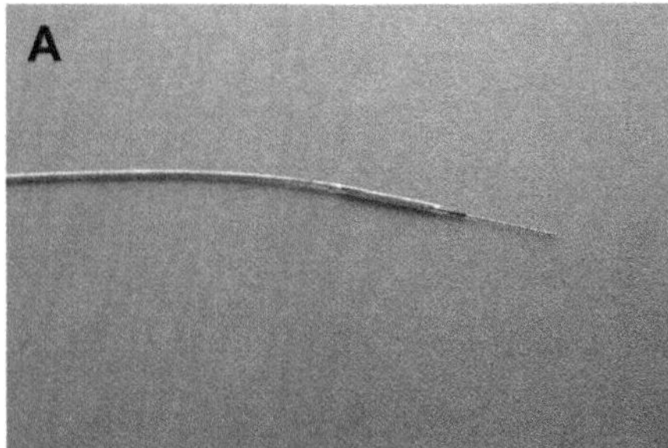

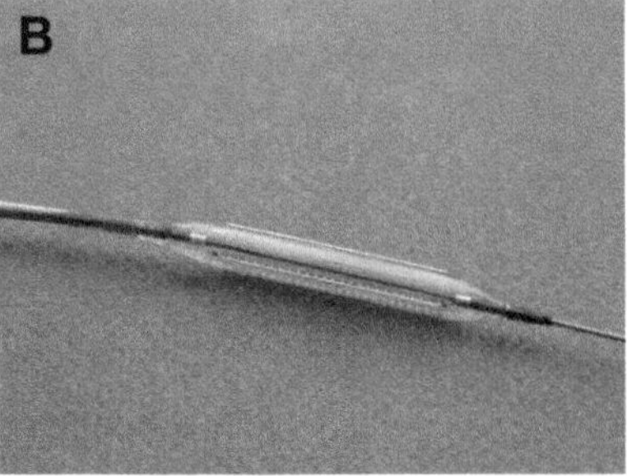

Fig. 4. (*A*) Cutting balloon catheter (deflated, as on insertion into the salivary duct). (*B*) Inflated cutting balloon showing microtome blades on the surface.

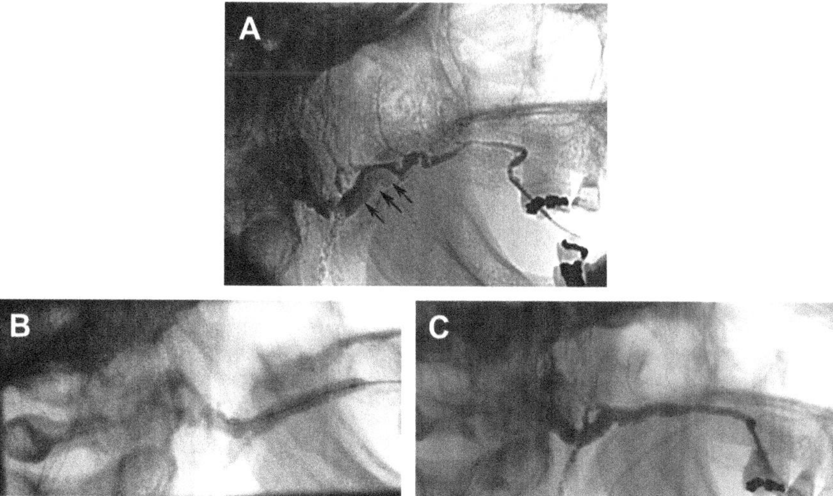

Fig. 5. Parotid ductoplasty; (*A*) Preoperative appearance showing a distally placed diffuse stricture with irregular dilation of the proximal duct, containing several mucous plug filling defects (*arrows*). (*B*) Balloon inflated within the stricture. (*C*) Postoperative sialogram showing elimination of stricture and dispersal of mucous plug debris.

atmospheres on inflation (eg, Symmetry Stiff Shaft Balloon, Boston Scientific Corporation, Natick, MA, USA). Once manipulated into position within the most proximal stricture, the balloon is inflated rapidly, held in place for 2 minutes, and deflated. The procedure can be repeated to eliminate all identifiable strictures, working stepwise distally toward the duct orifice. This technique has the advantage of minimal instrumentation. It involves only the insertion of a 3F angioplasty balloon catheter into the duct, and it is therefore a minimally invasive procedure. The position of the catheter can be monitored throughout the procedure by fluoroscopy. A dense point stenosis may be difficult to dilate fully, and on inflation, the balloon (which is filled with radiopaque contrast media, visible on the radiographic image) shows a "waist" where it is indented by the tight stenosis. The stricture should be dilated repeatedly until it is eliminated. Here, cutting balloons have an advantage.

Technique for endoscopically guided balloon sialoplasty

Preoperative sialography is strongly recommended, even for sialendoscopy, to identify the presence and position of all stenoses and help plan the depth required for insertion of the sialendoscope. As discussed earlier, local anesthesia can be delivered incrementally through the endoscope. The duct orifice is dilated manually until the endoscope can be inserted and advanced to the first stricture. The stricture may respond to pressure applied directly to it by the tip of the endoscope; otherwise, an angioplasty balloon, placed in parallel with the endoscope, can be advanced through the stricture and inflated under direct vision. However, the duct needs to be wide enough to accommodate the combined width of the instruments. The balloon is carefully positioned within the tightest part of the stricture and may be inflated several times. The endoscope is advanced stepwise, treating each stricture as it is encountered, and working proximally toward the hilum of the gland.[6] The process is thus the reverse of the radiologically guided technique.

OUTCOMES

Several studies have reported success in case series from 30 to 125 patients, most (75.3%) with parotid duct stenosis.[1,5,6,9,10] Balloon ductoplasty was found to be technically feasible in 87% to 95% cases of duct stenosis, and resulted in improvement or elimination of mealtime-related pain and swelling in 92% to 96% of cases. In a personal series of 249 salivary balloon ductoplasties, 230 have been undertaken in the parotid gland over a 10-year period, and 11% required bilateral parotid dilatations. On postoperative sialography, the stricture was judged to have been eliminated in 205 of 249 cases (82%); the stricture was shown to be partially eliminated in 33 (13%); and the procedure failed in 12 (5%). Follow-up is important in these cases as experience shows that stenosis can re-form over time. Sixteen patients have returned with re-stenosis of the salivary duct, which has required repeat balloon ductoplasty (mean interval, 31 months).

SALIVARY STONES

Problems and Aims of Treatment

Salivary stones commonly form in certain locations; treatment modalities are needed tailored to these presentations. The submandibular duct is notable for the marked curve or "genu" formed, as the duct passes over the posterior free margin of the mylohyoid muscle to descend into the gland. The parotid duct changes direction at 2 sites; it curves around the masseter muscle distally, and there is a right-angled bend proximally, as it descends into the deep aspect of the parotid. This is the point where the hilum and duct unite. Stones form in the hilum of the parotid and submandibular glands adjacent to these kinks. Clinically it seems that the anatomic shape of the duct system plays a part in stone formation (**Fig. 6**).

New Treatment Modalities

In the early 1990s, dedicated salivary lithotripters were developed (Minilith; Storz Medical AG, Tägerwilen, Switzerland). These lithotripters were modeled on the machines used in renal lithotripsy, but they were a miniaturized version with a small shockwave focus, ideal for use in the head and neck. Initially, they were deployed for all salivary stones, and it is based on this experience that current protocols have evolved.

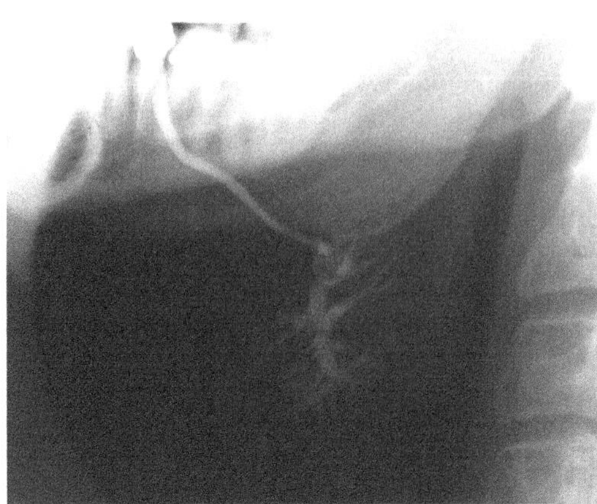

Fig. 6. Typical location for a submandibular duct stone lodged in the 'genu' region.

Salivary lithotripsy is simple to perform, requires no analgesia, and has low morbidity. Treatment of large stones is protracted (up to 15,000 shockwaves). Interventional sialographic or endoscopic techniques have been developed to compliment lithotripsy by offering solutions to the retention of small stone fragments and for the dilatation of duct strictures. The advent of sialoendoscopes produced new opportunities, but attempts at endoscope-guided intracorporeal laser and shockwave lithotripsy were not successful. The energy transferred was excessive and led to ductal damage and stricture formation. In contrast, simple endoscopic or radiologically guided basket retrieval of stones was effective and, to a lesser extent, microforceps proved effective at retrieving small stone fragments. A series of microinstruments in the form of tridents, graspers, and balloon catheters are now available for use with the endoscopes. It is with this selection of instruments that the protocol presented in **Table 1** has been adopted.

Interventional sialography and endoscopic therapy

Endoscopy and radiologically guided intervention are discussed together because the active agent (basket) is the same in each technique.

Endoscopes designed for salivary intervention range in size and faculty and are rigid or semirigid. Most endoscopic interventions are undertaken with a basket. Occasionally, a balloon is used, which can be inflated behind a stone to draw it forward to the duct ostium, as reported by Briffa and Callum[11] in the first radiologically guided extraction of a stone. Dormia baskets should be in the range of 2 to 3F gauge, with 3- to 12-wire designs, and may be tipped or tipless. Nitinol tipless baskets have great flexibility, can be opened and forced forward over impacted stones, but are not particularly radiopaque. Steel baskets have more rigidity and are easily identified on radiological images.

Pre-interventional assessment is by ultrasound or sialogram, to confirm the size (ideally <5 mm) and mobility of the stone and ensure no distally placed strictures are present. Most clinicians have used small Dormia baskets with a high degree of success.[12–15] The radiological technique includes a preoperative sialogram to visualize the obstruction. Under radiographic guidance, using fluoroscopy as in a vascular radiology suite, the basket is advanced past the stone, opened, and then drawn forward. Usually, the stone can be secured by rotating the wire basket as it comes into contact with the calculus. This technique has the advantage of requiring little

Table 1
Protocol showing the optimal application of minimally invasive techniques for the elimination of stones

	Management Protocol for Salivary Stones
Mobile stones <5 mm	
SMG and parotid	Endoscopic/radiological basket removal
Fixed stones >5 mm	
SMG	(1) Intraoral endoscope-assisted surgery (2) Lithotripsy ± basket removal (often used if (1) medically contraindicated)
Parotid	(1) Lithotripsy (2) Endoscope assisted surgery

Abbreviation: SMG, submandibular gland.

Data from Iro H, Zenk J, Escudier MP, et al. Outcome of minimally invasive management of salivary calculi in 4,691 patients. Laryngoscope 2009;119(2):263–8.

additional equipment, because it uses facilities normally available within the radiology department of a general hospital (**Fig. 7**).

With the endoscope, this action is carried out under direct vision (**Fig. 8**). The parotid duct is easy to cannulate. Usually, the submandibular duct ostium has to be incised for insertion of an endoscope. Once the stone is grasped, it cannot easily be disengaged and released. This situation would cause a basket to become lodged in the duct. Hence, the stone size limits this technique (**Fig. 9**). Tight strictures and long narrow duct segments, lying distal to the stone and needing prior dilatation with a balloon catheter, can be managed, ideally, within this same procedure. Once the stone is brought to the ostium, a small incision is made to retrieve the calculus. Using appropriate selection criteria, the success of the technique is high; in the authors' experience of 223 radiologically guided stone extractions, 75% were made completely stone-free and a further 9.4% had 1 or more stones removed, although residual stones remained in unreachable sections of the duct system (**Table 2**).[10] Stones positioned within the hilum, within diverticula or small secondary branches are difficult to retrieve because the basket cannot be advanced behind or around the stone to engage it.

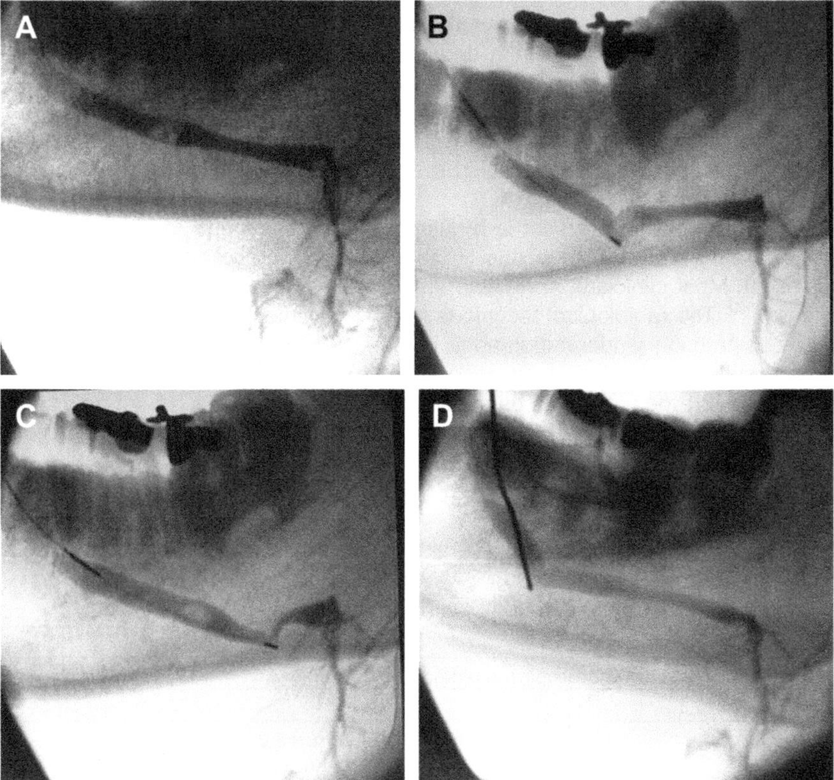

Fig. 7. Fluoroscopic sialogram images showing stages of radiologically guided stone removal. (*A*) Stone is identified as a filling defect within the mid one-third of the submandibular duct. (*B*) A closed Dormia basket is inserted up to the stone. (*C*) The basket is pushed beyond the stone, before opening the basket and drawing back to capture the stone. (*D*) The postoperative sialogram confirms that the stone has been removed and no further stones can be identified.

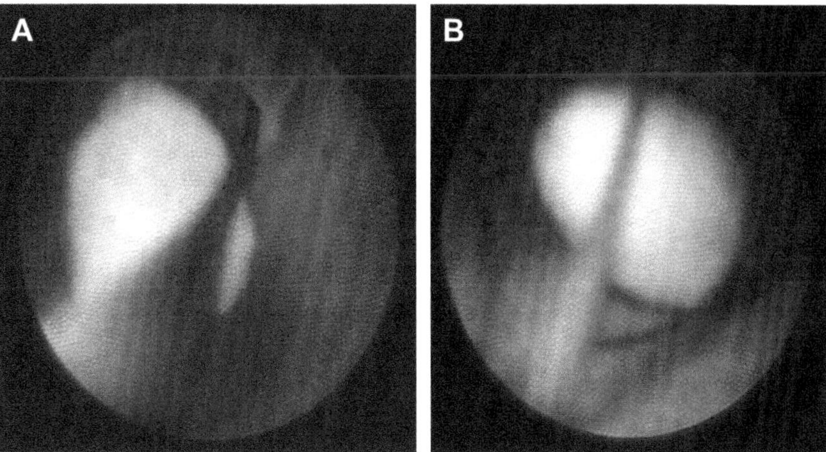

Fig. 8. Basket retrieval of stone under endoscopic control; (*A*) the stone is bypassed by the closed Dormia basket; (*B*) the basket is opened and withdrawn over the stone to capture it.

Morbidity

Complications The principal side effects are discomfort and swelling of the affected gland, and antibiotics are prescribed after extensive manipulation, to reduce the risk of infection. In one case, the basket became impacted and required surgical release from the parotid duct. In 2 further basket impactions, the duct was successfully dilated by angioplasty balloon insertion alongside the basket, which freed the impacted basket and stone. These experiences highlight the need for sound preparatory imaging to determine the size, location, and mobility of the stone.

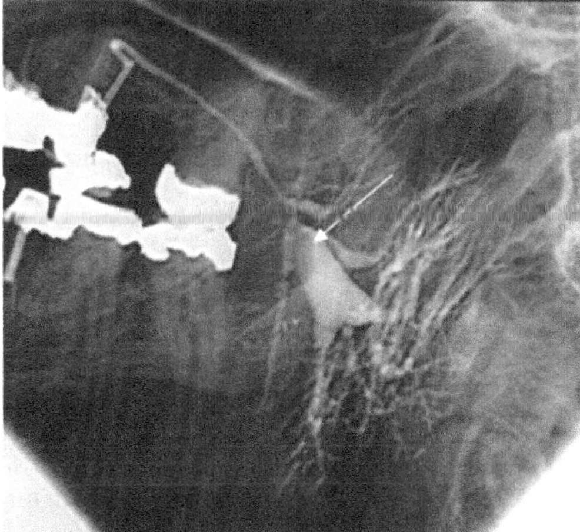

Fig. 9. Parotid sialogram showing a large stone (*arrow*) within the dilated hilum of the parotid gland but lying proximal to a dense stenosis. This stone would not be suitable for basket extraction, being too large to pass down the duct and would risk impaction of basket and stone within the duct. Prior balloon ductoplasty should be performed.

Table 2
The selection criteria for radiologically or endoscopically guided stone extraction

Submandibular Gland	Parotid Gland
Mobile stone	Mobile stone
Stone diameter no more than 25% > distal duct caliber (distally placed stenosis requires prior dilatation)	Stone diameter no more than 25% > distal duct caliber (distally placed stenosis requires prior dilatation)
Patent main duct	Patent main duct
Stone within lumen of main duct distal to mylohyoid bend	Stone within main duct distal to hilum

Summary of Salivary Stones

Basket and forceps retrieval of stones can be performed under endoscopic or radiological control. Using appropriate selection criteria, stone clearance rates are excellent (over 75%).[10,16] Morbidity of the procedure is minimal but local infiltration is advised. A minor surgical procedure may be necessary to gain endoscopic access to the submandibular gland, but not with the radiologically guided technique.

GLAND-PRESERVING SURGERY

Stones in the Submandibular Gland

The previous techniques deal with stones that are small and mobile. A significant number of submandibular stones are larger than 8 mm in diameter and are usually located in the hilum of the submandibular gland. Experience has demonstrated that these stone are not amenable to lithotripsy or basket retrieval.

Technique

Two gland preserving techniques have evolved.[17,18] Both are designed to be used under day-case general anesthesia or, in appropriate patients, under local anesthesia. The object is to remove the stone via an intraoral procedure and to preserve the salivary gland (**Fig. 10**). One technique entails opening the duct along its length until the stone is visible within the hilum of the gland. The stone is then delivered and the duct marsupialized to the floor of the mouth. This approach has the benefit of allowing traction to be applied to the duct, and by doing so, advancing the stone and hilum of the submandibular gland by approximately 1 cm. An alternative approach maintains the integrity of the duct. The floor of the mouth is opened and the duct traced posteriorly until the calculus is identified. The duct is incised only over the surface of the stone. The stone is released and the continuity of the duct restored with a 6.0 Vicryl suture (Prolene suture material should be avoided, because it facilitates calculus formation).

Selection criteria

The assessment is by ultrasound or sialogram, but the presence of a palpable stone is an important predictor of stone retrieval. Nonpalpable stones are situated within the gland and are difficult to remove. The endoscope is used to confirm complete clearance after surgery.

Success rates

The results of 11 studies, relating to the removal of 1058 transoral calculi, report overall success in 92.1% of cases.[19]

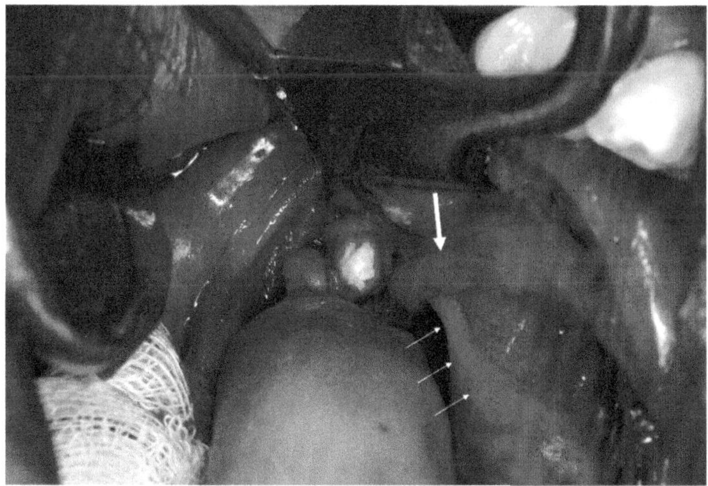

Fig. 10. Intraoral surgical removal of stone from hilum of the submandibular gland. The stone is seen through the incision made in the duct. Note the submandibular duct (*arrow*) and lingual nerve (*small arrows*).

Morbidity

Surgical exploration of the floor of the mouth leads to significant discomfort for 48 hours. The risk of injury to the lingual nerve is reported as 0.5%, but it is usually due to stretching and resolves over a 10-day period. Postoperative hemorrhage is uncommon. Reports of duct stenosis vary from no cases to 4.3% of cases. If the sublingual gland is violated, there is a risk of ranula (4%–7%); so at surgery, the sublingual gland is usually rotated out of the surgical field.[18]

Stones in the Parotid Gland

Patients have an understandable reluctance to submit to parotidectomy as the first-line treatment for a parotid stone. The high success rate of minimally invasive techniques (lithotripsy or basket retrieval) means that only 10% of cases remain symptomatic, and they are ideally suited to endoscope-assisted surgical removal of the stone. Selection criteria include large stones (>1 cm), glands with persistent sialoadenitis that are unsuitable for lithotripsy, and recalcitrant stones. The technique has been described previously (**Fig. 11**).[19] An endoscope is inserted into the duct, the stone visualized, and its position marked on the surface of the skin. The light emanating from the end of the endoscope is visible through the soft tissues. If the stone is large and superficial (anterior border of masseter), then it can be approached through a vertical incision directly over the stone. This approach is not suitable for proximal stones within the gland. In such circumstances, a limited preauricular incision is made under general anesthesia, the skin is elevated, and the endoscope tip light is used to identify and skeletonize the duct. The stone is then released by a longitudinal duct incision. The duct walls are reapposed and the tissues closed in layers. A pressure dressing reduces the risk of sialocele.

Success

Stone retrieval rates are greater than 95%. If the stone cannot be visualized preoperatively (endoscopically), then it is prudent to delay the operation for further assessment.

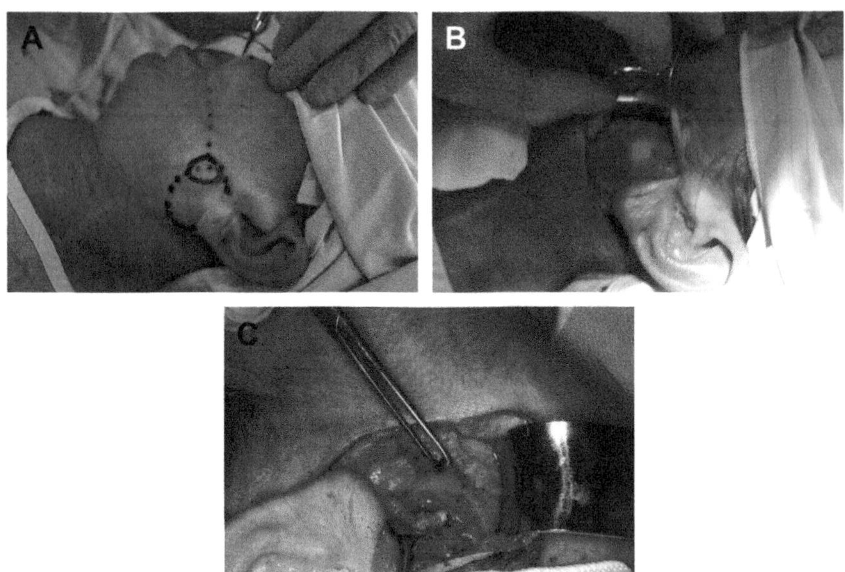

Fig. 11. (*A*) First stage in surgical endoscope-assisted stone removal from parotid gland, with the bright endoscope tip aligned against the parotid stone. (*B*) Endoscope-localized guidance of surgical approach onto parotid stone. (*C*) Identification and retrieval of stone.

Morbidity

Endoscope-assisted stone retrieval is much less invasive than the traditional superficial parotidectomy, with a significantly reduced threat to the facial nerve. In a series of over 60 cases, facial nerve injury was not encountered; however, this procedure is invasive and requires a general anesthetic. Patients are discharged and sent home on the day after surgery. In a consecutive series of 36 cases, 1 patient developed acute sialoadenitis in the immediate postoperative period and 1 patient developed a troublesome stricture that required duct ligation. In 2 further cases the duct was damaged and ligated. There were no long-term sequelae at follow-up after 3 years.

SUMMARY

Over a period of 20 years, the management of salivary obstruction has changed dramatically. The accumulating data suggest that the current standard of practice, which is gland resection, will not be tenable in the future. It is envisaged that, with time, small salivary gland centers will develop to serve populations of about 1 million. In a series of 4600 salivary calculi, stone clearance was 80%, with gland removal of only 3%.[16]

REFERENCES

1. Ngu RK, Brown JE, Whaites EJ, et al. Salivary duct strictures: nature and incidence in benign salivary obstruction. Dentomaxillofac Radiol 2006;35:1–8.
2. Buckenham TM, Page JE, Jeddy T. Technical report: interventional sialography–balloon dilatation of a Stensen's duct stricture using digital subtraction sialography. Clin Radiol 1992;45(1):34.

3. Buckenham TM, George CD, McVicar D, et al. Digital sialography: imaging and intervention. Br J Radiol 1994;67(798):524–9.
4. Roberts DN, Juman S, Hall JR, et al. Parotid duct stenosis: interventional radiology to the rescue. Ann R Coll Surg Engl 1995;77(6):444–6.
5. Brown AL, Shepherd D, Buckenham TM. Per oral balloon sialoplasty: results in the treatment of salivary duct stenosis. Cardiovasc Intervent Radiol 1997;20(5): 337–42.
6. Lari N, Chossegros C, Thiery G, et al. Sialendoscopy of the salivary glands. Rev Stomatol Chir Maxillofac 2008;109(3):167–71.
7. Tsetis D, Morgan R, Belli AM. Cutting balloons for the treatment of vascular stenoses. Eur Radiol 2006;16(8):1675–83.
8. Saad WE. Percutaneous management of postoperative anastomotic biliary strictures. Tech Vasc Interv Radiol 2008;11(2):143–53.
9. Drage NA, Brown JE, Escudier MP, et al. Balloon dilatation of salivary duct strictures: report on 36 treated glands. Cardiovasc Intervent Radiol 2002;25(5):356–9.
10. Brown JE. Interventional sialography and minimally invasive techniques in benign salivary gland obstruction. Semin Ultrasound CT MR 2006;27(6):465–75.
11. Briffa NP, Callum KG. Use of an embolectomy catheter to remove a submandibular duct stone. Br J Surg 1989;76(8):814.
12. Kelly IM, Dick R. Technical report. Interventional sialography: dormia basket removal of Wharton's duct calculus. Clin Radiol 1991;43(3):205–6.
13. Brown JE, Drage NA, Escudier MP, et al. Minimally invasive radiologically guided intervention for the treatment of salivary calculi. Cardiovasc Intervent Radiol 2002; 25(5):352–5.
14. Marchal F, Dulguerov P, Becker M, et al. Submandibular diagnostic and interventional sialendoscopy: new procedure for ductal disorders. Ann Otol Rhinol Laryngol 2002;111(1):27–35.
15. Nahlieli O, Nakar LH, Nazarian Y, et al. Sialoendoscopy: a new approach to salivary gland obstructive pathology. J Am Dent Assoc 2006;137(10):1394–400.
16. Iro H, Zenk J, Escudier MP, et al. Outcome of minimally invasive management of salivary calculi in 4,691 patients. Laryngoscope 2009;119(2):263–8.
17. Zenk J, Constantinidis J, Al-Kadah B, et al. Transoral removal of submandibular stones. Arch Otolaryngol Head Neck Surg 2001;127:432–6.
18. McGurk M. Surgical release of a stone from the hilum of the submandibular gland: a technique note. Int J Oral Maxillofac Surg 2005;34(2):208–10.
19. McGurk M, MacBean AD, Fan KF, et al. Endoscopically assisted operative retrieval of parotid stones. Br J Oral Maxillofac Surg 2006;44(2):157–60.

Treatment of Juvenile Recurrent Parotitis

Philippe Katz, MD[a,*], Dana M. Hartl, MD, PhD[b], Agnès Guerre, MD[a]

KEYWORDS

- Juvenile recurrent parotitis • Medical treatment
- Sialography • Sialendoscopy

Juvenile recurrent parotitis (JRP) is a nonspecific sialadenitis with recurrent inflammation of parotid glands in children. JRP is the second most common cause of parotitis in childhood, only after paramyxovirus (the mumps). Furthermore, chronic enlargement of the parotid gland with recurring infection may lead to mistaking this disease for other differential diagnoses such as Godwin's benign lymphoepithelial lesion,[1] chronic punctate sialectasis, Mikulicz disease, and Sjögren syndrome.[2]

Clinical symptoms of JRP include recurrent parotid inflammation with swelling or pain associated with fever. This pathology is usually unilateral, but bilateral can occur with symptoms usually more prominent on one side. The particular natural history of this disease is its recurrence. The first episode typically occurs between the age of 1 and 2 years and is most often not diagnosed, goes unnoticed, or is mistaken for the mumps, otitis, or pharyngitis.

The diagnosis, often made after the third or fourth episode, is suggested from the history of the disease, the clinical examination, and ultrasonographic findings. The interval between two acute episodes is variable, with an average from 15 days to 2 months, but the disease always recurs. The main criteria for establishing the severity of JRP is the frequency of the recurrences.[3]

The true severity of this disease is its inexorable progression leading to the destruction of the glandular parenchyma with a diminution of its functionality by 50% to 80%. Ultrasonographic findings then show vacuoles, a dilatation of Stensen's canal, and a wide-open ostium. The challenge is, thus, to diagnose JRP as early as possible, to provide treatment, and to avoid the ultimate destruction of the gland.

Many causes have been described as being responsible for JRP. The present consensus favors a multifactorial origin. However, the main cause is decreased salivary production with an insufficient salivary outflow through the ductal system, which favors ascending salivary gland infections via the oral cavity. Partial obstruction of the

[a] Institut d'Explorations Fonctionnelles des Glandes Salivaires, 7, Rue Theodore de Banville, Paris 75017, France
[b] Department of Otolaryngology Head & Neck Surgery, Institut Gustave Roussy, 39 rue Camille Desmoulins, 94805 Villejuif Cedex, France
* Corresponding author.
E-mail address: drkatz.philippe@gmail.com (P. Katz).

Otolaryngol Clin N Am 42 (2009) 1087–1091
doi:10.1016/j.otc.2009.09.002
oto.theclinics.com
0030-6665/09/$ – see front matter

ducts is gradually followed by retention and duct dilatation. Thus, further infection is facilitated by sialostasis.[4] Microbiological studies show the same mixed streptococcal and staphylococcal pathogens as found in the oral cavity.[5]

A diminution of local or general immunity has been suggested by several studies on genetic factors and immunoglobulin A deficiency. Allergy has also been incriminated, but not confirmed, as a predisposing factor.[6–8]

TREATMENT OF JRP

Medical Treatment

The treatment modalities range from conservative observation to invasive surgical procedures. Indeed, some investigators advocate abstention because of the habitually spontaneous disappearance of the signs in 95% of the cases before or at puberty.[9] These investigators use preventive therapy against recurrences such as massages, encouragement of fluid intake, warmth, and use of chewing gum or sialogogues. Antibiotic treatment is often proposed but with varying regimens. Cohen and colleagues[10] recommended long-term, low-dose prophylactic antibiotics when an immunoglobulin A deficiency is observed. Antibiotics, analgesics, mouth rinses, and sialogogues are considered the first line of treatment.

Surgery

Minor surgical procedures have been described. One is ligation of Stensen duct to create a pressure-induced atrophy of the secretory acinar cells. However, this method is rarely used because of frequent sialocele or abscess formation. According to the literature, another method of facilitating acinar cell atrophy is through denervation of the parasympathetic supply to the parotid by transecting Jacobson nerve in the middle ear cleft. Some investigators have proposed transecting the chorda tympani nerve, but the results have been unsatisfactory with recurrence of the salivary flow.

Major surgical approaches include superficial, subtotal, and total parotidectomy. Usually only radical methods resolve symptoms, but they are known to be associated with complications such as a high rate of facial nerve damage, Frey syndrome, earlobe numbness, traumatic neuroma of the greater auricular nerve, and unsatisfactory aesthetic results. Only total parotidectomy resolves symptoms, not partial parotidectomy.[11–13]

Sialography and Sialendoscopy

Many different types of intraglandular medical treatment have been described. Ductal injection of normal saline (0.9%) solution and manipulation with a lacrimal probe via the ostium of Stensen duct has been recommended. Tetracycline instillation into the parotid duct has also been described as having effective results through its sclerotic and cytotoxic effects in the gland.[14] Wang and colleagues[15] proposed intraductal injections of methyl violet, which induced widespread fibrosis and reduction of gland activity with resolution of clinical symptoms. However, it has been established that these dyes are capable of carcinogenic activity, so their intraglandular use should be discontinued.[16]

Galili and Marmary[3] were the first to use lavage to treat JRP with sialography, with good results in 13 of 15 children with unilateral swelling. Symptoms persisted in five of seven children with bilateral disease. Nahieli and colleagues[2,17] treated JRP by dilatation and abundant flushing (60 mL) under endoscopic control in a series of 26 cases (between 1993 and 2002) with a resolution of symptoms in 92% of the cases with a follow-up of 36 months.

Patients who are candidates for interventional endoscopic treatment are those who suffer from more than one acute episode per year. The justification of this treatment was the sialographic substantiation of multiple strictures of the ducts and the need to dilate them. Furthermore, endoscopic findings show multiple mucous plaques that may be washed away. Lavage with isotonic saline solution under hydrostatic pressure causes dilatation of the strictures and removal of the debris and mucus plaques through the ostium of Stensen duct. Nahieli and colleagues[2] described an adjunct to the procedure by introducing a high-pressure sialoballoon (2.5 French; 18 bars) to dilate the strictures. After the procedure, they injected hydrocortisone solution intraductally and, when possible, introduced a sialostent for 4 weeks to prevent recurrence of the strictures. The postoperative treatment was based on antibiotics, analgesics, and water intake. Sialendoscopy was always bilateral and performed under general anesthesia.

If the result seems to be effective, these reports do not comment on complications.[2,3,17] Furthermore, this type of treatment requires general anesthesia and is thus invasive in children. Finally, there is no information regarding the evaluation of glandular function after puberty, and intraglandular high pressure and invasive dilatations may definitively damage glandular function.

Quenin and colleagues,[9] and Faure and colleagues,[18] published preliminary reports of 10 cases using sialendoscopy to treat children with symptomatic JRP. They observed resolution of the symptoms in 89% of the cases with a follow-up of 11 months. Sialendoscopy was performed for patients suffering from at least two episodes of parotitis within a 6-month period. The procedure was bilateral in 7 of the 10 cases and performed under general anesthesia (average time of sialendoscopy 57 minutes) with a hospitalization of 24 hours. The investigators followed a protocol similar to that described by Nahieli and colleagues.[17] They concluded that the diagnosis of JRP is more sensitive with sialendoscopy than with ultrasonography and that sialendoscopy should be used regularly as a diagnostic tool. Concerning the therapeutic effects, they found that high-pressure saline solution was as effective as the sialoballoon for dilatation of the strictures. The main risk described was the possibility of swelling of the pharyngeal portion of the parotid gland, with partial upper airway obstruction, which may be avoided by performing unilateral sialendoscopy only. The investigators also described technical difficulties with endoscope diameter, which limits exploration only to the first branches of the salivary duct (seven cases).

According to the literature, sialendoscopy would seem to provide satisfactory results in the treatment of JRP. However, these reports are of relatively small cohorts (36 in 2 reports). The authors prefer a less invasive treatment method used in over 800 cases, described below.

Sialography with Iodinated Oil

Method

After the diagnosis is made, we always begin treatment with a prescription of antibiotics: macrolides (spiramycin) and nitroimidazoles (metronidazole) by mouth, with antispasmodics (phloroglucinol), with dose according to the weight of the child. Treatment is prescribed for at least 15 days. Corticosteroids (prednisolone, 1 mg per kilo per day) are associated with this treatment.

After this initial treatment, once the infection, inflammation, and pain cease, we perform sialography on an outpatient basis using iodinated oil (Lipiodol Ultra-Fluid ©Guerbet®) without any anesthesia of Stensen papilla. The procedure is atraumatic and painless with a very slow injection of only 0.1 to 0.2 mL of Lipiodol without applying any pressure.

We follow the patients in the clinic with clinical examination and ultrasound. In cases of recurrence, we perform the same procedure a second time, but with only one radiograph during the sialography, at a dose of 0.02 millisirven to limit radiation exposure.

RESULTS OF SIALOGRAPHY

From January 2000 to January 2007, the authors treated 840 children (403 girls and 437 boys, male-to-female ratio of 1:08) age 6 months to 14 years (average 4.5 years). Diagnosis was made on clinical history, clinical examination, and ultrasonographic findings. Clinically, all patients had unilateral or bilateral swelling and pain, redness of Stensen papilla, mucoid pus, and, often, fever and systemic signs of infection.

Standard and Doppler ultrasound were systematically performed to confirm the diagnosis. Ultrasound showed swelling of the parotid area and glandular parenchyma, vacuolization of the glandular tissue, increased vascularization, dilatations of the duct, and a widening of the Stensen papilla, on one side or bilaterally. All patients had a dominant affected gland. None of the children had comorbidity, particularly immunodeficiency.

The average follow-up was 5.5 years (range 2–9 years). Eighty-seven children (10.3%) were treated at the first episode of JRP. After one treatment, these 87 patients had a total disappearance of symptoms without any recurrence. The other 753 patients had already experienced a second recurrence or multiple recurrences. After one treatment, these patients did not present any other episode during the following 6 to 18 months, with an average symptom-free interval of 1 year. Symptoms recurred in 738 (98%) of these 753 patients, who were then treated again in the same manner. Again, the symptom-free interval was 6 to 18 months with an average of 1 year. During the follow-up, the number of recurrences ranged from one to four (average 2.5). Symptoms never recurred after puberty, however.

No complications or side effects were observed. The subjective evaluation of the procedure by the patient and by his or her parents was good or very good in all cases.

DISCUSSION OF SIALOGRAPHY METHOD

The authors' study with 840 patients followed for an average of 5.5 years is, to our knowledge, the largest study of JRP to date. The main advantage of sialography with iodinated oil is its simplicity and atraumatic nature. It is performed in an outpatient setting and may be repeated as necessary. An advantage of performing sialography is to confirm the diagnosis by visualizing punctate sialectasis and dilatation of the peripheral ducts, which create a sausage-like appearance. More important, sialography provides an in situ antibacterial effect using iodine at a high concentration (iodine 48%). Because of the sialostasis, the iodine remains within the gland and takes a very long time to be evacuated (an average of 10 days to 1 month), which increases its local antiseptic effect.

The authors' observed no complications with this treatment, as compared with the risks involved in more invasive types of treatment (pharyngeal swelling, risks of general anesthesia). Having observed 100% efficacy in the 87 patients treated after only one episode of parotitis, the authors' believe that this low-risk treatment is better adapted to JRP, which is a benign disease. Furthermore, the authors' believe that this treatment may allow better long-term preservation of glandular function than other, more invasive, procedures that involve high pressure within the gland. However, this needs confirmation.

SUMMARY

JRP is a common recurring bacterial infection of the parotid gland, with spontaneous resolution at puberty. In light of experience with 840 cases, the authors' propose, after antibiotic treatment for the acute infection, an in situ sterilization by sialography with high-concentration iodinated oil, as an outpatient procedure. In 87 patients treated at their first episode, we observed 100% effectiveness in preventing recurrence, and no complications or adverse effects in the 840 children treated. Early diagnosis seems to be a key to prevention of recurrence and physicians and pediatricians should be aware of this disease and treatment options.

REFERENCES

1. Godwin JT. Benign lymphoepithelial lesions of the parotid gland: adenolymphoma, chronic inflammation, lymphoepithelioma, lymphocytic tumor, Mikulicz disease. Cancer 1952;5(6):1089–103.
2. Nahieli O, Bar T, Shacham R, et al. Management of chronic recurrent parotidis: current therapy. J Oral Maxillofac Surg 2004;62:1150–5.
3. Galili D, Marmary Y. Juvenile recurrent parotitis: clinicoradiologic follow-up study and the beneficial effect of sialography. Oral Surg Oral Med Oral Pathol 1986; 61(6):550–6.
4. Mandel L, Witek EL. Chronic parotitis: diagnosis and treatment. J Am Dent Assoc 2001;132:1707–25.
5. Brook I. Diagnosis and management of anaerobic infections of the head and neck. Ann Otol Rhinol Laryngol Suppl 1992;155:9.
6. Ericson S, Zetterlund B, Ohman J. Recurrent parotitis and sialectasis in childhood. Clinical, radiologic, immunologic, bacteriologic and histologic study. Ann Otol Rhinol Laryngol 1991;100:527–35.
7. Reid E, Douglas F, Crow Y, et al. Autosomal dominant juvenile recurrent parotitis. J Med Genet 1998;35:417–9.
8. Fazekas T, Wiesbauer P, Schroth B, et al. Selective IgA deficiency in children with recurrent parotitis of childhood. Pediatr Infect Dis J 2005;24(5):461–2.
9. Quenin S, Plouin-Gaudon I, Marchal F, et al. Juvenile recurrent parotitis. Arch Otolaryngol Head Neck Surg 2008;134(7):715–9.
10. Cohen HA, Gross S, Nussinovitch M, et al. Recurrent parotitis. Arch Dis Child 1992;67:1036–7.
11. Moody AB, Avery CME, Walsh S, et al. Surgical management of chronic parotid disease. Br J Oral Maxillofac Surg 2000;38:620–31.
12. Sadeghi N, Black MJ, Frenkiel S. Parotidectomy for the treatment of chronic recurrent parotitis. J Otolaryngol 1996;25:305–17.
13. O'Brien C.J Murrant NJ. Surgical management of chronic parotitis. Head Neck 1993;15:44–58.
14. Bowling DM, Rauch SD, Goodman ML. Intraductal tetracycline therapy for the treatment of chronic recurrent parotitis. Ear Nose Throat J 1994;73:267–74.
15. Wang S, Li J, Zhu X, et al. Gland atrophy following retrograde injection of methyl violet as a treatment in chronic obstructive parotitis. Oral Surg Oral Med Oral Pathol 1998;85:276–87.
16. Vachalkova A, Novotny L, Blesova M. Polarographic reduction of some triphenylmethane dyes and their potential carcinogenic activity. Neoplasma 1996;43: 113–22.
17. Nahieli O, Shacham R, Shlesinger M, et al. Juvenile recurrent parotitis: a new method of diagnosis and treatment. Pediatrics 2004;114:9–12.
18. Faure F, Froehlich P, Marchal F. Pediatric sialendoscopy. Curr Opin Otolaryngol Head Neck Surg 2008;16:60–3.

Sialendoscopy Strategies for Difficult Cases

Michael H. Fritsch, MD, FACS

KEYWORDS

- Salivary • Stones • Stenosis • Sialendoscopy
- Microvascular • Cosmetic

Salivary gland surgery has progressed to the point where many pathologies that once required gland resection are now removed worldwide with endoscopes and extracorporeal lithotriptors. Nevertheless, patients can present to their physician with extraordinary salivary duct pathologies. The diagnosis and treatment for these difficult cases can lie outside the usual clinical treatment algorithms for endoscopes and lithotriptors. At first, the best treatment for these difficult problems might seem to be surgical gland resection. However, the goal of achieving physiologically intact salivary glands after treatment runs contrary to gland removal. The physician is placed in the challenging position of finding ways to overcome salivary duct problems without removing the gland. As an additional complicating factor, in North America, extracorporeal shock-wave lithotripsy (ESWL) for the salivary gland is not yet governmentally approved; the published algorithms for physicians and patients from other countries depart from the North American experience. Therefore, some alternative treatment options have been developed for difficult cases of salivary duct obstruction in North America, of which several are applicable to patients anywhere.

ENDOSCOPIC SEGMENTAL-OPEN APPROACH

Some patients with larger stones cannot be treated effectively solely by intraductal approaches. Nahlieli,[1] in 2002, and McGurk[2] in 2004, described parotid procedures combining endoscopic intraductal transillumination of the skin, as a surgical target locator, with an open-surgical approach, to gain direct access to the stone and deliver it from the duct. After removal of the stone, the duct is closed over a stent. These 2 approaches work well for Stensen duct or hilum stones, but they do not address the "intraparenchymal" stone located in the secondary and tertiary duct or the diseased salivary drainage basin proximal to the stone. In the author's institution, experience has shown that the so-called intraparenchymal stones are probably

Department of Otolaryngology-Head and Neck Surgery, Indiana University Medical Center, 702 Barnhill Drive, Suite 0860, Indianapolis, IN 46202, USA
E-mail address: mfritsch@iupui.edu

Otolaryngol Clin N Am 42 (2009) 1093–1113
doi:10.1016/j.otc.2009.08.006
oto.theclinics.com
0030-6665/09/$ – see front matter

intraductal, with the actual duct being expanded until transparently thin and the stone appearing to be in the parenchyma. In these proximal areas, no stent can be placed for postoperative conservation of the duct. In addition, the wedge-shaped drainage-basin of the gland proximal to these stones is often already chronically diseased with severe ductal ectasia. Conversely, the uninvolved ducts and their attached gland tissue may be normal. Therefore, a parotidectomy would needlessly remove normal tissue along with diseased gland. For cases of a stone within an isolated duct that blocks a diseased drainage basin, Endoscopic Segmental-Open parotidectomy is introduced.

Segmental Parotidectomy

The patient is prepared for surgery as per McGurk, with the addition of a nerve integrity monitoring system (NIMS; NIM-Response 2.0, Medtronic, Inc, Jacksonville, FL, USA) facial nerve monitor. The stone is endoscopically located where it is lodged in the specific secondary or tertiary duct. Through the gland tissue, the stone is dissected free of the duct and parenchyma and removed. Thereafter, the remaining diseased duct and drainage basin are resected by performing a wedge-shaped partial parotidectomy. The partial parotidectomy targets only the diseased gland segment. The other normal ducts and gland tissue are left intact. By removing the stone and the specifically involved ducts and gland tissue, a repetitive cycle of sialadenitis is avoided.

Regarding cosmesis, the real effect of a parotidectomy is seen when resected areas cause a facial depression and create areas of shadow. Most noticeable is the "eye-catcher" shadow located below the zygomatic arch. The parotid gland in the zygomatic area is rarely found to have stone pathology or other problems; its duct and parenchyma can usually be spared to great cosmetic advantage for the patient. The residual normal gland effaces the light shadow and leads to markedly improved cosmesis.

Sometimes, there may be areas of zygomatic parenchyma that have no duct connections but are left for cosmetic reasons. If the isolated gland tissue is bulky, it can be injected with botulinum toxin type A to render the tissue inactive and prevent sialocele, until the raw tissue bed heals and scar tissue obliterates the surgical planes.

Another advantage of the segmental parotidectomy using an endoscope is that the possibility of a sialocele is greatly reduced by meticulous closure of the circumscribed surgical field. Any open ducts and raw gland tissue are given attention. Because the endoscope is already positioned within the duct, after the resection of parotid tissue is completed, back-pressure testing of the duct with saline solution is performed. It allows the surgeon to find and oversew even the smallest ducts that were crosscut in the dissection. To help protect against Frey syndrome, a pie-shaped wedge of a collagen matrix barrier material (Duragen, Integra Lifesciences Corporation, Plainsboro, NJ, USA) is sewn into the corresponding wedge of parotid bed.

Patient 1

An 11-year-old female patient, with recurrent left parotid swelling for 4.5 years, underwent sialography showing an 11.6 by 8.0 mm stone in a secondary duct. Sialendoscopy could visualize the stone, but not reach it for intraductal instrumentation treatment. No ESWL lithotriptor was available. A Transfacial approach through the cheek was not allowed by the family for cosmetic reasons, which would also not have been able to address the proximal gland drainage basin and facial nerve. Because the stone was in a secondary duct, the possibility of duct stenoses, with future surgery needed to treat residual gland problems, was a major consideration. The Endoscopic-Open approach, with endoscopic transillumination and NIMS facial nerve monitoring, was used to find and remove the stone through a modified-Blair incision (**Fig. 1**). The stone "socket"

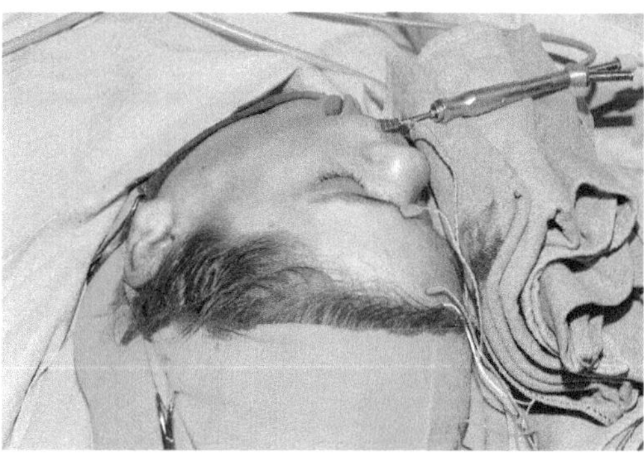

Fig. 1. The Endoscopic-Open approach is demonstrated in this view of the left face. The key feature is that the endoscope transilluminates the skin at the duct obstruction point. Facial nerve monitoring equipment is also seen.

with its specific salivary drainage basin was then segmentally removed (**Fig. 2**). The unaffected upper half of the superficial lobe was preserved. The remaining crosscut ducts were back-pressured with saline solution and oversewn with 5-0 chromic sutures. The remaining upper and lower parts of the anterior gland parenchyma were loosely closed in a "V to Y" fashion. A collagen barrier was placed. The remaining zygomatic area parotid gland provided sufficient tissue to offset a cosmetic parotid defect; a smooth transition between the zygoma and the cheek contours was achieved (**Fig. 3**). Postoperatively, the parotid orifice showed clean saliva when "milking" the remaining gland. A 5-year follow-up showed the patient to be asymptomatic, with a functioning residual gland on physical examination.

ENDOSCOPIC DOUBLE-OPEN APPROACH

At times, the anteriorly positioned Stensen duct and the posterior-most parotid gland may be simultaneously diseased. In these difficult cases, anterior duct structures may need to be surgically accessed, in combination with surgical work on the posterior

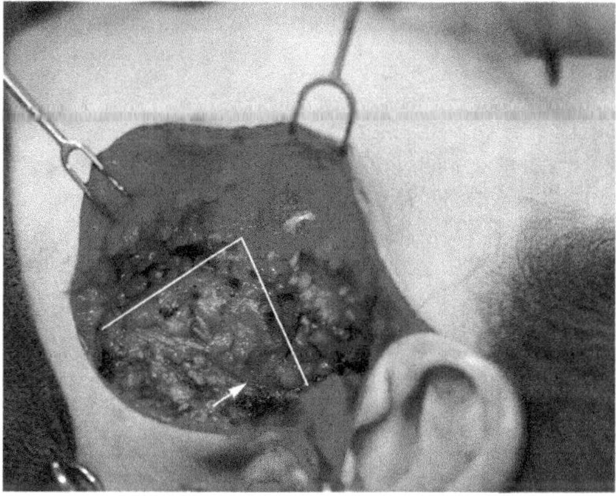

Fig. 2. The wedge-shaped segmental salivary drainage basin, proximal to the large stone, has been segmentally resected. The facial nerve is seen in the parotid bed (*arrow*). Sometimes, removal of only a small segment of the parotid tail is necessary.

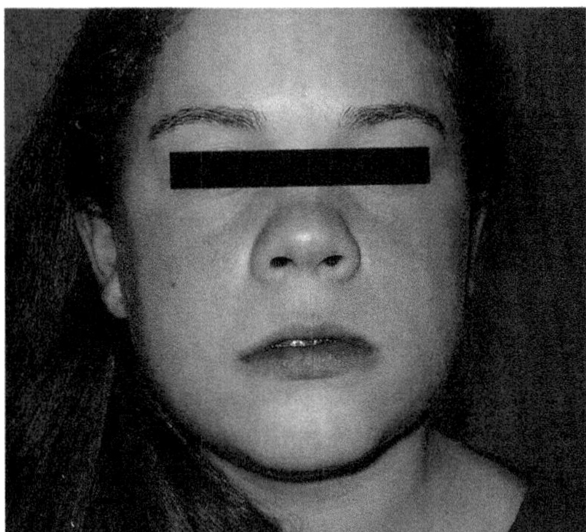

Fig. 3. This frontal face view shows how preservation of the unaffected parotid gland helps to efface the depression left behind from the resected gland. The parotid gland immediately inferior to the zygoma is especially important.

gland and the facial nerve. Therefore, access to the entire length of the parotid duct and gland is needed.

The classic preauricular parotidectomy incision, with undermining in an anterior direction, does not allow for dissection of the anterior parotid duct and facial nerve branches. An increasingly narrow surgical field is found in the anterior acute angle between parotid gland and skin. Visualization of the anterior nerve and duct is poor. The main facial nerve branch that overlays the Stensen duct is the buccal branch; however, other nerve arborizations can be prolific and only direct transfacial access provides a surgical field for reliable nerve preservation. Conversely, if a transfacial incision is made at a midmasseter muscle location, then dissection over the posterior parotid gland and facial nerve is not possible; a preauricular approach is also needed.

To achieve effective surgical exposure over the entire parotid gland and duct, the "Endoscopic Double-Open" approach is introduced. The transfacial and modified-Blair incisions are used during the same procedure. The transfacial incision allows the facial nerve main buccal branch, the cobweblike facial nerve arborizations, and the anterior duct to be readily visualized and surgically operated. The preauricular incision allows surgical access to the posterior portion of the parotid gland and facial nerve that are beyond the posterior limits of the transfacial incision. With the endoscope in the duct and the 2 external incisions, the surgeon can feel confident of having complete surgical exposure from inside and outside, and from the anterior duct to the posterior duct and gland. This technique gives the surgeon complete access to the parotid duct and gland.

Patient 2

A 24-year-old man presented with a progressive 3-year history of a 6.0 by 3.0 cm subcutaneous tubular mass of the right cheek. A magnetic resonance scan showed the appearance of a giant sialocele (**Fig. 4**). The gland itself had ectasias. The other major salivary glands were normal. Using the endoscopic technique, the duct showed a complete, nondistensible, "hard" stenosis at the anterior border of the masseter muscle. The holmium laser was used to penetrate the stenosis and the sialocele

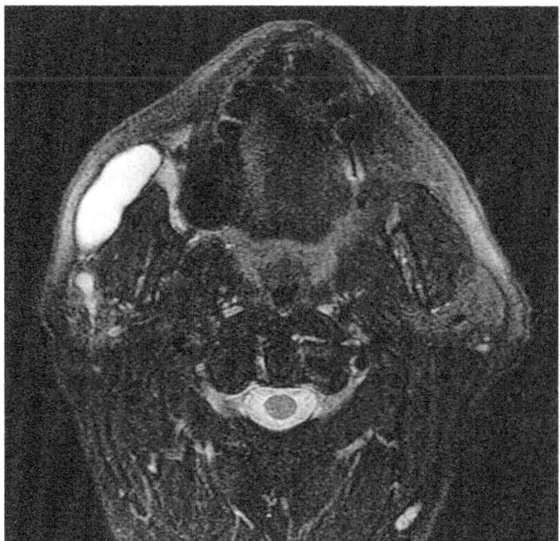

Fig. 4. A magnetic resonance imaging scan shows a hyperintense right parotid duct sialocele on this T2 axial section. Because of ductal obstruction, a slowly progressive tissue expansion of the duct has taken place. It measures approximately 6.0 by 3.0 cm.

was entered. Much turbid, green-colored, salivary mucus with thickly particulate sediment was encountered inside the sialocele (**Fig. 5**). The walls became heavily rugated as the sialocele was decompressed. Large sedimentary flakes of green matter detached from the walls. The proximal end of the sialocele led into the hilum and stenotic duct branches. It was clear that a hollow stent would become recurrently plugged. Also, an intraoral sialocelostomy would probably be prone to retrograde infection because of the cavernous size of the sialocele and poor condition of the gland. A vein graft replacement appeared to have a poor chance of success, because of the dilated hilum deep within the gland and multiple intraglandular duct stenoses.

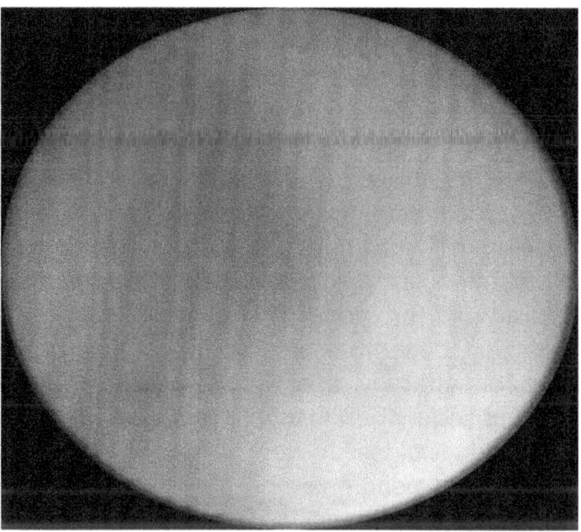

Fig. 5. An endoscopic view of the sialocele interior. The rugose walls and green particulate sediment are seen; the darker lumen is visible in the center.

Also, the patient wanted a "cure" at one surgical sitting, rather than recurrent attempts to rehabilitate a chronically diseased gland. Rather than continue a chronic parotid problem, the decision was made to segmentally resect the gland and the sialocele duct using the Endoscopic Double-Open approach. The endoscope was used to transilluminate the decompressed sialocele and the skin, and help mark the course of the duct and locate the Transfacial incision. The NIMS monitor was in place and a microscope was used to carefully transfacially dissect the anterior-most facial nerve branches. The duct was dissected forward into the mouth and freed up to the parotid hilum posteriorly (**Fig. 6**). Through the preauricular incision, a Segmental parotidectomy with facial nerve preservation was performed; the segment of gland tissue abutting the zygoma was left in place to atrophy and help the cosmetic effacement of the defect. A collagen barrier was placed over the raw tissue bed to help prevent Frey syndrome. The incisions were closed using plastic technique (**Fig. 7**). The patient is asymptomatic 2 years after surgery, without facial nerve or cosmetic deficits.

ENDOSCOPIC-STAGED APPROACH

Extraordinarily large stones or multiple stones, with associated granulation tissue within a salivary gland, may initially be thought to be sialadenectomy candidates. However, except for the duct sialolith problem, the rest of the gland is often normal, and many glands may return to normal function once the obstruction is removed. Preservation of one or more glands has significant value, especially if more than one gland is diseased.

The chronic coliclike pain and swelling associated with stones in the duct is relieved by removal of the stone. However, complete removal may not be possible during one endoscopic procedure. The main reasons for this are (1) the stone "rind" may remain inaccessible or impacted into and immoveable from the duct wall; (2) the size and number of stones may prolong surgery; and (3) perforation of the duct, with progressive endoscopic irrigation fluid extravasating into subcutaneous tissues, may require termination of the procedure. The lack of a lithotriptor means that the full monolithic size of the stone will be the object of treatment. The Endoscopic-Staged approach is well suited and now introduced.

If two or more endoscopic intraductal treatments are used serially, preservation of the duct and gland is possible, while also avoiding open surgery complications or scars. Resumption of treatment where the previous procedure left off can take place after 3 to 4 weeks of healing time, sometimes with a stent in place. During the intersurgical period, the patient may have the same or fewer symptoms as before the procedure, depending on stone integrity. It is known from ESWL treatments that a large stone may not be necessarily removed with one treatment. Rather, ESWL may create fissures and cracks within the stone and allow the gland to decompress through the cracks, until further ESWL completely destroys the stone and renders a cure. Indeed, some patients have been known to have fractured stones in situ for years without symptoms. Until the point of colic, all stones allow for some salivary decompression by fluid pressure relief around the stone. Thus, by perforating or fracturing a stone during the initial endoscopy, decompression of the gland and partial relief of symptoms is likely (**Fig. 8**). This strategy is especially important for physicians without access to ESWL. With subsequent endoscopic procedures, further progress on the obstruction will bring the duct closer to normal patency or will completely remove the duct obstruction. The duct becomes more resilient and dilated with each endoscopic procedure, giving better access for follow-up procedures. Compared with open surgery, the additional endoscopy time is offset by the short patient recovery time and the avoidance of a facial scar or nerve complications.

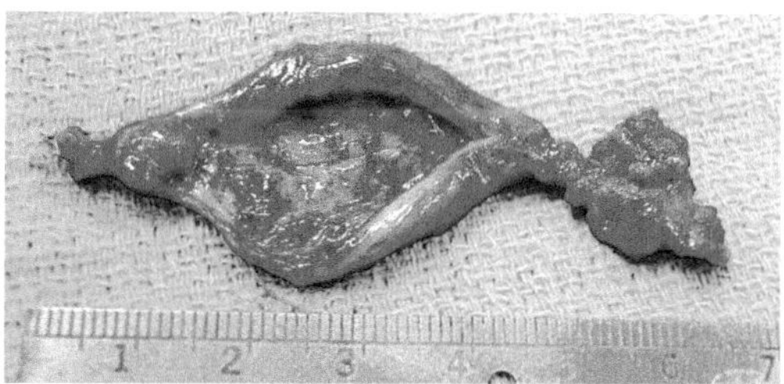

Fig. 6. The resected sialocele specimen showing the total duct stenosis (*left*) and attachment into the parotid gland (*right*).

Patient 3

A 43-year-old man presented with a 4-cm long chain of unilateral parotid stones, branching into several ducts, with episodic cheek pain (**Fig. 9**). Endoscopic treatment proceeded with use of holmium laser, wire baskets, and mini-forceps under general anesthesia. Both granulation polyps and stones were encountered (**Fig. 10**). After approximately 2 hours, the duct had been traumatized to the point that further endoscopy could have caused duct stenosis. The procedure was terminated as an "outpatient" case, with the patient returning to normal activity. After 3 weeks, the same procedure was repeated; the distal duct had healed and re-epithelialized without stent usage; again polyps and stones were encountered in the more proximal duct and were endoscopically treated. After 2 hours, a similar circumstance to the first procedure occurred. Again, the procedure was terminated and a 3-week hiatus for healing was allowed. During the third procedure, work was progressing on the terminal stones and polyps, but it required considerable pressure and "snaking" of the endoscope to reach the obstructed area in the parotid tail. After 45 minutes of work, the endoscope shaft dissociated from the endoscope body, which necessitated ending the procedure. After 1 month, the final stones and polyps were removed with a new endoscope and the duct was cleared of obstructions (**Fig. 11**). The patient, who had had progressively fewer symptoms after each procedure, became asymptomatic and remains so 5 years after surgery. In this patient, it is probable that ESWL would not have been effective as a sole treatment modality because of the soft-tissue polyps, although ESWL use may have lessened the difficulties encountered by endoscopic treatment of the sialolith components.

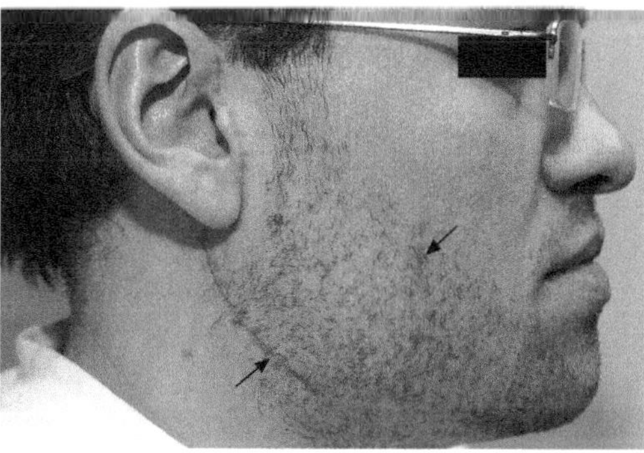

Fig. 7. Right side of the face showing the 2 healing Double-Open approach incisions from which the sialocele was resected.

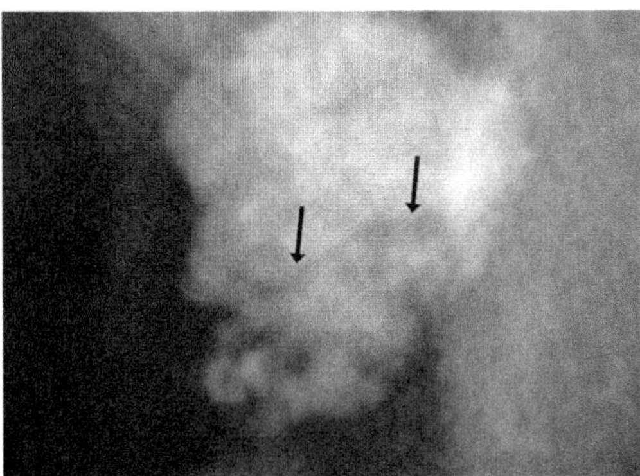

Fig. 8. A radiograph of a stone that has received ESWL. Note the cracks and fissures that allow for decompression of salivary pressure despite continued presence of the stone (*arrows*).

MICROVASCULAR END-TO-END DUCT ANASTOMOSIS AND VEIN REPLACEMENT SURGERY

Although endoscopic surgery can overcome many obstacles, intractable duct problems do occur. The most problematic is probably a "hard" stenosis or stricture. These fibrous lesions resist dilation. Although a small 0.4 mm guidewire may be passed into some of these stenoses, the larger diameter of the endoscope and the soft- or high-pressure balloons prevents them from entering into the stenoses; also, due to duct curvature, a stiff laser fiber is of little use. Conventional treatment would be gland resection; however, the entire gland and duct are often normal except for the hard stenosis or stricture problem. In these cases, a resection of the narrowed duct segment, with either microvascular end-to-end anastomosis or duct replacement by vein graft interposition, can be performed to conserve the gland.

Patient 4: End-to-end Anastomosis

A 44-year-old woman presented with progressive pain during eating. A 1.0-cm long stenotic duct segment was seen on intraoperative sialogram in the midmasseteric

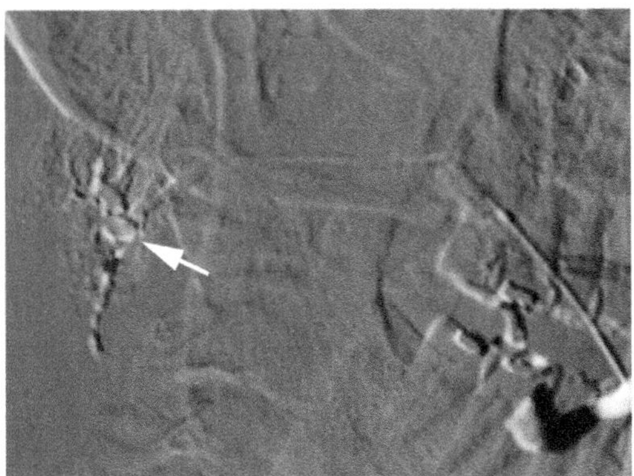

Fig. 9. A fluoroscopic sialogram of the parotid duct showing tightly packed stones and polyps (*arrow*) that branch into several secondary ducts over a course of multiple centimeters.

duct (**Fig. 12**). Sialendoscopy revealed a 0.6-mm diameter hard stenosis that failed all attempts to dilate it. An Endoscopic-Open Transfacial approach, with resection of the stenotic duct segment, was planned. Endoscopic skin transillumination was used to precisely locate the duct obstruction and accurately mark the facial incision. A 2.0-cm incision in a vertical relaxed skin tension line was made just behind the light. The skin mobility gave adequate anterior-posterior surgical field exposure. The NIMS facial nerve monitor was used. The buccal branch of the facial nerve was first isolated by spreading the parotid tissue just lateral and superior to the light (**Fig. 13**). After confirmatory facial nerve stimulation, a vessel loop retractor around the nerve helped duct exposure. The overall outside diameter of the duct varied between 3.0 and 5.0 mm, but no external sign of a stenosis was visible. The duct was circumferentially dissected and a vessel loop was placed around it. A cut into the duct 1.2 cm posterior to the endoscope tip entered normal duct. The duct was resected up to the location of the endoscope. There was no tension on the anastomosis because of prior duct dissection in both directions. Using microvascular clips, an end-to-end microscopic anastomosis was performed using 9-0 Prolene sutures (Ethicon Inc, Somerville, NJ, USA) with 6 stitches placed (**Figs. 14** and **15**). The advential layers were closed with 5-0 Vicryl sutures (Ethicon Inc, Somerville, NJ, USA). A 4F stent was placed over a guidewire through the mouth and into the proximal duct. Plastic skin closure ensued. The stent was sewn into the oral mucosa using two 5-0 silk sutures, for a planned 4-week placement. After 10 days, the stent was accidently removed by the patient and was not replaced because of lack of symptoms. The patient remains asymptomatic 4 years after surgery.

Patient 5: Vein Graft Replacement, Duct-to-mouth

A 47-year-old white woman presented with a symptomatic unilateral 2-cm Stensen duct stricture in the midanterior masseteric area. The papilla was a pinpoint opening. Sialogram was confirmatory and the magnetic resonance imaging scan result was negative for other pathologies. Sialendoscopy could only advance 1 cm until a hard

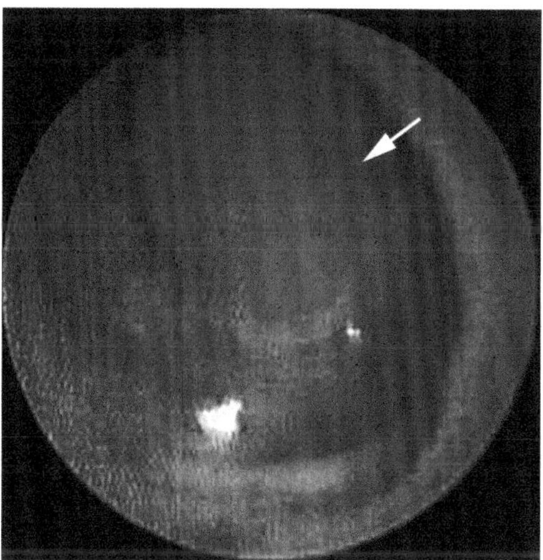

Fig. 10. An endoscopic view of the parotid duct with a granulation polyp seen (*arrow*). The inflammatory reaction to some stones is severe and can generate purulent exudates and polyps.

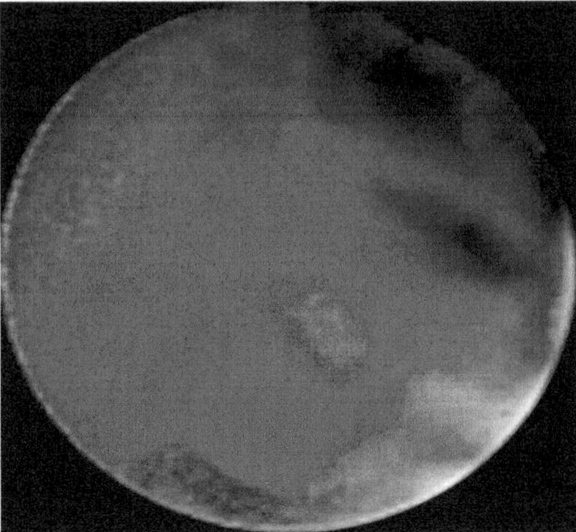

Fig. 11. An endoscopic view of a secondary duct after all stones and polyps were removed. Four endoscopic sessions were needed. Tertiary ducts can be seen entering this secondary duct in the upper right corner. A laser fiber is seen in the lower center.

stenosis of 0.5-mm diameter was encountered that was completely resistant to dilation. An Endoscopic-Open Transfacial approach was undertaken. After isolation of the duct within the cheek, it was partially transected 1.5 cm from the light source and in 2.0-mm increments proximally, until a normal lumen was found. The pathologic anterior duct was detached from the oral mucosa. A vascular loop was used as a retractor from the mouth through the cheek incision (**Fig. 16**). An ipsilateral dorsal hand vein graft was harvested using atraumatic microvascular technique (**Fig. 17**). The graft was placed over a 4F hollow stent. Through the transfacial incision, the stent was inserted about 1 cm into the proximal duct (**Fig. 18**). A 6-0 chromic suture was used to anchor the stent into the proximal duct, to prevent it from slipping out during the anastomosis. Using microvascular technique, 8-0 Ethibond sutures (Ethicon Inc, Somerville, NJ, USA) were used for a vein-to-duct anastomosis with 7 stitches (**Fig. 19**).

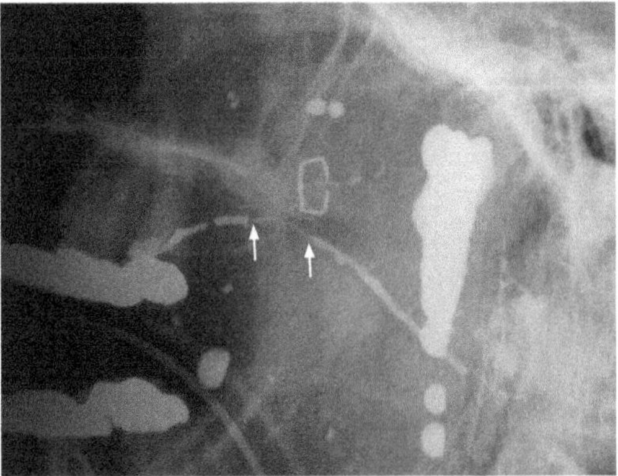

Fig. 12. An intraoperative sialogram of the left parotid with a 1.0-cm stenotic segment seen (*between arrows*). The metal clip was placed on the cheek just above the site where the patient pointed to maximal symptoms.

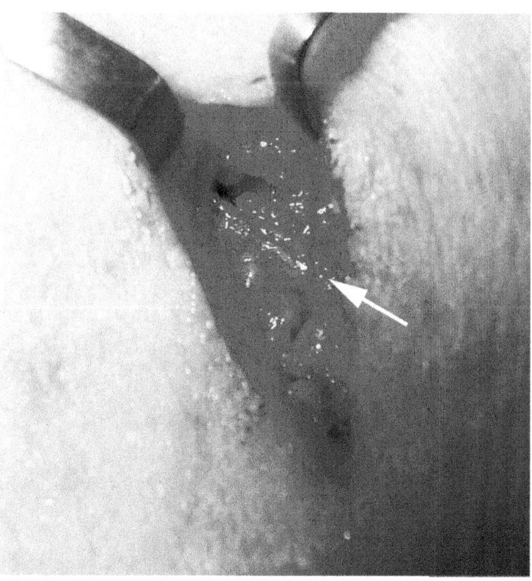

Fig. 13. The left facial nerve main buccal branch lies superficial and just superior to the parallel-running Stensen duct in this Endoscopic-Open Transfacial approach (*arrow*).

Attention was turned to the oral cavity, where the stent was protruding through the papilla resection area. The vein was advanced to the oral mucosa and seven 8-0 Ethibond sutures were placed; the stent was sewn to the oral cavity mucosa with two 5-0 silk sutures through the stent (**Fig. 20**). The stent was left in place for 6 weeks. The patient is asymptomatic 8 months after surgery.

Patient 6: Vein Graft Interposition, Duct-to-duct

A 43-year-old white woman presented with a symptomatic unilateral 1.6-cm Stensen duct stricture in the midmasseteric area. Sialendoscopy revealed a nondilating "hard" stricture with a 0.45-mm opening. An Endoscopic-Open Transfacial approach was

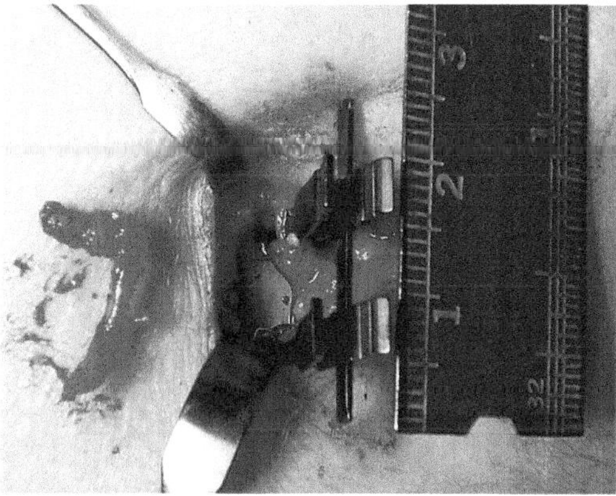

Fig. 14. A microvascular anastomosis using clips to help approximate the Stensen duct ends is shown; a blue plastic microvascular background is seen. Circumferential dissection of the duct loosens its attachments and allows for enough length to provide a tension-free closure. The resected duct is seen to the left of the surgical field.

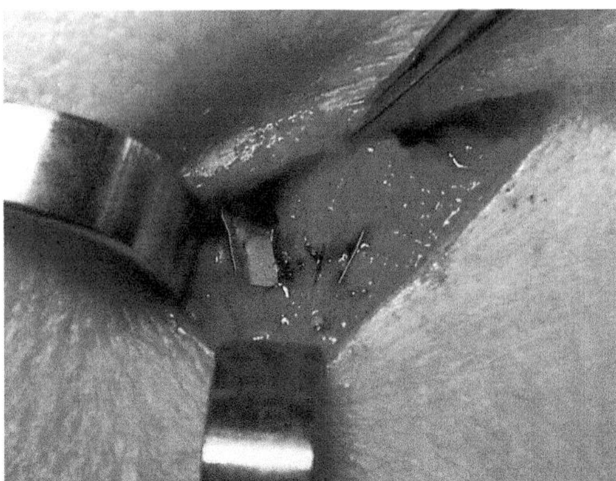

Fig. 15. The finished end-to-end duct anastomosis is seen. Blue 9-0 Prolene suture was used. Within the duct, a 4F hollow stent remains for 4 to 6 weeks while complete healing occurs.

used, with transillumination of the cheek, to help locate the incision site. NIMS monitoring was used. After isolation of the facial nerve buccal branch, the duct was dissected free from the surrounding tissue. The duct was partially transected at a distance of 1.5 cm from the light, and every 2.0 mm, until normal lumen was encountered. A 2.0-cm dorsal hand vein graft was harvested. The graft was placed over a 4F hollow stent with a guidewire through the stent. The guidewire was placed through the transfacial incision into both duct ends. Then the stent was inserted approximately 1 cm into both duct ends. The proximal duct end was dilated to allow for introduction of the stent. Using microvascular technique, six 8-0 Ethibond stitches were placed to achieve a watertight seal at each duct end, with the vein as an interposition graft (**Fig. 21**). The stent extended for 1 cm beyond the proximal anastomosis and into the mouth at the distal end **Fig. 22**. Saline irrigation showed the stent to be patent. The soft tissues were closed using 4-0 Vicryl to cover the vein, and a plastic technique skin closure ensued. The stent was left in place for 6 weeks before removal (**Fig. 23**).

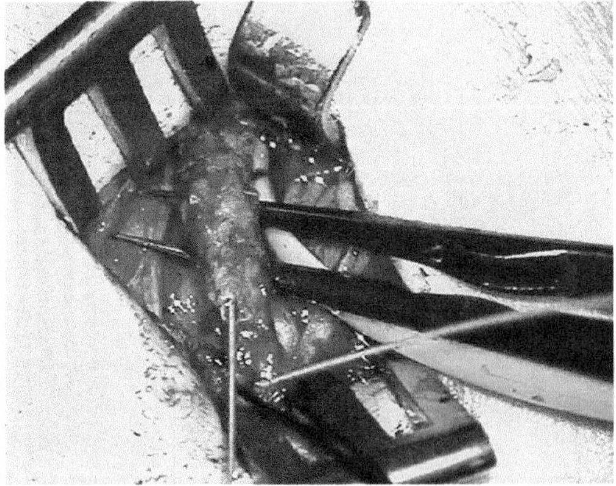

Fig. 16. This view of a duct stenosis for a right Endoscopic-Open Transfacial approach shows how the pathologic duct was isolated and then resected into the mouth. A blue vessel loop cheek retractor is seen going from the cheek incision into the mouth.

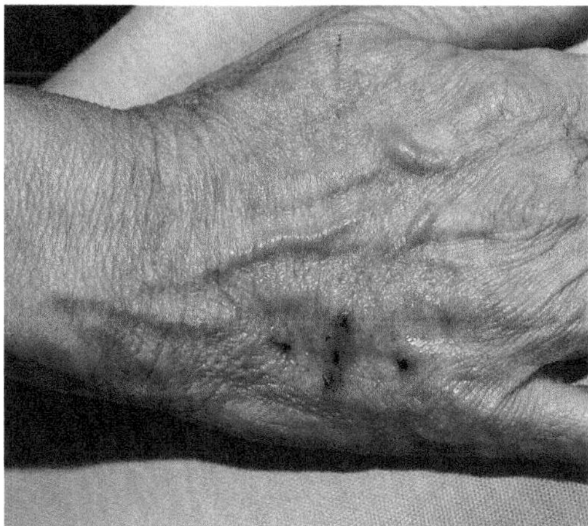

Fig. 17. A dorsal hand vein graft was used in this case. More robust veins are found as tributaries to the superficial saphenous vein around the medial malleolus of the foot.

FLOOR-OF-MOUTH MUCOSAL FLAP INTRAORAL APPROACH

Multiple techniques have been put forward for stone removal and duct repair of the submandibular gland through an intraoral approach.[3,4,5] These techniques center on identification of the duct, removal of duct pathology, and closure of the duct for reconstitution of the salivary flow. However, in one technique, a Sialo Drain (TM) (Sialo Technology , Ashkelon, Israel) is placed into the duct and sewn to the anterior floor of mouth (FOM).[6] Sometimes the stone is excessively large, or there is a chronic inflammatory reaction with profuse granulation tissue around the stone with an active gland. In such cases, the proximal duct is completely obscured from view, with or without use of the endoscope. There is no visible duct to close or into which to insert a drain. When the sialolith is delivered in these cases, on viewing the inflamed hamburgerlike tissue bed,

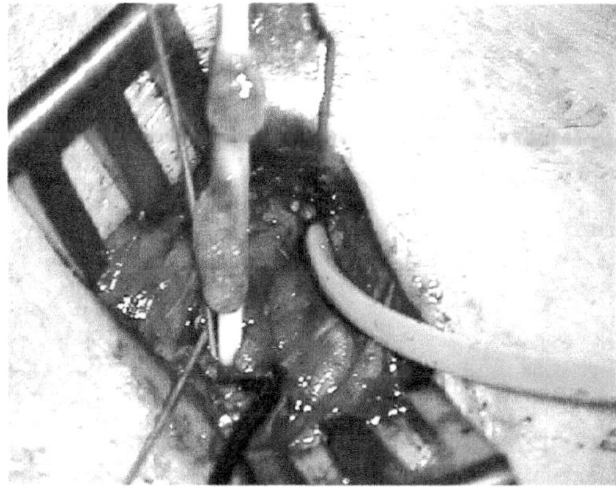

Fig. 18. To allow the anastomosis to heal without salivary leakage, the hollow white stent is placed approximately 1.0 cm into the proximal duct. It allows the gland to function normally, yet protects the anastomosis from salivary flow pressures. The graft has already been placed over the stent at this point.

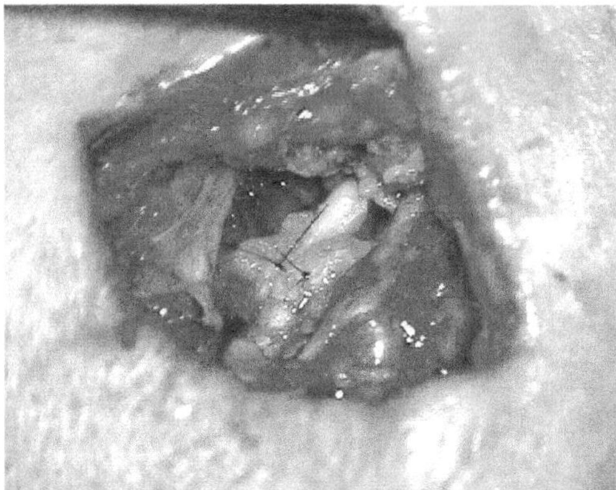

Fig. 19. A watertight proximal anastomosis is required to prevent a sialocele with progression to a fistula or abscess. The stenotic right duct has been resected. The vein-covered stent is visible in the center. Buccal branches of the facial nerve can be seen on both sides of stent.

no confidence is gained that a severe stenosis can be avoided or that the wound bed will heal without creating a purulent sialocele. There remains only an empty socket from which the stone was delivered. In such difficult cases, it would be usual to perform an adenectomy. Another alternative is the "FOM mucosal flap," introduced here. A posteriorly based 2.0-cm wide and 5.0-cm long mucosal flap is freed from the ipsilateral FOM. The flap runs parallel to the tongue. It is taken from the loose mucosa between the tongue and alveolus. The lateral flap incision line begins with the initial sialolithotomy incision. After elevation, the flap is rotated and sewn into the depths of the submandibular gland empty socket. It is sewn to the medical aspect of the socket to prevent occlusion of the proximal nonviewable duct (**Fig. 24**). In this way, a reliable mucosa-lined fistula is created between the unrecognizable hilum-duct granulation bed and the oral cavity. The remaining duct is left intact. The donor site FOM is closed by undermining and with a linear suture line. If there is duct stenosis or obliteration, only the fistula will drain saliva. In other cases, the fistula and the duct

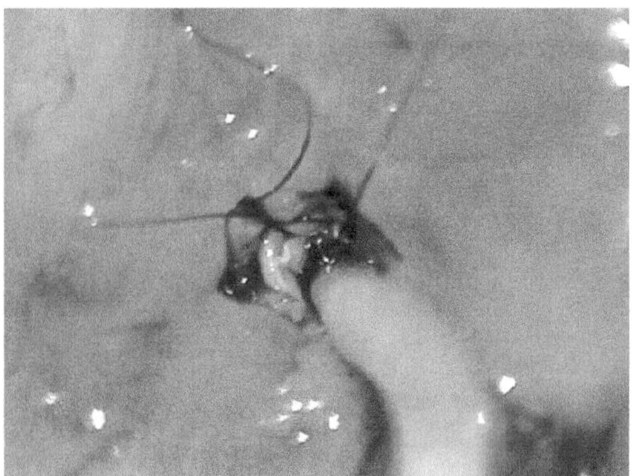

Fig. 20. In this intraoral view, the vein graft is sewn watertight to the oral mucosa with 8-0 nylon sutures. The distal anastomosis is sewn in place after the proximal side is completed. The white 4F hollow stent is seen supporting the anastomosis.

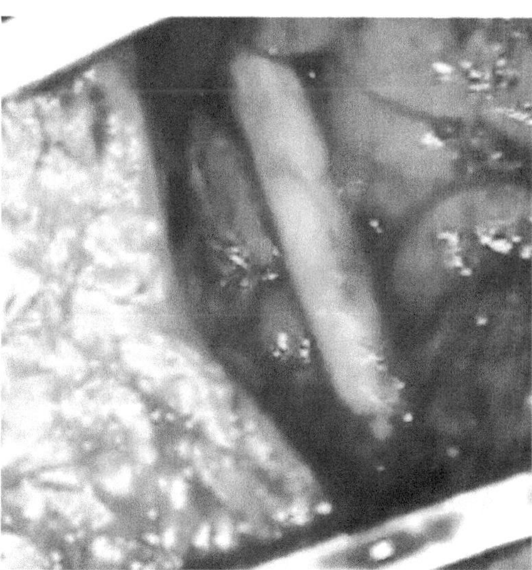

Fig. 21. The proximal and distal Stensen duct anastomoses are seen in this view of a left Endoscopic-Open Transfacial vein graft replacement of a Stensen duct stricture. The vein graft is supported by a white hollow stent.

punctum show salivary flow simultaneously. In edentulous patients, the inner surface of the denture needs to be trimmed to prevent abrasions to the new FOM topography and flap.

Patient 7: FOM Mucosal Flap

A 52-year-old man with a 1.5-cm stone of the submandibular gland had recurrent infections of the gland with associated cellulitis and intraprandial pain and swelling. An outside institution had recommended conventional submandibular adenectomy. Under general anesthesia, sialendoscopy was performed up to the enormous stone at the hilum and the scope was withdrawn. Then the FOM was observed and, at the same time, the submandibular gland was elevated using external digital pressure.

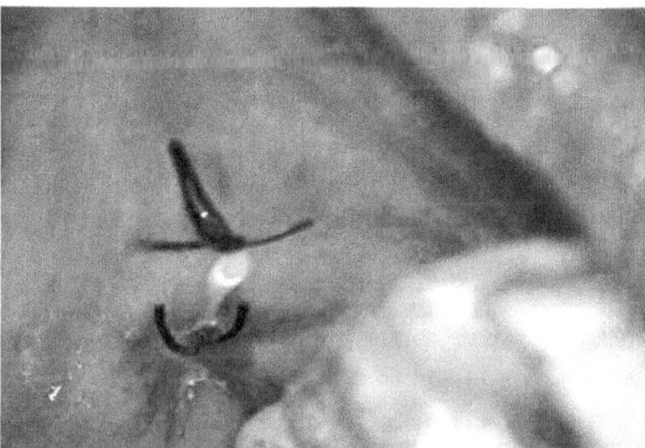

Fig. 22. The stent continues through the anastomosis site to be anchored intraorally with two 5-0 silk sutures. Salivary flow is confirmed exiting from the stent, as seen in this view. The stent will stay in place for 4 to 6 weeks.

The stone was palpated from inside the oral cavity. Without regard to the duct, a mucosal incision was placed directly over the stone inflammatory "ball." Blunt and sharp dissections were used to identify the lingual nerve and to avoid branches of the lingual artery. The stone was palpable through the inflammatory tissues. The tissues over the stone were incised and the yellow stone was removed piecemeal, followed by irrigations. The resulting tissue bed socket had no identifiable landmarks and was bleeding mildly from the granulation tissue. No duct or salivary stream landmarks were seen. Sialendoscopy through the duct could be brought into the empty socket, but no proximal ducts could be found. The gland was still functional as shown by the preoperative symptoms. With no guarantee of salivary drainage through the natural duct, the possibility of sialocele formation was high. A permanent drainage pathway was needed. For this reason, a FOM mucosal flap of 2.0 by 5.0 cm was created, rotated into the socket, and sewn into the friable tissue depths with two 3-0 Vicryl sutures (**Fig. 24**). Further anchoring sutures were placed, creating a U-shaped tract, and the donor site was linearly closed with absorbable sutures. Two years postoperatively, the patient is asymptomatic. Saliva flows from the mucosal lined fistula and the natural duct (**Fig. 25**).

DISCUSSION

In the course of examining and treating salivary gland duct obstruction problems, various pathologies will present to the physician. Within each of the pathologies, a broad spectrum of severity will be seen. Most patients have less severe problems and can be treated with conventional endoscopic instruments and algorithms, as described in the literature. However, some cases lie outside the "usual and customary" presentation for endoscopic treatment and are affected by difficult problems. The problems may arise for several reasons, including lack of lithotriptor availability, proximal intraparenchymal location of the pathology, nondilating strictures, numerous or advanced pathologies, giant sialoceles, and cosmetic considerations.

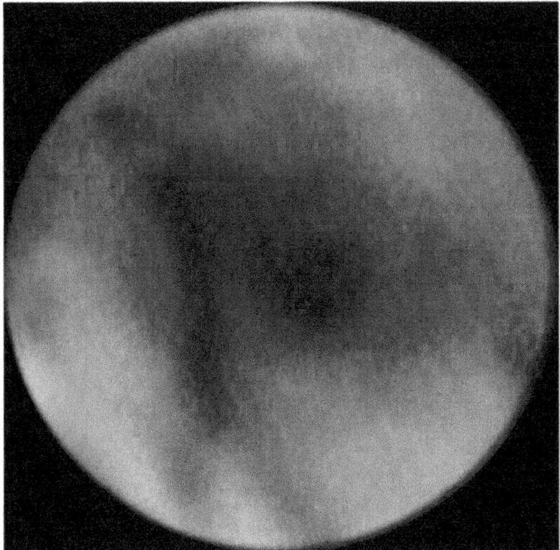

Fig. 23. Endoscopic view of a Stensen duct microvascular anastomosis with the black 8-0 nylon sutures visible intraductally at the healed incision line. Laser lysis is used to remove the remaining sutures.

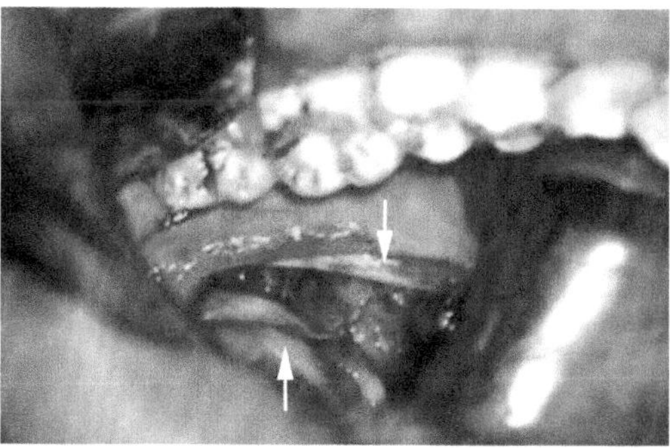

Fig. 24. A left FOM flap is seen sewn in place from the posteriorly based pedicle into the "hamburger" depths of the empty stone socket (*upper arrow* on lingual nerve, *lower arrow* on flap). The mucosal flap allows egress of saliva along a planned fistula tract.

For these cases, the conventional treatment position is gland resection. By resecting the gland, the pathology is completely removed. However, the function of that resected gland is lost to the patient, even if the obstruction was due to a circumscribed problem, such as a 5.0-mm long duct stenosis. In these circumstances, the gland is potentially salvageable, which is worth the time and effort. By applying operative methods such as the Endoscopic-Segmental parotidectomy, Endoscopic Double-Open or Staged approaches, Endoscopic-Open duct resection with duct reanastomosis or vein graft interposition, and FOM mucosal flaps, many of the glands that were once routinely removed may be preserved. Some glands are still beyond the reach of present-day treatment and will need to be resected until other strategies are found.

Apart from the operative methods so far described, there are other circumstances encountered during endoscopic treatment, where technical challenges can become difficult obstacles. Advance awareness of these problems and their remedies can facilitate progress for the treating physician.

Extravasation of saline irrigation into the surrounding tissues can occur during either submandibular or parotid endoscopy, if the duct is violated. Usually, this occurs during laser treatments of large stones, dilation of strictures, or usage of duct dilators in narrow-diameter ducts. In parotid cases, extravasation is revealed by a steadily enlarging subcutaneous knot in the cheek at the point of the duct perforation. When

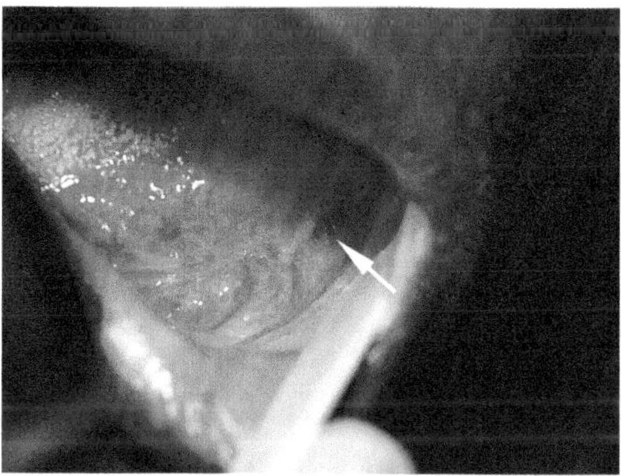

Fig. 25. A view into the oral cavity showing a left FOM flap fistula after healing (*arrow*).

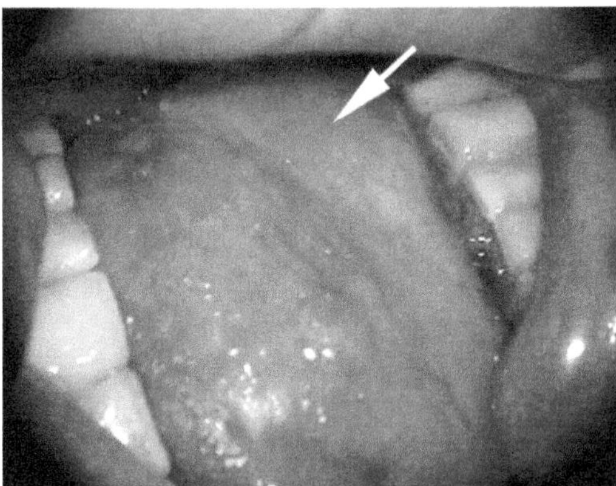

Fig. 26. If intraoperative endoscopic saline extravasation occurs, a Pseudo-ranula is formed under the tongue (*arrow*). If left unattended, the entire FOM may become elevated and airway compromise is a possibility.

a parotid saline infiltration happens, several options exist. In the case of a small opening, the endoscope can be advanced past the opening so that the irrigation pressure head is proximal to the opening. The low-pressure outflowing saline will exit the duct punctum and the uncorked instrument channel. Intermittent irrigation use is advised. Alternately, the surgeon can terminate the procedure and wait for 3 weeks of healing time before restarting endoscopy. For the FOM, the loose areolar tissue may distend very quickly forming a gray-blue boggy mass that elevates the tongue as a Pseudo-ranula (**Fig. 26**). As the FOM becomes swollen and edematous, an airway compromise is possible. If this pseudoranula occurs, an incision through the mucosa, with further blunt dissection into the areolar "water balloon," quickly allows decompression of the saline, which runs into the mouth (**Fig. 27**). The physician may continue the procedure, being vigilant of the FOM.

During sialography, a poppy seed oil–based iodine solution (Ethiodol) is often used. Sialography of a partially obstructed duct could cause the duct to rupture, with contrast extravasation under routine injection pressures. In such cases, the oil

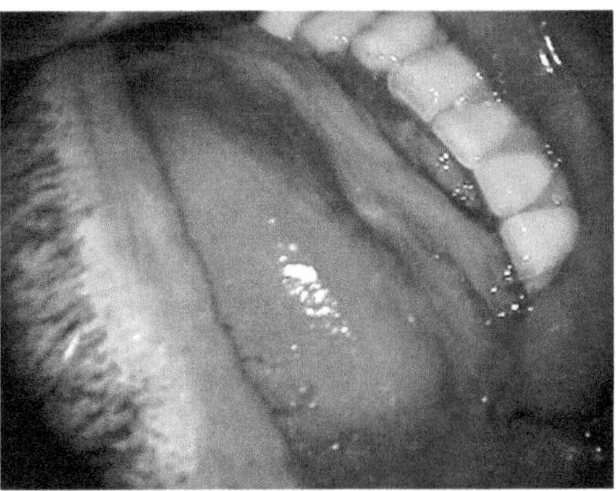

Fig. 27. The Pseudo-ranula is immediately relieved by incising the FOM mucosa and bluntly dissecting into the loose areolar tissue to drain the saline accumulation.

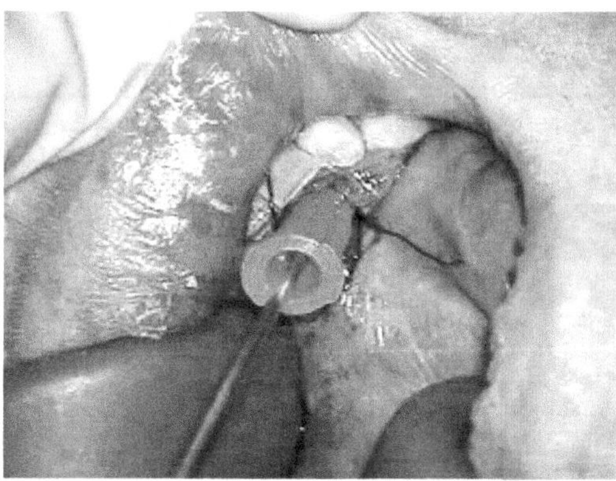

Fig. 28. A 14-gauge (or larger) angiocatheter is seen, placed as a temporary stent within the right submandibular duct. It serves to permit endoscopic entry and removal without repeatedly traumatizing the papilla and duct. A 4F stent can be threaded through it.

preparation in the tissues will initiate a progressive inflammatory reaction around the oil globules. Multiple subcutaneous abscesses may form, which will release oil if drained. Conservative treatment with antibiotics has not proven useful except to prevent outright abscess formation. Drainage is most accurate when an inflammatory nodule presents subcutaneously.

During any part of a sialendoscopy procedure, the punctum can dislocate from the mucous membrane and submerge below the surface. If this happens, a "cut-down" to the duct may be necessary to reattach it to the mucous membrane surface. For the submandibular gland, the most distal 5.0 mm of the duct is often narrow. To allow endoscopic access at the start of the case, the duct may be resected and followed with an advancement dochoplasty. At other times, due to repetitive entry with the endoscope, the duct attachments to the mucosa can become fragile. In these cases, a 14-gauge angiocatheter (Insyte, Becton Dickinson, Sandy, UT, USA) is placed over the endoscope before entering the duct, and it is advanced into the duct with the

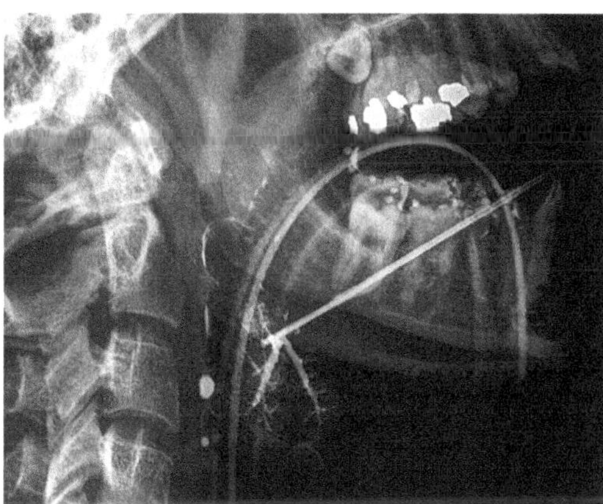

Fig. 29. A submandibular intraoperative transendoscopic sialogram, showing an endoscope in place with contrast medium injected through the endoscope. The entire duct system or just an isolated duct branch segment can be chosen with this sialogram technique.

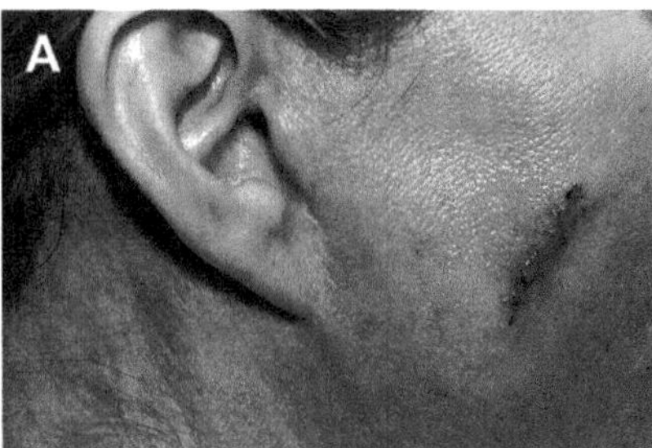

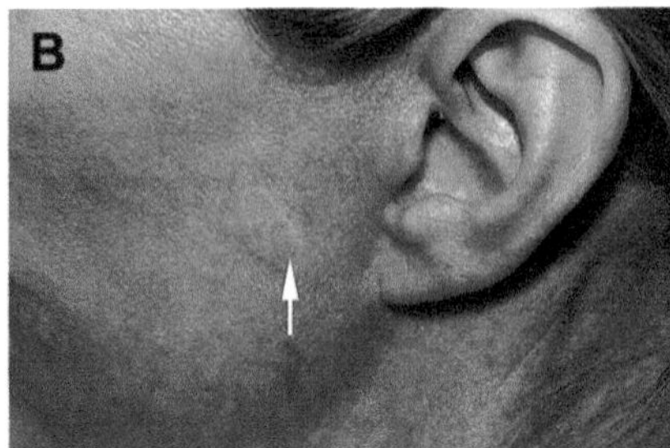

Fig. 30. The initial impression of where the duct and the previous repair are located could be assumed to be at the location of a previous transfacial scar (*A*). However, a facelift cosmetic procedure will misleadingly displace the scar into a posterior direction from its original position (*B*).

endoscope. After the first pass, the angiocatheter stays in place as a temporary operating stent. Multiple passes with the endoscope are easily made through the Stensen and Wharton ducts, lined with the protective angiocatheter (**Fig. 28**).

In the same way as segments of the parotid gland are addressed by Segmental parotidectomy, diagnosis with Segmental sialograms can also be made. If a stone is in a distal branch of the parotid, sialographic contrast can be placed directly through the endoscope to check for the duct status, or the entire duct system can be injected through the endoscope. This is particularly useful when a tight stenosis has been dilated with the endoscope. The same type of transendoscopic sialogram can be performed for the whole or part of the submandibular gland (**Fig. 29**).

If a patient with a prior transfacial incision undergoes a facelift, the original scar may be pulled in a posterior direction by 3.0 cm. In such cases, any further work on a duct problem would need to take place anteriorly to the Transfacial incision, possibly needing a second ipsilateral transfacial incision for access (**Fig. 30**).

SUMMARY

Difficult cases require thought and effort to save a physiologically intact gland. Saving the nondiseased parts of a salivary gland may require new strategies of treatment. Sparing part or all of a gland is a major benefit for the patient. Techniques that are therapeutic for the affected parts of the gland, while leaving the remaining normal gland unchanged, can provide a more physiologic result for the patient. The techniques presented in this article help to fulfill these goals and provide guidance for various difficult case presentations.

ACKNOWLEDGMENTS

The author wishes to thank Rebecca Colson, administrative assistant, for her assistance in the preparation of the manuscript; also Philippe Katz, MD, Urban Geisthoff, MD, and Oded Nahlieli, DMD, Professor, for their support.

REFERENCES

1. Nahlieli O, London D, Zagury A, et al. Combined approach to impacted parotid stones. J Oral Maxillofac Surg 2002;60:1418–23.

2. McGurk M, MacBean A, Fan KF, et al. Conservative management of salivary stones and benign parotid tumours: a description of the surgical techniques involved. Ann R Australas Coll Dent Surg 2004;17:41–4.
3. McGurk M, Escudier M. Removing salivary gland stones. Br J Hosp Med 1995;54:184–5.
4. Zenk J, Iro H. Die Sialolithiasis und deren Behandlung. Laryngol Rhinol Otol 2001;80:115–36 [in German].
5. Capaccio P, Bottero A, Pompilio M, et al. Conservative transoral removal of hilar submandibular salivary calculi. Laryngoscope 2005;115:750–2.
6. Nahlieli O, Shacham R, Zagury A, et al. The ductal stretching technique: an endoscopic-assisted technique for removal of submandibular stones. Laryngoscope 2007;117:1031–5.

Extracorporeal and Intracorporeal Lithotripsy of Salivary Gland Stones: Basic Investigations

Johannes Zenk, MD*, Michael Koch, MD, Heinrich Iro, MD

KEYWORDS

- Salivary glands • Salivary stones
- Intracorporeal and extracorporeal lithotripsy
- Laser • Shockwaves

Although less common than in the urinary or biliary tracts, calculus formation in the major salivary glands can also cause unpleasant symptoms with pain and swelling of the affected organ (salivary colic).[1] Analysis of postmortem specimens led Rauch and Gorlin[2] to the conclusion that some 1.15% of the population has stones in the salivary glands. Escudier and McGurk[3] estimated that the incidence of symptomatic disease is 27 to 56 cases per 1 million inhabitants in the United Kingdom. Assuming that it is valid to extrapolate epidemiologic data, this figure related to the 300 million inhabitants of the United States means that 8100 to 16,800 patients are treated each year. The traditional treatment for sialolithiasis was extirpation of the affected gland. This was performed not just because of the symptoms but also for fear of recurrence and because of the residual loss of function of the affected salivary gland. Since van den Akker and Busemann-Sokole[4] published their findings in 1983, however, it has been known that salivary gland function can recover completely after stone extraction alone. This provided one of the basic principles and prerequisites of the concept of minimally invasive surgery with conservation of function in the treatment of sialolithiasis. A second important aspect is the possibility of complications, such as nerve damage (facial, lingual, and hypoglossal nerves), cosmetically unacceptable scarring, and Frey syndrome, which may occur with complete resection of the gland.

Since the mid-1980s, much thought has been given to treating sialolithiasis with extracorporeal or intracorporeal shock waves in a manner similar to that used for urinary tract or biliary tract stones, and this has been implemented successfully.

Department of Otorhinolaryngology, Head and Neck Surgery, University of Erlangen Nuremberg, Waldstrasse 1, D-91054 Erlangen, Germany
* Corresponding author.
E-mail address: johannes.zenk@uk-erlangen.de (J. Zenk).

Otolaryngol Clin N Am 42 (2009) 1115–1137
doi:10.1016/j.otc.2009.08.005
oto.theclinics.com
0030-6665/09/$ – see front matter

This article provides an overview of the various methods of extracorporeal and intracorporeal lithotripsy that have been used or proposed for salivary calculi to date, considering the advantages and disadvantages of each of the techniques.

HISTORY

The word "lithotripsy" means "stone fragmentation" and was first proposed in 1813 by Gruithuisen, a Bavarian surgeon.[5] He suggested that a urinary stone could be grasped in the bladder by an instrument introduced by way of the urethra, so that holes could be drilled in the stone to pulverize the stone. The underlying principle was that the small stone fragments produced would pass out of the body through the outflow tracts (ureter-urethra for urinary stones, the bile ducts for biliary calculi) without any adverse effects.

New instruments were developed over the next few years and the first successful lithotripsy was performed in 1824, in public, at the French Academy in Paris. The procedure avoided the need for surgical incisions and replaced lithotomy in five out of every six cases over the following decades. At the same time, the mortality associated with treating the condition fell from 15% to 7%.[5]

Despite these early successes, the development of general anesthesia and the advent of surgical asepsis led to a return to surgical removal of the stones from the affected organs by the late nineteenth century. This could be difficult in the case of kidney stones, but the advent of cholecystectomy for gallstones in 1882 rendered these highly amenable to treatment.

The first reports of attempts to destroy gallstones and bladder calculi by noncontact sonic techniques came from Berlinicke and Schenetten 1951,[6] Mulvaney 1953,[7] and Coats in 1956.[8] Using ultrasound with an intensity of about 5 W/cm^2 and exposure times of up to 30 minutes, slight degradation rates for the stones could be achieved. These attempts were stopped, however, because of serious tissue damage and lack of effectiveness.

The possibility of destroying stones without contact, from a certain distance, arose from advances made in high-speed physics.[9] In 1975, urinary calculi placed in a beaker of water were completely disrupted using focused shock waves, without any direct contact with the appliance; 1980 saw the first successful fragmentation of renal calculi in humans, using shock waves from an external source focused within the body.[10] This revolutionized the treatment concept for renal stones and the first reports of gallstone lithotripsy using a modified kidney lithotripter were published in 1983.[10] At the end of 1985, Sauerbruch and colleagues[11] successfully treated the first patients with gallstones by extracorporeal shock wave lithotripsy. Extracorporeal lithotripsy of biliary tract and pancreatic duct stones followed.[12,13]

Parallel to the development of extracorporeal methods, intracorporeal techniques were also tested and established in various organ systems. These include intracorporeal electrohydraulic methods, various laser lithotripsy systems, and pneumatic lithotripsy. The development and diversification of the individual techniques in different organ systems is beyond the scope of this article but studies on the lithotripsy of salivary gland stones are mentioned in the relevant sections.

EXTRACORPOREAL LITHOTRIPSY

Definition and Mechanism of Action of Extracorporeal Shock Waves

Extracorporeal shock waves are compression waves propagated through a medium at supersonic speed. Although the behavior of shock waves is physically similar to that of ultrasound waves, there are great differences in physical characteristics and energy between the two.[10,14] Although shock waves come from a single pressure pulse rising steeply to a peak and then decaying slowly, ultrasound waves are characterized by sinusoidal pressure variation, with successive compressive and tensile phases (**Fig. 1**). When passing through biologic tissue, high-frequency waves lose energy to a much greater extent than low-frequency waves, so that shock waves with lower-frequency components are much less attenuated and penetrate to greater depths than ultrasound waves.[10,15]

If when passing through biologic tissue a shock wave strikes a body of different impedance (eg, a stone), it is reflected as a compressive and tensile wave, depending on the acoustic properties of the interface. Mechanical damage occurs when the pressure exceeds the compressive or tensile strength of the material.[16] Fragmentation of the stone can be explained as follows: an externally induced shock wave penetrates the body and is propagated uninterruptedly because there is basically no difference between the impedance of water and tissue. At the tissue-stone interface (ie, the anterior border of the stone) partial reflection of the shock wave causes compression forces to develop and act on the stone here. That part of the shock wave that travels through the stone is again reflected, this time from the posterior wall, creating a further compressive and tensile wave. The stone breaks up when the pressure exceeds the compressive or tensile strength of its material. The center of the stone is initially not affected, so it must be exposed to repeated shock waves.[17] Every effort is made to focus the shock wave as narrowly as possible, to minimize the burden on the tissues as the waves pass through. In this way, maximum pressure amplitude is achieved in the focal area with only slight compressive stress distant from the focus.[18] The shock waves have to be transmitted into the body from a medium with acoustic impedance similar to that of biologic tissue. Because biologic tissue is composed of about 70% water, water is used as the coupling medium. This prevents troublesome reflections and resultant stress or damage at the body surface.[15,18] To be more specific, three different systems have been developed to date, and are now discussed (**Fig. 2**).

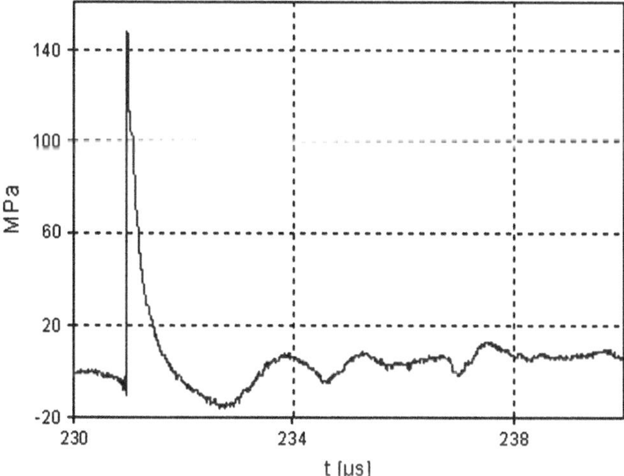

Fig. 1. Progression of pressure versus time of a typical shock wave. Note the rapid increase to very high pressure values.

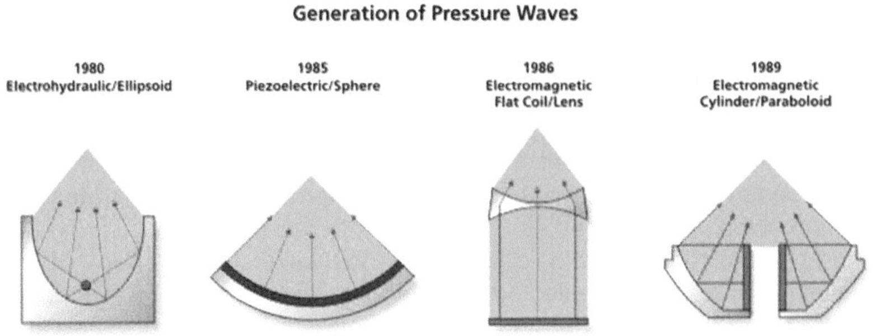

Fig. 2. Generation of extracorporeal shock waves: electrohydraulic, piezoelectric, and electromagnetic.

Generation of Extracorporeal Shockwaves

Electrohydraulic principle

The shock wave originates from the discharge of an underwater electrical spark. First, energy stored in a capacitor is released within a very short time. An arc forms between the electrodes; within about a microsecond, this explosively vaporizes the fluid surrounding the arc path, generating plasma-like conditions. The rapid vaporization and expansion generates a shock wave in the surrounding fluid, with spherical propagation of the wave. The shock wave is focused by generating it at the focal point of a reflector with rotational symmetry; it is reflected at the ellipsoid wall and the reflections produced convene at a second focal point (see **Fig. 2**).[18,19]

Piezoelectric principle

The main component of a piezoelectric shock wave generator is a piezoelectric acoustic radiator consisting of a large number of ceramic elements arranged as a mosaic on the concave surface of a spherical recess. The structure is self-focusing. A high-frequency, high-voltage impulse from a pulse generator stimulates all of the individual ceramic elements simultaneously and causes their sudden expansion (piezoelectric principle). Water is used as the coupling medium to transmit the targeted shock wave. The hollow spherical structure allows a reflection-free, self-focusing system without aberrant acoustic wave components (see **Fig. 2**).[20]

Electromagnetic principle

An electrical impulse from a generator is conducted to a flat coil. This induces changes in an adjacent metallic membrane and a shock wave of increasing intensity is propagated in a water container connected upstream. The shock wave is focused through an acoustic lens.[21,22] A cylinder coil together with a paraboloid construction can also be used for focusing the shock waves (see **Fig. 2**).

Lithotripters Used and Basic Investigations

The first report of the in vitro use of an electrohydraulic lithotripter (Dornier MedTech Europe GmbH, Wessling, Germany) to treat a salivary gland calculus was in 1986.[23] The study used a large sialolith (1.5 $\times$ 0.5 cm), which had been removed from the hilum of a submandibular gland. The stone was put in a plastic bag filled with water and immersed in the water-bath of a renal lithotripter. Under radiograph guidance, the stone was placed at the focus and a series of 50 shock waves applied. The stone fragmented. Nevertheless, the authors went on to say that the existing lithotripter would need to be modified to facilitate treatment in patients. They were aware of possible complications and wanted to ensure precise focusing and keeping the mandible out of the focus.

A further in vitro case report[24] used an electromagnetic lithotripter (Siemens AG Company, Medical Solutions, Erlangen, Germany). The aim of the experiment was to determine whether it was possible to position a patient so as to allow fragmentation of a stone without damaging the surrounding structures. Although the eyes, brain, and larynx could be protected, it was not possible to protect the teeth. In vitro, a stone disintegrated very quickly (200 shocks at 16 kV). The application of shock waves to an extracted tooth resulted in the fracture of the amalgam filling after 200 impulses and significant damage to the tooth enamel. The authors concluded that a special device with a small focus volume would have to be created for lithotripsy of submandibular stones.

This led to in vitro and in vivo experiments with the piezoelectric lithotripter from Wolf (Knittlingen, Germany). In comparison with electrohydraulic and electromagnetic systems, this system has the highest focusing gain "G" because of the generator aperture (**Table 1**). "G" is defined as the ratio of the maximum pressure at the focus to the maximum pressure at the source.[19] With G less than 20, it is usually necessary to give the patient an anesthetic, because a relatively large part of the shock wave energy is released on the surface. The focus dimensions of the piezoelectric system are considerably smaller and the probability of expected collateral damage is less (**Table 2**). Because of the prerequisites, appropriate in vitro and in vivo testing was performed before using salivary lithotripsy in humans to establish whether it was possible to use shock wave therapy for salivary gland stones.[25,26] Of 100 salivary gland stones treated in vitro by piezoelectric shock waves, 80% disintegrated completely. Complete disintegration was defined as the maximum diameter of the fragments being less than 1.5 mm.

It was assumed that stone fragments of this magnitude would pass out of the body spontaneously through the normal outflow channels. Later anatomic investigations confirmed this hypothesis.[27] Neither the mineral composition nor the size, weight, or volume of the stone had any effect on whether the stone could be fragmented. The greater the size of the stone, the greater the mean number of shock waves required to fragment the stone completely. With respect to the fragmentation rate and treatment time, about 3000 shock waves seemed to be worthwhile for later use in patients.

Further in vitro studies on human tissue and in vivo studies in 30 rabbits (shock waves applied to the parotid area) were intended to identify acute and chronic damage to the tissues. They showed that bleeding into the tissues was caused by the opening of only the smallest blood vessels, irrespective of the impulse intensity of the shock wave in the experiment (**Fig. 3**). No permanent tissue damage was observed. Nevertheless, shock waves applied directly to the eye with conduction across the superior orbital fissure led to detectable clinical and morphologic changes.[25]

On the basis of these results, using shock wave systems with correspondingly small focus volumes and the physical properties mentioned previously, and assuming the precise positioning of the patient and reliable ultrasound (or alternatively radiograph)

Table 1
Gain of focus for different lithotripters

System	Gain of Focus (G)
Electrohydraulic (eg, Dornier HM 3)	5
Electromagnetic (eg, Siemens Lithostar plus)	19
Piezoelectric (eg, Wolf Piezolith 2300)	250

Table 2
Dimension of the focus zone for different lithotripters

	Dimension of Focus	
System	Axial (in mm)	Lateral (in mm)
Electrohydraulic (eg, Dornier HM 3)	90	15
Electromagnetic (eg, Siemens Lithostar plus)	40	11
Piezoelectric (eg, Wolf Piezolith 2300)	5	3

localization of the stone, serious adverse effects are not to be expected with salivary stone lithotripsy.

Based on these results, two systems proved to be suitable for clinical use: the Piezolith 2300 model and its successors, the Piezolith 2500 and 2501 (**Fig. 4**) (Richard Wolf, Knittlingen, Germany); and the Modulith and Minilith electromagnetic systems (**Fig. 5**) (Storz Medical, AG, Tägerwilen, Switzerland). Both systems have the corresponding protocols and presettings for the treatment of salivary calculi.

In the piezoelectric system, the water path is closed tightly with a latex membrane. This membrane can be adjusted by changing the pressure, so that during treatment the patient can be positioned comfortably on this device, which is like a soft cushion.

The shock wave generator can be moved in three planes to find the stone, so that the shock waves can be focused precisely on the sialolith under ultrasound guidance. The pulse frequency of the shock waves can be increased in three steps from 1 to 2.5 Hz; the maximum pressure development in the focus volume for salivary calculi lithotripsy is approximately 80 MPa.[28,29]

The Minilith electromagnetic system consists of a miniature generator, which is fixed to a hinged bracket that can be moved though all spatial planes. This appliance has an

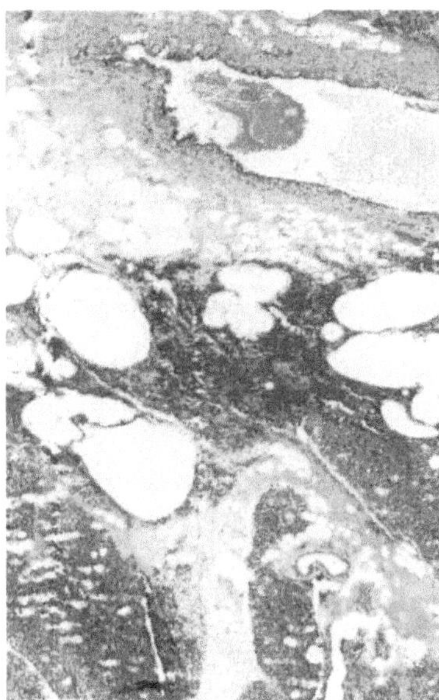

Fig. 3. Subfascial bleeding within the parotid gland of a rabbit in animal experiments after extracorporeal shock wave application (HE, ×25).

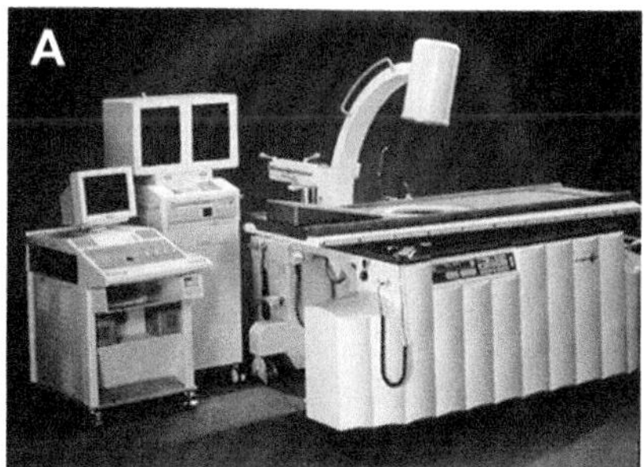

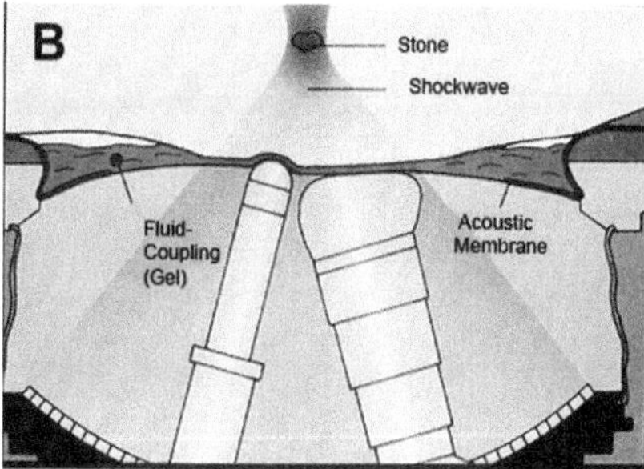

Fig. 4. (*A*) Piezoelectric device Piezolith 2500 (Wolf Company, Germany), which is used for salivary stone lithotripsy. (*Courtesy of* Wolf Company, Germany.) (*B*) Scheme of shock wave application with the Piezolith 2500. Piezocrystals (*yellow*) in a self-focusing arrangement. Water-filled basin with integrated ultrasound scanner and radiograph covered by an acoustic membrane. Stone within the focus of the shock waves.

integrated ultrasound localization system and a small water path. The system is mobile. The construction of the transducer with a rotary arm also allows lithotripsy to be performed with the patient in various positions.[30,31] A comparative study of the two lithotripters found no significant differences between the in vitro effects or clinical results.[32] Animal studies on the use of shock waves around the face, however, are available only for the piezoelectric system.[25]

Patient Preparation

Although no dangerous adverse effects have occurred to date, patients should be informed of the following risks before they are given shock waves to the head and neck: bleeding; infection; abscess formation; subsequent removal of the gland; hearing loss or tinnitus; and potential damage to the teeth and injury to the eye (with incorrect application). Absolute contraindications are patients with cardiac pacemakers, the presence of coagulation disorders and acute infections of the gland.[33]

Routine ultrasound B-scans are performed on the affected gland 1 hour before and 1 day after shock wave lithotripsy. In addition, all patients should have an audiogram performed before treatment and 24 hours afterward, to determine any possible iatrogenic hearing loss.[34] Administration of oral analgesics before treatment is not usually necessary unless the patient has a very low pain threshold. Children under the age of 10 years are usually given a general anesthetic.[35]

Before the stone is positioned in the focus, an ear plug is inserted into the external auditory meatus to protect the inner ear from injury caused by the acoustic shock when the shock wave is generated.[36]

After setting the appliance under ultrasound guidance, shock waves are initially applied at the lowest intensity. Under continuous ultrasound monitoring, the intensity of the waves is increased and treatment continued until the maximum number of shock waves has been given (piezoelectric, 3000 pulses[26]; electromagnetic, 1300–7500 pulses).[31,37,38] Treatment is stopped earlier if the stone has fragmented completely and can no longer be located with ultrasound, or if shock wave application is no longer safe because the patient is not cooperative.

If the shock waves fragment the salivary stone, it must be ensured that the fragments are flushed out through the natural outflow ducts of the gland. This can be encouraged by supportive measures performed by the patient or the treating physician.

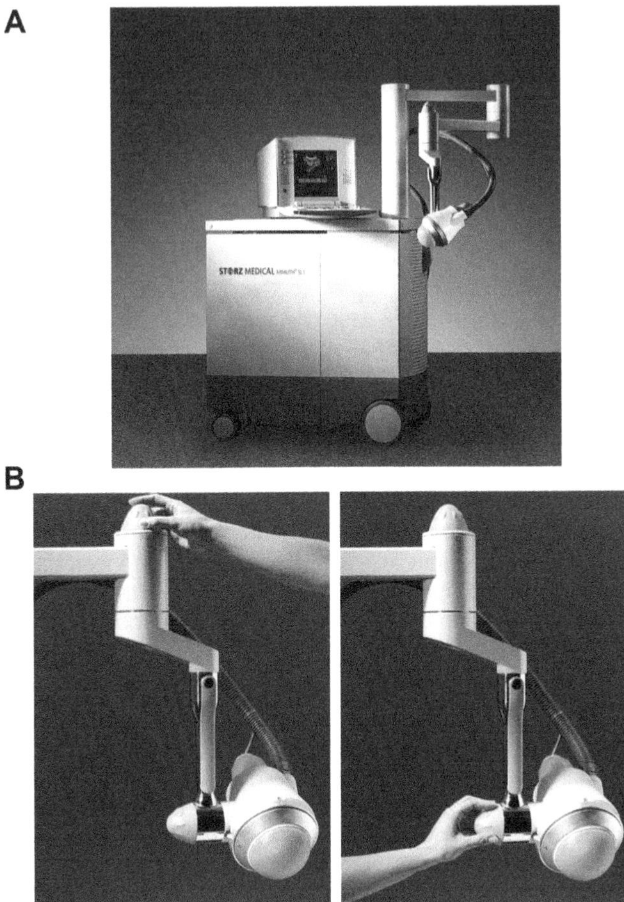

Fig. 5. (*A*) Electromagnetic lithotripter Minilith SL 1 (Storz Medical, Switzerland) with integrated ultrasound localization. (*B*) Small electromagnetic generator of the Minilith (covered by a membrane), which can be moved within all dimensions for lithotripsy of salivary stones. (*Courtesy of* Storz Medical, Switzerland.)

Sialagogues and gland massage ensure a continuous flow of saliva. In addition, excretion of the stone can be facilitated by bouginage of the natural ostium, the narrowest part of the outflow tract. If individual fragments are palpable in the distal ducts near the ostium, or can be identified on ultrasound, these fragments can be extracted using a Dormia basket. Prophylactic oral antibiotics and anti-inflammatory drugs are given to all patients on the day of treatment and for 2 days afterward.

If symptoms persist or residual stones are identified on ultrasound scanning, a second treatment is given 2 months after the first treatment session, with a third session after 4 months if necessary.[29]

INTRACORPOREAL LITHOTRIPSY

The intracorporeal lithotripsy of salivary gland stones had its first flush of popularity at the beginning of the 1990s, when laser, electrohydraulic probes, and pneumatic lithotripsy were evaluated and tested in a way similar to other specialties (urology and gastroenterology). Shock waves were usually applied under endoscopic control. As a rule, endoscopes at that time had a relatively large diameter, and a poorer imaging quality than the miniaturized sialoscopes now available. This is certainly one of the main reasons that intracorporeal lithotripsy has not yet become routine clinical practice in the treatment of salivary gland stones. Nevertheless, the semiflexible and smaller endoscopes available today are greatly improved, and there are new laser systems that may possibly be used for this purpose.

Laser Lithotripsy

Basic principles

"Laser" stands for light amplification by stimulated emission of radiation. To produce laser light (= energy) electrons of a particular substance or element have to be stimulated by an external source and raised to a higher energy level. This means that there is amplification of monochromatic, coherent light waves.[39–41] The principle of light amplification is explained in **Fig. 6**.

The amplification medium may be a gas (eg, CO_2, excimer, argon), liquid (eg, fluorescent alcoholic solutions, dyes), or solid (eg, neodymium:yttrium-aluminum-garnet [Nd:YAG], holmium:YAG [Ho:YAG], erbium:YAG [Er:YAG], chrysoberyl [alexandrite]), which can be stimulated to photon emission. The laser power in watts, the irradiation exposure in seconds, the emitted energy (watt or joule), the power density (watt per square centimeter), and the energy density (joule per square centimeter) are all important for calculating the laser effects.[39]

Principle of shock wave generation with lasers

It has been postulated that the absorption of the laser pulse causes plasma to form on the surface of the calculus (plasma is a rapidly expanding cavity of ions and electrons that collapses rapidly after the laser pulse). This action produces a mechanical shock wave. The saline solution used for irrigation confines the shock wave and concentrates its effect on the stone. The high pressure created by the shock wave then causes the calculus to fragment. The absorption properties depend greatly on the material; there is generally an increase in absorption at shorter wavelengths. Between 300 and 800 nm, the absorption of typical human calculi is so high that a shock wave can be generated by the process described previously, with moderate energy (20–100 mJ) and impulse duration in the microsecond range.[42] About 60% of the generated shock wave energy penetrates the stone and causes effective fragmentation, whereas the remaining 40% is partially reflected at the surface of the stone or causes adverse thermal effects.[13]

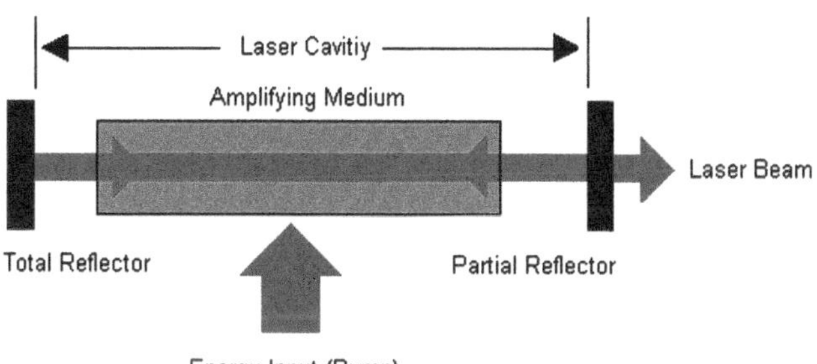

Fig. 6. Laser principle.

Although each pulse may remove only a small fragment, the multihertz transmission rate and the multiple shock waves produced result in laser fissures. These fissures promote rapid crumbling of the stone. The combination of wavelength, pulse duration and frequency, pulse energy, and fiber diameter determines the size of the fragments produced by the laser.[5]

Basic investigations: laser lithotripsy

The first in vitro laser lithotripsy of salivary calculi was reported in 1990,[44] using a pulsed dye laser (cumarine, 504 nm) with a pulse duration of 1.5 μs. The initial light pulses were focused into a 600-μm fiber, with maximum impulse energy of 250 mJ produced at the end. It was shown that the average number of 50-mJ pulses applied at 10 Hz required to fragment stones was far higher in salivary calculi than in urinary or biliary stones. A later in vitro study by Sterenborg and colleagues[44] compared a pulsed dye laser (Candela Laser GmbH, Neu-Isenburg, Germany); a Ho:YSGG laser (Laser 1-2-3; Schwartz Electrooptics, Orlando, Florida); and an electrohydraulic apparatus. All three devices produced a shock wave but also generated expanding and quickly imploding gas bubbles (cavitation), which could damage the duct wall. In addition, the high cost, large size of the equipment, and need for special safety procedures were believed to be contraindications to laser lithotripsy.

A further in vitro study by Gundlach and colleagues[45] considered carbon dioxide, Nd:YAG, and XeCL excimer lasers. These lasers were used to investigate the photo-absorption and reflective properties of 18 salivary calculi. The pulsed excimer laser with a wavelength of 308 or 351 nm was judged to be the best, and a pulse duration of 60 ns proposed for use.

In 1992, the authors' working group performed structured in vitro and the first in vivo experiments using five different laser systems with integrated stone-tissue recognition:[29,46] (1) alexandrite laser (Lithotripter Impact, 755 nm [Dornier MedTech Europe GmbH, Wessling, Germany]); (2) Nd:YAG laser (Lasolith, 1024 nm [Lasag AG, Gwatt, Switzerland]); (3) cumarine dye laser (Pulsolith, 504 nm [Technomed International Inc, Danvers, Massachusetts, USA]); (4) excimer laser (MAX 10, 308 nm [Technolas GmbH, Munich, Germany]); and (5) rhodamine 6G dye laser (Lithognost, 595 nm [Telemit/Baasel LaserTechnik, Starnberg, Germany]).

The underlying principle of this patented stone-tissue recognition is based on the different radiograph fluorescence generated by the laser pulse on tissue and stone. After only 200 ns, before the shock wave is generated, the target can be recognized as either a stone or soft tissue. A rapid optical shut-off is activated if tissue is identified, and this reduces the energy of the laser pulse by almost 90%.

All systems were first tested in vitro to find out whether fragmentation of salivary stones was in principle possible. The stones kept in normal saline were divided into groups according to size, and treated with different powers and frequencies. Complete fragmentation was defined as all particles measuring less than 1.5 mm; the stone was partially fragmented when the maximum particle size was greater than 1.5 mm.

With maximum energy and laser pulse of 80 mJ and pulse repetition rate of 10 Hz, the alexandrite laser only partially fragmented 2 out of 12 stones of different sizes (2–15 mm). The Nd:YAG and the cumarine dye laser were used to treat 18 and 21 sialoliths, respectively. Despite maximum energy (60 mJ and 160 mJ) and different pulse frequencies (2–13 Hz and 2–10Hz) none of the stones in any of the groups showed signs of sufficient fragmentation even after the maximum 2500 pulses.

Using the excimer laser on a total of 27 sialoliths (nine stones in each size group), 13 (48%) were completely fragmented and 14 (52%) partially fragmented with a maximum energy of 60 mJ. Fragmentation clearly depended on the size, weight, and volume of the stones: whereas 89% of stones measuring less than 5 mm disintegrated completely, the corresponding figure for the group measuring up to 10 mm was only 56%, and no stone up to 15 mm was completely fragmented.

There was no relation to the composition of the stone (organic or inorganic components). All completely disintegrated stones were treated with energies up to 20 mJ and 2700 to 24,000 pulses. Even using higher energy did not result in complete fragmentation.

Using the rhodamine 6G dye laser with a frequency of 10 Hz, 10 stones (33%) out of 30 sialoliths were completely fragmented, 12 stones (40%) partially fragmented, and 8 stones not fragmented. The fragmentation rate was not dependent on the size of the stones (27%). Complete fragmentation was achieved with an energy of 60 to 80 mJ after 220 to 1240 pulses. All partially or nonfragmented stones were treated with a maximum energy of 120 mJ and up to 2500 shock waves.

On the basis of the in vitro results, the last two systems were considered potentially suitable for salivary stone lithotripsy. Appropriate in vivo experiments were performed on rabbits before any possible use on humans. The first step consisted of ligating the parotid duct of rabbits according to the method described by Wallenborn and coworkers[47] under intramuscular anesthesia with xylazine and ketamine. Stensen duct was then dilated from a maximum original diameter of 0.2 mm to more than 2 mm, so that a laser fiber could be introduced. The acute experiment with the laser could be performed in vivo after 14 to 18 days. The laser parameters were selected according to the values obtained in vitro and the shock waves applied both parallel and at an angle of 45 degrees to the duct epithelium, and to such structures as the parotid gland, the facial nerve, and the masseter muscle.

Even when the probe was positioned strictly parallel to the tissue, shock waves applied with the excimer laser caused perforation of the parotid duct (**Fig. 7A**). Interestingly, this occurred after only 650 pulses at 10 mJ and 400 pulses at 20 mJ. Bleeding occurred, and thermal damage in the surrounding tissue (**Fig. 7B**). In addition, typical changes caused by heat could be seen in the tissues on microscopy: tissue defects at the point of direct application, followed by a narrow zone of charred tissue and a coagulation zone.

The rhodamine 6G dye laser also caused duct perforation after 300 pulses at 100 mJ and similar damages to the tissue (**Fig. 8**). Thanks to the energy reduction, no macroscopic or microscopic damage was seen in the parotid duct, even after the application of 1000 pulses, if the "stone recognition" mode was preselected. Bombarding the

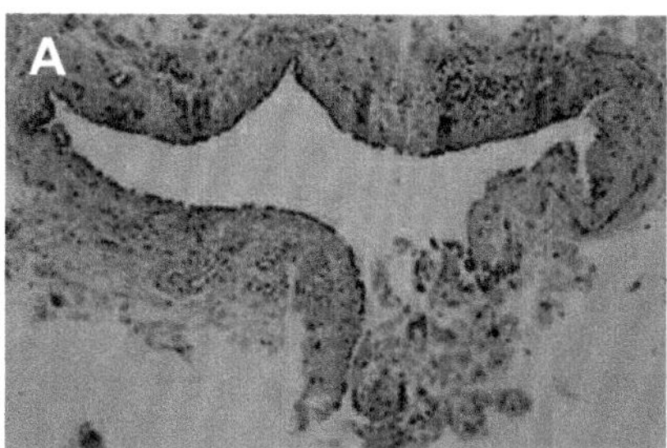

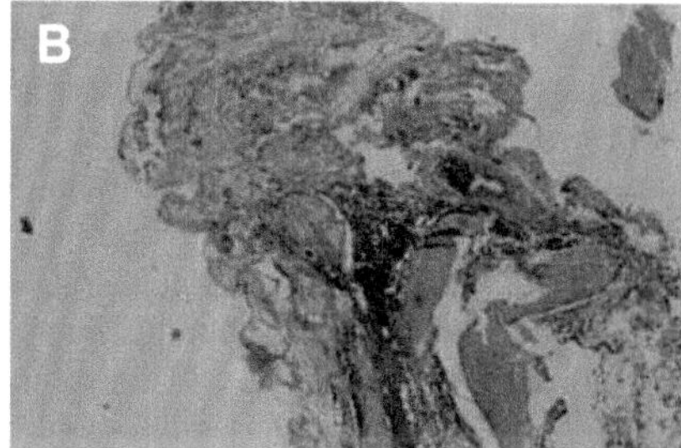

Fig. 7. (*A*) Microscopically visible duct perforation after application of an excimer laser (HE, ×100). (*B*) Microscopic damage to the facial nerve in rabbits after direct application of an excimer laser (HE, ×100).

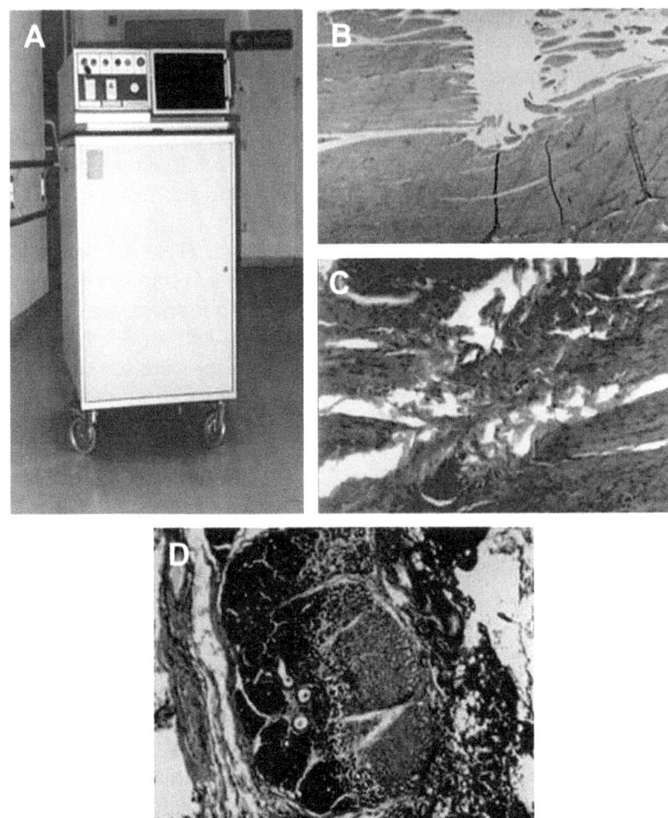

Fig. 8. (*A*) Rhodamin-6G-dye-Laser Lithognost. (*B, C*) Damage of muscles after direct application of laser energy without the stone-detection mode. No damages occurred when the stone-tissue detection mode was switched on (HE, ×100). (*D*) Direct mechanical and thermal damage to the facial nerve after application of shock waves with the Lithognost laser (stone-tissue detection mode was switched off) (HE, ×25). No damage with the mode switched on.

masseter and the salivary gland parenchyma caused bleeding with subsequent failure of the automatic energy reduction and then similar changes to those described previously.

Kerr and colleagues[48] reported treating two patients successfully with the Ho:YAG laser. In a recent study of 17 cases treated with this laser, the authors reported that all stones were completely fragmented.[49] This study was part of a larger one using several different techniques with limited data on the protocol used, however, both in terms of selection criteria and the treatment provided. One reported disadvantage of this laser is its inability to sustain the beam to the center of the stone. As a result, the cut is at the periphery of the stone, which increases the risk of duct wall damage.

The use of the Er:YAG laser was initially limited by the lack of appropriate delivery systems. This problem was addressed by the development of hollow metal wave guides optimized for Er:YAG laser transmission, end-sealed with a polished sapphire rod of 0.63-mm diameter.[50] Using an endoscope and the Opusdent laser (Lumenis Ltd, Yokneam, Israel) with a pulse energy of 150 to 300 mJ (10 Hz), fragmentation rates of 1.8 mm^3/s were achieved; 21 stones in 18 glands were treated. Where complete fragmentation was not possible, preparation for forceps retrieval and separation of the surrounding tissue to facilitate endoscopic or surgical removal were performed. The technique was successful in only five (24%) cases.

Siedek and colleagues[51] reported the latest in vitro study of the effects induced by the frequency doubled Q-switched–double pulse Nd:YAG (FREDDY) laser (532 nm/1064 nm, W.O.M. World of Medicine AG, Ludwigsstadt, Germany) and the Ho:YAG laser (2100 nm, AURIGA, StarMedTec GmbH, Starnberg Germany) on 15 salivary calculi and on salivary gland tissue.

Stones treated with the Ho:YAG were vaporized in a milling-like process, whereas the FREDDY laser cracked the stones into pieces, although fragmentation failed in two cases. The fragmentation rates achieved by the FREDDY laser were greater than those of the Ho:YAG laser, but the fragments were mainly bigger. Results did not depend on the composition of the stones. Laser pulse effects on soft tissue were found slightly beyond the mucosa and epithelium of the duct walls.

Histologic sections of the salivary duct specimens showed laser damage to the tissue for both FREDDY and Ho:YAG laser applications. With contact laser light application, the epithelium of the duct was disrupted and the submucosal layer showed damage up to the muscularis propria. Although the FREDDY laser induced more punched-out, circular lesions with minor lateral thermal changes, the Ho:YAG laser caused eruption of the superficial tissue layer and a visible lesion.

Overall, the study clearly demonstrated the different processes of destroying salivary calculi using two different laser systems. Although both laser systems posed little direct risk to the surrounding tissue, it still has to be shown whether cracked and accelerated particles harm soft tissue. A complete overview and summary for lasers used in vitro and in vivo for the treatment of salivary stones is listed in **Table 3**.

INTRACORPOREAL ELECTROHYDRAULIC LITHOTRIPSY

History

In the early 1950s, Yutkin discovered the principle of electrohydraulic shock waves.[52] Electrolithotripsy was then used in industry to fragment rock in mines. After Reese, an engineer in Riga, had undergone successful surgery for a ureteral stone, he had the idea of using the industrial technique for medical purposes.[53] He developed the prototype of the Urat 1 lithotripter, which was used for the first successful tests on fragmenting bladder calculi in vitro in 1960. The appliance was presented to the western world at Expo 67 in Montreal, where it aroused great interest, because it offered another physical principle in addition to mechanical stone fragmentation.

Voltage built up in a generator, with the help of capacitors, discharges within a fraction of a second. This causes a spark across the gap between the otherwise insulated anode and cathode at the tip of a thin probe, with resultant thermal expansion of the spark plasma (T>10,000 K) and surrounding fluid. This generates a spherically propagated shock wave. Intracorporeal electrohydraulic lithotripsy also has to be applied in contact with surrounding fluid. The intensity of the shock waves depends on the diameter of the probe and the voltage applied.

First reports of basic investigations and use on bladder and ureteral stones followed swiftly. Complications, however, such as bladder and ureteral perforation, were reported.[53–56] The later development of miniaturized probes and generators with lower power and direct endoscopically guided application reduced the complication rate and allowed the use of intracorporeal lithotripsy in the common bile duct and ureter. Nevertheless, here too there were soon reports of perforation and complications, so

Table 3
Lasers designated or used for intracorporeal lithotripsy of salivary stones up do date

Laser	Wavelength in nm	Energy/Pulse in mJ/s	Frequency in Hz	Diameter of Fiber in mm	Stone Fragmentation in Vitro	Tissue Reactions in Vivo	Authors
Dye (cumarine)	504	50	10	600	+ (53 shots per mg stone)	Duct wall damages possible	Sterenborg et al 1990 and 1991[44]
Excimer	308/351	10–15	20–40	400	++ (1 cm stone in 10 min)	No side effects in patients reported	Gundlach et al 1990[45]
Alexandrite	755	60	10	200	(+) case report about 1 stone	No side effects reported	Arzoz et al 1994[67]
Alexandrite	755	80	10	400	– 2/12 stones fragmented		Iro et al 1995[46]
Neodymium:YAG	1024	60	2–13	400	– No fragmentation		Iro et al 1995[46]
Dye (coumarine)	504	160	2–10	320	– No fragmentation		Iro et al 1995[46]
Excimer	308	10–20	20–40	400	+++ (all stones fragmented)	Duct perforations and tissue coagulation	Iro et al 1995[46]

Rhodamine-6G dye without tissue detection	595	60–80	10	400	++ (73% of stones fragmented)	Duct perforations and tissue coagulation	Iro et al 1995[46]
Rhodamine-6G dye with tissue detection	595	60–80	10	400	++ (73% of stones fragmented)	No severe tissue damage	Iro et al 1995[46]; Zenk et al 1994[29]
Holmium:YAG	2100	500 (300–800)	3	230	++ 24.5 – 66.6 mg/min, total disintegration in all stones	Duct damages visible, thermal changes	Kerr et al 2001[48] Papadaki et al 2008[49] Siedek et al 2008[51]
Erbium:YAG	2940	150–300	10	630	(+) fragmentation rate 1.8 mm^3	No early complication	Raif et al 2006[50]
FREDDY	532/1064	120–160	1	230	++ 3–640 mg/min, no tall stones fragmented	Superficial duct damages, smaller thermal-induced changes of epithelium	Siedek et al 2008[51]

Abbreviation: YAG, yttrium-aluminum-garnet.

that intracorporeal electrohydraulic methods have to be used with certain precautions (stone secured in a basket, expanding device to protect duct walls).[57–60] In 1989, Cook and coworkers[61] reported the first case where intracorporeal electrohydraulic lithotripsy was used to treat a salivary calculus under general anesthetic. Königsberger and colleagues[62] used this method on a small patient population and did not report any major complications.

Basic Investigations

In 1993, Iro and colleagues[63] published the first systematic in vitro and in vivo tests using all the electrohydraulic generators available at the time (Lithotron, Walz, Germany; Riwolith, Wolf, Germany; Calcutript, Storz, Germany). Of 58 salivary gland stones treated in vitro with various sizes of probe and intensities, 53 (91%) could be fragmented; 39 (67%) of these had fragments less than 1.5 mm. The number of impulses required fell with increasing diameter of the probe, intensity, and decreasing size of the stone. The mineral composition of the stone and the type of generator had no effect on fragmentation. The stones that were not fragmented or only partially disintegrated were all treated with probes of diameter less than 3F catheter (1 mm).

In vitro tests on surgically removed human salivary glands and their duct systems showed tissue destruction and duct perforation after the application of only two to five single pulses (**Fig. 9**A, B). The same effects were seen with in vivo application in blocked duct systems in rabbits (**Fig. 9**C), and application in the vicinity of the facial nerve, muscles, and salivary glands if the probe tip was less than 2 mm from the tissue in each case. This was also true when the probe was positioned parallel to the tissue (**Fig. 10**). It can be said for intracorporeal electrohydraulic lithotripsy that, even though

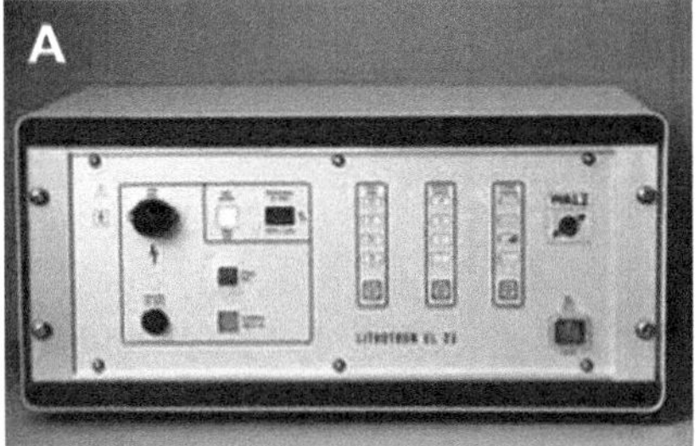

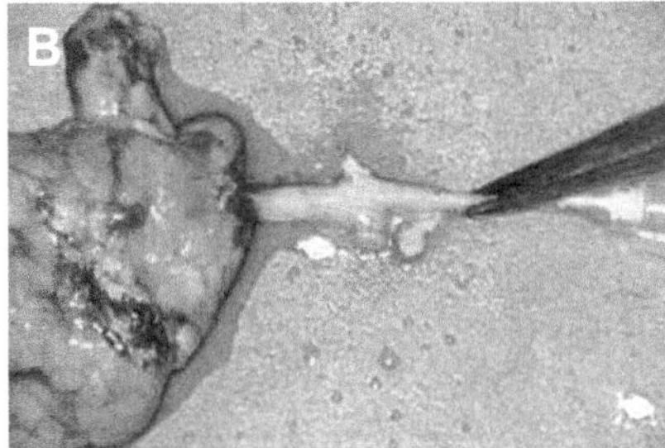

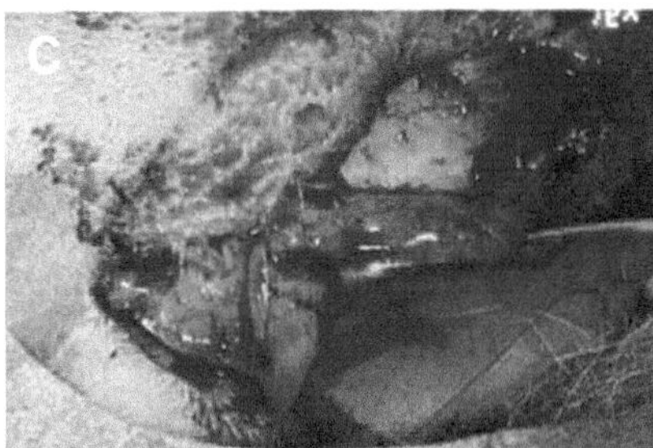

Fig. 9. (*A*) Electrohydraulic intracorporeal device (Lithotron, Walz Company, Germany). (*B*) Direct visible damage to the submandibular duct during application of electrohydraulic intracorporeal shock wave in vitro. (*C*) Duct perforation in vivo in rabbits after application of a single-pulse electrohydraulic intracorporeal lithotripsy fiber with 1.6F catheter. Duct perforation clearly visible together with the electric spark of a subsequent impulse.

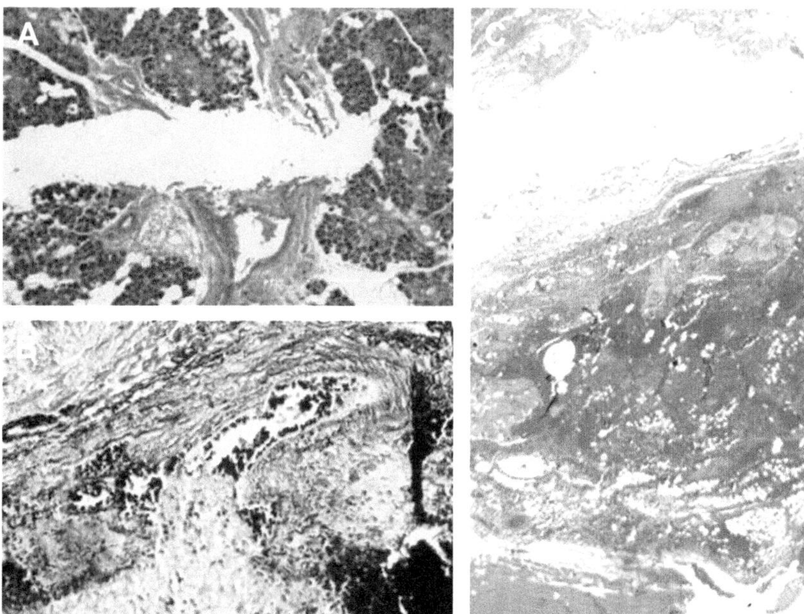

Fig. 10. (*A*) Damage of the parotid tissues after direct application of electrohydraulic intracorporeal shock waves (HE, ×100). (*B*) Bleeding out of a vessel after application of electrohydraulic lithotripsy (trichrome ×200). (*C*) Nerve damage and hematoma near the nerve fibers after electrohydraulic lithotripsy in vivo in rabbits (HE, ×100).

good fragmentation of stones is possible in vitro, a certain minimum energy has to be applied to disrupt the stone sufficiently for it to fragment. Using the smallest 1.6F catheter probes, only two out of seven sialoliths were fragmented therapeutically. In addition, serious tissue damage occurred in the corresponding in vitro and in vivo tissue experiments; this method should not be put into clinical use. Apart from a small number of case reports, such as from Marchal and colleagues 2001,[64] there have been no reports on larger patient populations.

PNEUMATIC LITHOTRIPSY

A new method of lithotripsy under endoscopic guidance was introduced in urology in the 1990s: intracorporeal pneumatic lithotripsy.[65] This system works with ballistic energy and is similar to a biologic "pneumatic hammer." A prerequisite for using this appliance is the connection to a compressed air line. A semiflexible rod with a movable inner "hammer" component is brought directly up to the stone. The relatively low initial outlay for this equipment was a distinct advantage of the method, but the 0.8-mm external diameter of the probe made endoscopic guidance difficult.

Nevertheless, attempts to use this minimally invasive method in the treatment of human sialolithiasis seem to allow the clinical application of pneumatic lithotripsy because of the small diameters of the probes involved. Iro and colleagues[66] investigated the method with in vitro and animal experiments. The Lithoclast (EMS SA, Nyon, Switzerland) pneumatic lithotripter (**Fig. 11**A) was used to treat stones and tissue. Thirty salivary calculi were treated in this way. Four submandibular salivary glands and their ducts were surgically removed and exposed to the pneumatic probes. In two cases a salivary stone was implanted before pneumatic lithotripsy. In

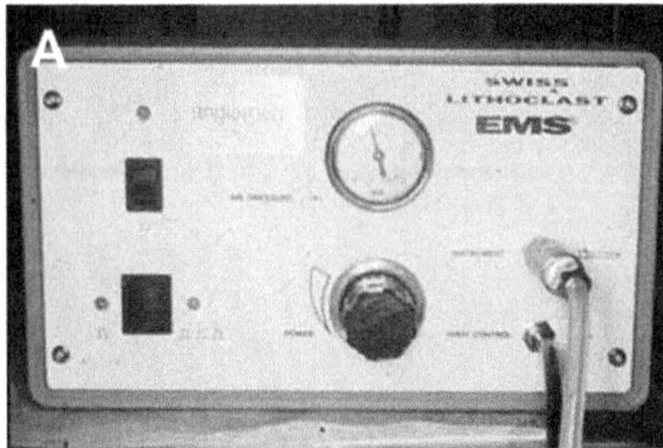

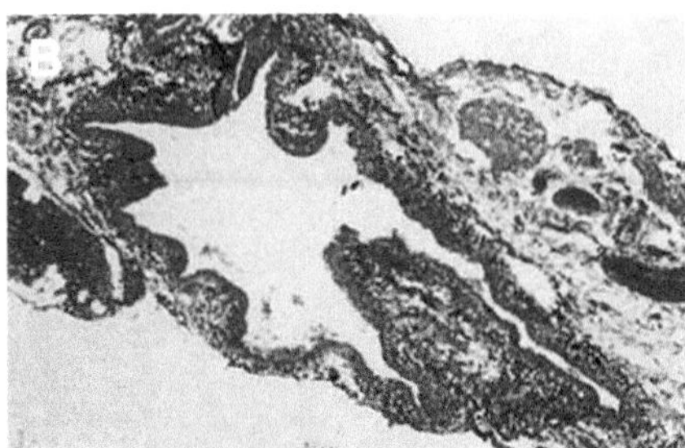

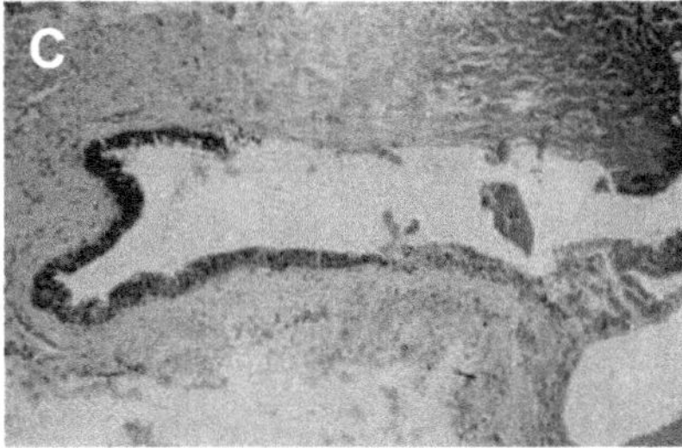

Fig. 11. (*A*) Lithoclast device for pneumatic lithotripsy. (*B*) Regular duct and duct epithelium of Stensen duct (HE, ×100). (*C*) Microscopically visible duct perforation and loss of epithelium after applying pneumatic lithotripsy within the ducts (HE, ×100).

two rabbits, the ducts of the parotid glands were ligated for 2 weeks, stones were placed in two of the four salivary ducts, the pneumatic probes were inserted along the ducts, and lithotripsy was performed.

All of the 30 salivary calculi were reduced to particles smaller than 1.5 mm in diameter. No macroscopic or microscopic damage was detectable while the probe was in a duct. In both the cases with implanted calculi, however, retropulsion of fragments occurred with subsequent perforation of the ducts (**Fig. 11**B, C). After applying ballistic pulses along the duct, small periductal hematomas without perforation could be seen macroscopically. Microscopically, only little bleeding was observed along the submucosa, with partial loss of the epithelium. In contrast, pulse application to the implanted stones led to their destruction, with perforation of the ducts and hemorrhage in the surrounding tissue.

Although the pneumatic lithotripsy method used in this study sufficiently destroyed the salivary calculi, the in vivo and in vitro tissue results showed that the clinical use of this technique does not seem to be justified in the treatment of sialolithiasis in humans.

The only report on pneumoballistic lithotripsy in patients is from Arzoz and colleagues[67] who compared it with laser lithotripsy in a group of 39 patients. Nine patients were treated with the Lithoclast and three with laser. Complete fragmentation was achieved in all cases, without undue trauma to the surrounding tissue.

SUMMARY

Whether a method succeeds in making the transition from technical development to clinical use depends on many factors. First, centers have to work on the development and refinement of the systems and basic investigations, which lead to clinical studies. In this respect, the guiding principle for the treating physician is "nihil nocere," do no harm. In keeping with this principle, extracorporeal lithotripsy has lent itself first and foremost as one of the least invasive methods for the treatment of salivary gland stones and has become well established in Germany and in the arbeitsgemeinschaft der wissenschaftlichen medizinischen fachgesellschaften e.V. guidelines for the treatment of sialolithiasis. Because of the high initial outlay for a mobile lithotripter (about EUR 120,000), its use can be justified only at high patient volume centers. The primary indications for extracorporeal lithotripsy are parotid gland stones, irrespective of their anatomic position in the duct system or size, as long as they cannot be removed endoscopically, and small stones less than 8 mm in the intraparenchymal duct system of the submandibular gland. Apart from a certain experience on the part of the person performing the treatment, important prerequisites for successful stone fragmentation are a generator approved for treating sialolithiasis (appropriate focus volumes and shock wave intensities) and application systems with integrated stone localization (eg, ultrasound). Systems without localization or possibilities for different patient positions, or systems meant for stones other than of the salivary glands, are to be considered obsolete. Interestingly, the development of extracorporeal shock wave lithotripsy has been mainly in European centers. The method has not been approved in the United States by the Food and Drug Administration.

Given the possible adverse effects, it is clear from the literature that both intracorporeal electrohydraulic and pneumoclastic lithotripsy are not suitable for the treatment of salivary gland stones. Taking into account the staff required, the investment and maintenance costs, and efficacy of the method, the indications for intracorporeal laser lithotripsy may be limited compared with the extracorporeal lithotripter. An ideal system (ie, a laser that has a good fragmentation rate, no adverse effects, and causes no tissue damage) does not exist at the present time. Even the rhodamine 6G dye laser with integrated stone-tissue recognition, which the authors used, did not meet expectations in clinical tests.[46] It is also questionable whether the Ho:YAG or the FREDDY laser[51] fulfill the ideal requirements. The clearly improved image quality of the new generation of endoscopes will make the use of lasers safer.

Laser lithotripsy of parotid gland stones has to be measured against the results of extracorporeal lithotripsy and endoscopic transcutaneous stone extraction. For stones in the submandibular gland, this treatment is in direct competition with transoral stone extraction, which gives excellent results.[68,69] There is almost a complete overlap of the indications for the treatment of stones located in the distal duct up to the hilum. When used in combination with extracorporeal shock wave lithotripsy, niches for laser lithotripsy are small stones in the submandibular gland, which cannot be removed transorally but can be endoscopically localized in the second or third order ducts; small sialoliths in the central duct system of the parotid gland, which can be reached with the endoscope; and stones that have proved resistant to extracorporeal shock wave lithotripsy.

REFERENCES

1. Zenk J, Constantinidis J, Kydles S, et al. Clinical and diagnostic findings of sialolithiasis. HNO 1999;47:963–9 [in German].
2. Rauch S, Gorlin R. Diseases of the salivary glands. In: Gorlin RJ, Goldman HM, editors. Oral pathology. St Louis (MO): CV Mosby Company; 1970. p. 997–1003.
3. Escudier MP, McGurk M. Symptomatic sialoadenitis and sialolithiasis in the English population, an estimate of the cost of hospital treatment. Br Dent J 1999;186:463–6.
4. van den Akker HP, Busemann-Sokole E. Submandibular gland function following transoral sialolithectomy. Oral Surg Oral Med Oral Pathol 1983;56:351–6.

5. Escudier MP. The development of salivary lithotripsy: it's role in the management of salivary calculi department of oral medicine. London: University of London; 2008. p. 289.
6. Berlinicke ML, Schenetten F. Effect in vitro of ultrasonic frequencies on gallstones. Klin Wochenschr 1951;29:390 [in German].
7. Mulvaney WP. Attempted disintegration of calculi by ultrasonic vibrations. J Urol 1953;70:704–7.
8. Coats EC. The application of ultrasonic energy to urinary and biliary calculi. J Urol 1956;75:865–74.
9. Schall R. Kurzzeitphysik. In: Vollrath K, Thomer G, editors. Detonationsphysik. Wien (Austria): Springer Verlag; 1976.
10. Chaussy C, Brendel W, Schmiedt E. Extracorporeally induced destruction of kidney stones by shock waves. Lancet 1980;2:1265–8.
11. Sauerbruch T, Delius M, Paumgartner G, et al. Fragmentation of gallstones by extracorporeal shock waves. N Engl J Med 1986;314:818–22.
12. Kerzel W, Ell C, Schneider T, et al. Extracorporeal piezoelectric shockwave lithotripsy of multiple pancreatic duct stones under ultrasonographic control. Endoscopy 1989;21:229–31.
13. Sauerbruch T, Stern M. Fragmentation of bile duct stones by extracorporeal shock waves: a new approach to biliary calculi after failure of routine endoscopic measures. Gastroenterology 1989;96:146–52.
14. Brendel W. Shock waves. A new therapeutic principle in medicine. MMW Munch Med Wochenschr 1984;126:1–3 [in German].
15. Hüter J. Messung der Ultraschallabsorption im tierischen Gewebeund ihre Abhängigkeit von der Frequenz [Measurements of the ultrasound-absorption in animal tissue and its dependence on the frequency]. Naturwissenschaften 1948;35:285–96 [in German].
16. Chaussy C, Eisenberger F, Wanner K, et al. The use of shock waves for the destruction of renal calculi without direct contact. Urol Res 1976;175:175–83.
17. Delius M, Brendel W, Heine G. A mechanism of gallstone destruction by extracorporeal shock waves. Naturwissenschaften 1988;75:200–8.
18. Forssmann B, Hepp W, Chaussy C, et al. Eine Methode zur berührungsfreien Zertrümmerung von Nierensteinen durch Stoßwellen [A method of non contact fragmentation of Kidney Stones by shockwaves]. Biomed Tech 1977;22:164–9 [in German].
19. Coleman A, Saunders J. Comparison of extracorporeal shockwave lithotripters. In: Coleman A, Saunders J, editors. Lithotripsy II. London: BDI Publishing; 1987. p. 121–35.
20. Riedlinger R, Ueberle F, Wurster H, et al. Disintegration of kidney calculi by piezoelectrically generated high-energy sound waves. Physical principles and experimental studies. Urologe A 1986;25:188–92 [in German].
21. Folberth W. A universal lithotripter for interdisciplinary use: the Lithostar plus. In: Carlsson P, Tiselius H, editors. Extracorporeal shock wave lithotripsy: medical, technical, economic and policy implication. Stockholm (Sweden): Almquist and Wiksell periodical company; 1989. p. 136–55.
22. Wilbert D, Hutschenreiter G, Schärfe T, et al. Zweite Gerneration der berührungslosen Nierenstinzertrümmerung - klinische Ergebnisse der lokalen Stoßwellenlithotripsie [Second generation of non contact fragmentation of kidney stones]. Akt Urol 1988;19:93–7 [in German].
23. Marmary Y. A novel and non-invasive method for the removal of salivary gland stones. Int J Oral Maxillofac Surg 1986;15:585–7.

24. Brouns JJ, Hendrikx AJ, Bierkens AF. Removal of salivary stones with the aid of a lithotriptor. J Craniomaxillofac Surg 1989;17:329–30.
25. Iro H, Wessel B, Benzel W, et al. Tissue reactions with administration of piezoelectric shock waves in lithotripsy of salivary calculi. Laryngorhinootologie 1990;69: 102–7 [in German].
26. Iro H, Nitsche N, Meier J, et al. Piezoelectric shock wave lithotripsy of salivary gland stones: an in vitro feasibility study. J Lithotr Stone Dis 1991;3: 211–6.
27. Zenk J, Hosemann WG, Iro H. Diameters of the main excretory ducts of the adult human submandibular and parotid gland: a histologic study. Oral Surg Oral Med Oral Pathol Oral Radiol Endod 1998;85:576–80.
28. Iro H, Nitsche N, Schneider HT, et al. Extracorporeal shockwave lithotripsy of salivary gland stones. Lancet 1989;2:115.
29. Zenk J, Benzel W, Iro H. New modalities in the management of human sialolithiasis. MIT 1994;275–84.
30. Kater W, Meyer WW, Rachel U, et al. Lithotripsy of salivary calculi as a noninvasive treatment alternative to surgical removal of calculi. Biomed Tech (Berl) 1990; 35(Suppl 3):239–40 [in German].
31. Ottaviani F, Capaccio P, Campi M, et al. Extracorporeal electromagnetic shock-wave lithotripsy for salivary gland stones. Laryngoscope 1996;106: 761–4.
32. Benzel W, Zenk J, Iro H. Vergleich verschiedener Stoßwellensysteme zur extrakorporalen Lithotripsie von Submandibularissteinen 66. Jahresversammlung der Deutschen Gesellschft für HNO-Heilkunde, Kopf- udn Halschirurgie. Karlsruhe, 1995.
33. Iro H, Zenk J, Waldfahrer F, et al. Extracorporeal shock wave lithotripsy of parotid stones: results of a prospective clinical trial. Ann Otol Rhinol Laryngol 1998;107: 860–4.
34. Schlick R, Hessling K, Djamilian M, et al. ESWL in patients suffering from sialolithiasis. MIT 1993;2:129–33.
35. Iro H, Zenk J, Waldfahrer F, et al. Current status of minimally invasive treatment methods in sialolithiasis. HNO 1996;44:78–84 [in German].
36. Iro H, Schneider T, Nitsche N, et al. Extracorporeal piezoelectric lithotripsy of salivary calculi. Initial clinical experiences. HNO 1990;38:251–5 [in German].
37. Kater W, Meyer WW, Wehrmann T, et al. Efficacy, risks, and limits of extracorporeal shock wave lithotripsy for salivary gland stones. J Endourol 1994;8: 21–4.
38. Katz P. Nouvelle approche therapeutiques calculus salivaires. la lithotripsie extra corporelle- a propos de 200 cases [A new therapautic approach for salivary stones: extracorporeal lithotripsy–report about 200 cases]. Rev Stomatol Chir Maxillofac 1998;99:109–11 [in French].
39. Harten H. Physik für Mediziner. Berlin: Springer Verlag; 1987.
40. Tradowsky K. Laser-Grundlagen, Technik und Basisanwendungen. Würzburg (Germany): Vogel-Buchverlag; 1983.
41. Weber H, Herziger G. Laser-Grundlagen und Anwendung. Weinheim (Germany): Physik Verlag; 1978.
42. Reidenbach H. Hochfrequenz- und Lasertechnik in der Medizin. Berlin: Springer Verlag; 1983.
43. Mulvaney WP, Beck CW. The laser beam in urology. J Urol 1968;99:112–5.
44. Sterenborg HJ, de Reijke TM, Wiersma J, et al. High-speed photographic evaluation of endoscopic lithotripsy devices. Urol Res 1991;19:381–5.

45. Gundlach P, Scherer H, Hopf J, et al. Endoscopic-controlled laser lithotripsy of salivary calculi. In vitro studies and initial clinical use. HNO 1990;38:247–50 [in German].
46. Iro H, Zenk J, Benzel W. Laser lithotripsy of salivary duct stones. Adv Otorhinolaryngol 1995;49:148–52.
47. Wallenborn WM, Sydnor TA, Hsu YT, et al. Experimental production of parotid gland atrophy by ligation of Stensen's duct and by irradiation. Laryngoscope 1964;74:644–55.
48. Kerr PD, Krahn H, Brodovsky D. Endoscopic laser lithotripsy of a proximal parotid duct calculus. J Otolaryngol 2001;30:129–30.
49. Papadaki ME, McCain JP, Kim K, et al. Interventional sialoendoscopy: early clinical results. J Oral Maxillofac Surg 2008;66:954–62.
50. Raif J, Vardi M, Nahlieli O, et al. An Er:YAG laser endoscopic fiber delivery system for lithotripsy of salivary stones. Lasers Surg Med 2006;38:580–7.
51. Siedek V, Betz CS, Hecht V, et al. Laser induced fragmentation of salivary stones: an in vitro comparison of two different, clinically approved laser systems. Lasers Surg Med 2008;40:257–64.
52. Frimberger E, Kuhner W, Weingart J, et al. A new method of electrohydraulic cholelithotripsy (lithoklasia) (author's transl). Dtsch Med Wochenschr 1982;107:213–5 [in German].
53. Gellissen H, Reuter HJ. First experience with electrohydraulic lithotripsy of ureteral calculi. Z Urol Nephrol 1974;67:81–7 [in German].
54. Kierfeld G, Mellin P, Daum H. Lithotripsy using hydraulic waves in animal experiments. Urologe 1969;8:99–102 [in German].
55. Mitchell ME, Kerr WS Jr. Experience with the electrohydraulic disintegrator. J Urol 1977;117:159–60.
56. Rouvalis P. Electronic lithotripsy for vesical calculus with Urat-:1: an experience of 100 cases and an experimental application of the method to stones in the upper urinary tract. Br J Urol 1970;42:486–91.
57. Koch H, Stolte M, Walz V. Endoscopic lithotripsy in the common bile duct. Endoscopy 1977;9:95–8.
58. Liguory CL, Bonnel D, Canard JM, et al. Intracorporeal electrohydraulic shock wave lithotripsy of common bile duct stones: preliminary results in 7 cases. Endoscopy 1987;19:237–40.
59. Raney AM. Electrohydraulic lithotripsy: experimental study and case reports with the stone disintegrator. J Urol 1975;113:345–7.
60. Mo LR, Hwang MH, Yueh SK, et al. Percutaneous transhepatic choledochoscopic electrohydraulic lithotripsy (PTCS-EHL) of common bile duct stones. Gastrointest Endosc 1988;34:122–5.
61. Cook HP, Borrows DJ, Milroy EJ. Lithotripsy of inaccessible salivary duct stone. Lancet 1988;2:213–4.
62. Konigsberger R, Feyh J, Goetz A, et al. Endoscopically-controlled electrohydraulic intracorporeal shock wave lithotripsy (EISL) of salivary stones. J Otolaryngol 1993;22:12–3.
63. Iro H, Zenk J, Hosemann WG, et al. Electrohydraulic intracorporeal lithotripsy of salivary calculi: in vitro and animal experiment studies. HNO 1993;41:389–95 [in German].
64. Marchal F, Dulguerov P, Becker M, et al. Specificity of parotid sialendoscopy. Laryngoscope 2001;111:264–71 [in German].
65. Denstedt JD, Eberwein PM, Singh RR. The Swiss Lithoclast: a new device for intracorporeal lithotripsy. J Urol 1992;148:1088–90.

66. Iro H, Benzel W, Gode U, et al. Pneumatic intracorporeal lithotripsy of salivary calculi. In vitro and animal experiment studies. HNO 1995;43:172–6 [in German].
67. Arzoz E, Santiago A, Esnal F, et al. Endoscopic intracorporeal lithotripsy for sialolithiasis. J Oral Maxillofac Surg 1996;54:847–50 [discussion: 851–2].
68. Zenk J, Constantinidis J, Al-Kadah B, et al. Transoral removal of submandibular stones. Arch Otolaryngol Head Neck Surg 2001;127:432–6.
69. Iro H, Zenk J, Escudier MP, et al. Outcome of minimally invasive management of salivary calculi in 4,691 patients. Laryngoscope 2009;119:263–8.

Extracorporeal Lithotripsy Techniques for Salivary Stones

Pasquale Capaccio, MD*, Sara Torretta, MD, Lorenzo Pignataro, MD

KEYWORDS

- Salivary stones • Salivary gland disease • Lithotripsy
- ESWL • Sialendoscopy

Sialolithiasis accounts for approximately 50% of major salivary gland disease.[1] It is the most common cause of salivary obstruction and its estimated prevalence in the general population is 1.2%.[2,3] More frequently, and mainly unilaterally, it affects the submandibular gland (80%–90%),[4] with most of the stones located in the distal third of the duct or at the glandular hilum, whereas intraparenchymal sites are infrequent.[5] Only 5% to 10% of salivary stones involve the parotid gland.[6] Sublingual and minor salivary glands are involvement is unusual.

Ultrasonography (US) has an accuracy of 99% for stones with a diameter of more than 1.5 mm in experienced hands.[7] It can detect stones, whether or not they are radiopaque or nonradiopaque, and evaluate their size and relationship with the surrounding tissues.[8] The opportunity of distinguishing parenchymal and ductal locations by means of US makes it feasible to plan the best therapeutic option for each patient. Moreover, US examination together with color Doppler monitoring provides useful information about the structural features of the affected gland; it detects the possible concomitance of inflammation and can differentiate vascular and ductal structures.[9] It is an operator-dependent procedure, however, which may lead to difficulties in identifying the distal portion of Wharton's duct inside the floor of the mouth and may be responsible for undetected stones; in this case, the use of endoral radiographs and standard dental radiographs is diagnostically helpful.

The traditional therapeutic approach to stones is surgical duct dissection in the case of salivary stones located in the distal and middle portion of the ductal system and sialadenectomy in the case of proximal, hilar, and intraparenchymal stones.[10]

Over the past 20 years, new minimally invasive gland-preserving techniques have been introduced in the management of sialolithiasis, including shock wave lithotripsy, sialoendoscopy, interventional radiology, and endoscopic video-assisted transoral and transcervical stone retrieval.[11]

Department of Specialist Surgical Sciences, Fondazione I.R.C.C.S. Ospedale Maggiore Policlinico, Mangiagalli e Regina Elena, University of Milan, Via Francesco Sforza 35, 20122 Milano, Italy

* Corresponding author.

E-mail address: pasquale.capaccio@unimi.it (P. Capaccio).

Otolaryngol Clin N Am 42 (2009) 1139–1159
doi:10.1016/j.otc.2009.08.003
oto.theclinics.com

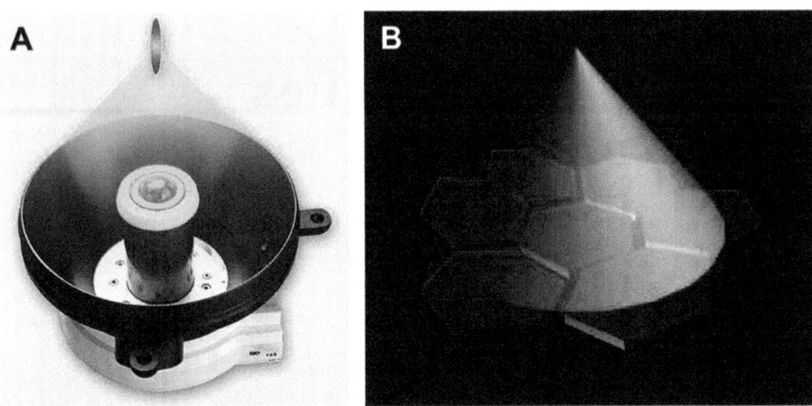

Fig. 1. Shock waves production by means of electromagnetic (*A*) and piezoelectric (*B*) sources.

Shock wave lithotripsy fragments stones so that they can be flushed out by physiologic saliva flowing out the duct. The shock waves may be produced by extracorporeal (electromagnetic or piezoelectric) sources (**Fig. 1**) or intracorporeal (electrohydraulic, pneumatic, or laser endoscopic) sources.[12–20] The former are performed under US

Table 1
Results of electromagnetic extracorporeal shock wave lithotripsy in the treatment of salivary calculi

Author	Year	Site	Number	Complete Stone Clearance (%)
Wehrmann et al[13]	1994	P	29	
		SM	44	
		All	73	38 (52)
Kater et al[26]	1994	P	29	14 (48)
		SM	75	26 (35)
		All	104	40 (38)
Ottaviani et al[14]	1996	P	16	9 (56)
		SM	36	15 (42)
		All	52	24 (46)
Ottaviani et al[27]	1997	P	24	14 (58)
		SM	56	23 (41)
		All	80	37 (46)
Escudier et al[15]	2003	P	32	13 (40)
		SM	84	27 (32)
		All	122	40 (33)
Capaccio et al[28]	2004	P	88	61 (69)
		SM	234	84 (36)
		All	322	145 (45)
McGurk et al[29]	2005	P	88	42 (48)
		SM	130	42 (32)
		All	218	84 (38)
Schmitz et al[30]	2008	P	59	18 (39)
		SM	126	33 (26)
		All	167	51 (30)

Abbreviations: P, parotid; SM, submandibular.

Table 2
Results of piezoelectric extracorporeal shock wave lithotripsy in the treatment of salivary calculi

Author	Year	Site	Number	Complete Stone Clearance (%)
Iro et al[31]	1992	P	16	9 (56)[a]; 13 (81)[b]
		SM	35	13 (37)[a]; 14 (40)[b]
		All	51	22 (43)[a]; 27 (53)[b]
Aïdan et al[32]	1996	P	3	1 (33)
		SM	12	4 (33)
		All	15	5 (33)
Iro et al[33]	1998	P	76	38 (50)
Külkens et al[34]	2003	P	42	26 (62)
Zenk et al[35]	2004	SM	197	58 (29)

Abbreviations: P, parotid; SM, submandibular.
[a] Four weeks after treatment.
[b] Twenty weeks after treatment.

control, which allows stone identification and targeted administration of the shock wave with real-time visualization of the fragmentation process, avoiding any iatrogenic lesions of the surrounding tissue; the latter mainly uses a laser beam brought to the stone by means of an endoscope and fiberoptics.

The most frequently used extracorporeal shock wave lithotripsy (ESWL) energy source is electromagnetic as it is minimally invasive and can be used on an outpatient basis without anesthesia. It was introduced in the 1980s for treatment of renal calculi and gallstones.[21,22] Electromagnetic and piezoelectric sources exploit the compressive and expansive waves generated by the difference in impedance at the stone-water interface and cause stone cavitation.[23] After encouraging results with multiple animal and in vitro experiments, the first successful ESWL for human sialolithiasis

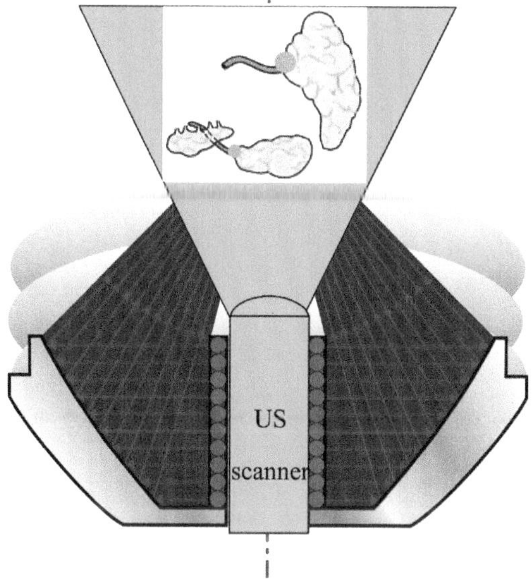

Fig. 2. US focusing shock waves on salivary stones.

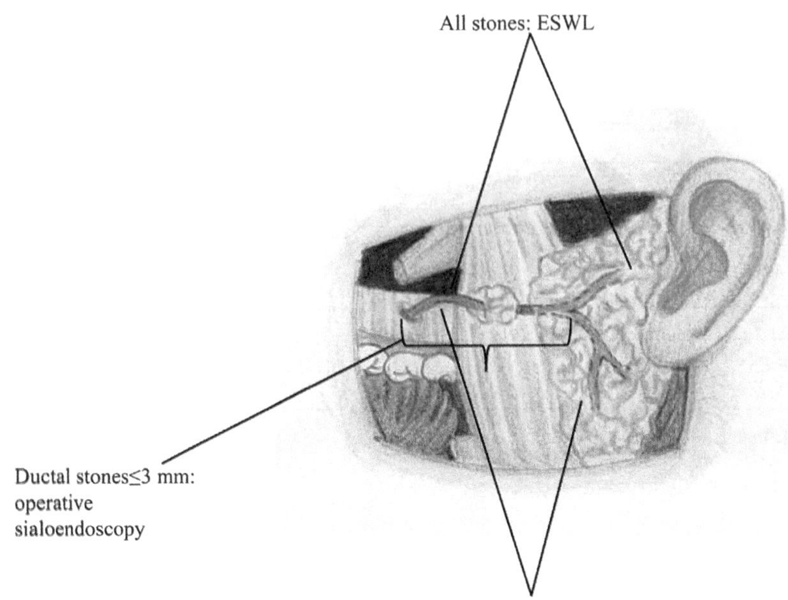

Fig. 3. Current minimally invasive management of parotid stones according to their site and size.

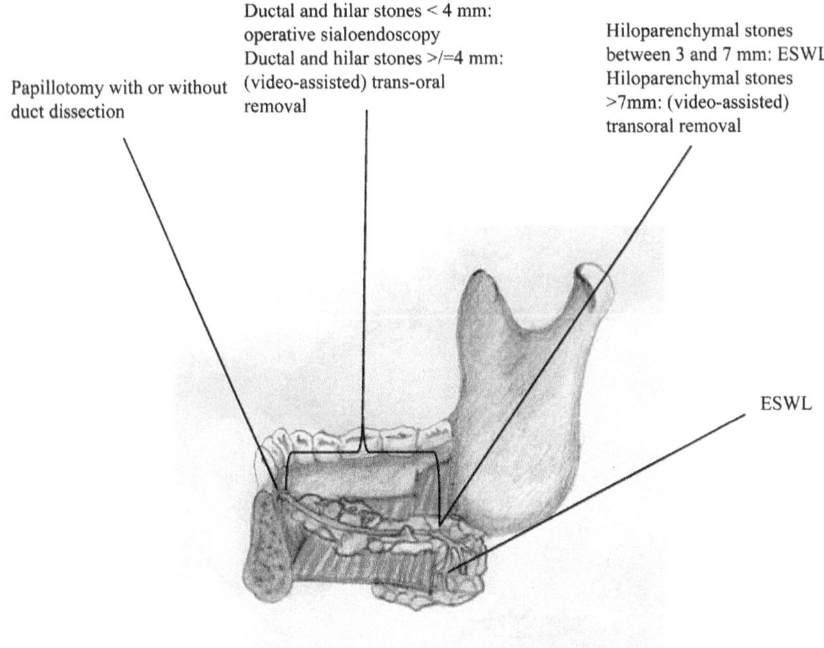

Fig. 4. Current minimally invasive management of submandibular stones according to their site and size.

was performed by Iro and colleagues[24,25] in 1989 using a device designed for renal lithotripsy. Since then, dedicated instruments have been designed and the use of ESWL has become increasingly widespread (**Tables 1** and **2**).[9,13–15,26–35]

US is used to focus the shock waves on the stone (**Fig. 2**). All of the stones that can be identified ultrasonographically and have a diameter of at least 2.4 mm are potentially amenable to treatment.[27] The minimal size of the electromagnetic focus is 2.4 mm. In the case of proximal locations or mobile intraductal stones, however, other therapeutic procedures should be preferred, such as dilatation/dissection of the proximal duct tract and retrieval by means of sialoendoscopy or interventional radiology

Table 3
Untoward effects of extracorporeal shock wave lithotripsy in the treatment of salivary calculi

Untoward Effects	Author	Year	Technique	Total Treated	Number (%)
Pain	Iro et al[31]	1992	P	51	51 (100)
	Wehrmann et al[13]	1994	E	56	56 (100)
	Ottaviani et al[14]	1996	E	52	8 (15)
	Yoshizaki et al[38]	1996	P	18	17 (94)
	Iro et al[33]	1998	P	76	53 (70)
	Capaccio et al[28]	2004	E	322	254 (79)
Swelling	Iro et al[31]	1992	P	51	1 (3)
	Ottaviani et al[14]	1996	E	52	5 (10)
	Capaccio et al[28]	2004	E	322	113 (35)
	Zenk et al[35]	2004	P	197	4 (2)
Ductal bleeding	Wehrmann et al[13]	1994	E	56	4 (71)
	Ottaviani et al[14]	1996	E	52	9 (17)
	Iro et al[33]	1998	P	76	30 (40)
	Escudier et al[15]	2003	E	122	49 (40)
	Capaccio et al[28]	2004	E	322	126 (39)
	Zenk et al[35]	2004	P	197	108 (55)
Cutaneous petechiae	Iro et al[31]	1992	P	51	7 (14)
	Wehrmann et al[13]	1994	E	56	11 (20)
	Ottaviani et al[14]	1996	E	52	3 (6)
	Yoshizaki et al[38]	1996	P	18	4 (22)
	Iro et al[33]	1998	P	76	30 (40)
	Capaccio et al[28]	2004	E	322	74 (23)
	Zenk et al[35]	2004	P	197	108 (55)
Acute sialadenitis	Escudier et al[15]	2003	E	122	7 (6)
	Zenk et al[35]	2004	P	197	4 (2)
	Schmitz et al[30]	2008	E	167	5 (3)
Temporary hearing	Kater et al[26]	1994	E	104	2 (2)
impairment	Iro et al[33]	1998	P	76	2 (3)
Temporary tinnitus	Kater et al[26]	1994	E	104	2 (2)
	Capaccio et al[28]	2004	E	322	2 (1)
	Schmitz et al[30]	2008	E	167	1 (1)
Tooth filling loss	Schmitz et al[30]	2008	E	167	2 (1)

Abbreviations: E, electromagnetic; P, piezoelectric.

Table 4
Demographic features, clinical data, and outcomes of treated patients

		Group A		Group B	
First level: demographic and clinical data		Number: 322 Males (%): 172 (53.4) Mean age ± SD: 6.6 ± 0.9 Submandibular (%): 234 (72.7) Intraductal (%): 112 (47.9) Hiloparenchymal (%): 122 (52.1) Parotid (%): 88 (27.3) Intraductal: 58 (65.9) Hiloparenchymal: 30 (34.1)		Number: 93 Males (%): 43 (46.2) Mean age ±SD: 5.1 ± 0.4 Submandibular (%): 45 (48.4) Intraductal (%): 19 (42.2) Hiloparenchymal (%): 26 (57.8) Parotid (%): 48 (51.6) Intraductal: 27 (56.2) Hiloparenchymal: 21 (43.8)	
Second level: treatment		Mean duration ±SD: 30 minutes ± 2.3 Mean number of shock waves ± SD: 1779 ± 3.4 Mean number of treatments ± SD: 6 ± 0.4		Mean duration ±SD: 31 min ± 2.7 Mean number of shock waves ± SD: 1829 ± 2.9 Mean number of treatments ± SD: 6 ± 0.8	
Third level: outcomes		Submandibular		Submandibular	
		D (%)	HP (%)	D (%)	HP (%)
	Complete stone clearance	52 (64.4)	32 (26.2)	12 (63.1)	10 (38.5)
	Residual fragments ≤2 mm	30 (26.8)	34 (27.9)	4 (21.1)	6 (23.0)
	Residual fragments >2 mm	30 (26.8)	56 (45.9)	3 (15.8)	10 (38.5)
	Total	112	122	19	26
		Parotid		Parotid	
		D (%)	HP (%)	D (%)	HP (%)
	Complete stone clearance	41 (70.7)	20 (66.7)	19 (70.4)	14 (66.7)
	Residual fragments ≤2 mm	15 (25.9)	9 (30)	7 (25.9)	4 (19.0)
	Residual fragments >2 mm	2 (3.4)	1 (3.3)	1 (3.7)	3 (14.3)
	Total	58	30	27	21

Fourth level: untoward effects	Local pain (%): 256 (79.5) Glandular swelling (%): 113 (35.2) Ductal hemorrhage (%): 124 (38.6) Cutaneous petechiae (%): 73 (22.7) Tinnitus (%): 2 (0.6)	Local pain (%): 75 (80.6) Glandular swelling (%): 30 (32.2) Ductal hemorrhage (%): 32 (34.4) Cutaneous petechiae (%): 22 (23.6) Tinnitus (%): 0 (0.0)
Fifth level: other required treatments	Recurrence (%): 4 (1.2) Papillotomy procedure (%): 26 (8.1) Sialadenectomy (%): 10 (3.1) — —	Recurrence (%): 2 (2.1) Papillotomy procedure (%): 9 (9.7) Sialadenectomy (%): 1 (1.1) Sialoendoscopy (%): 9 (9.7) Transoral removal (%): 8 (8.6)

Abbreviations: D, ductal; HP, hiloparenchymal.

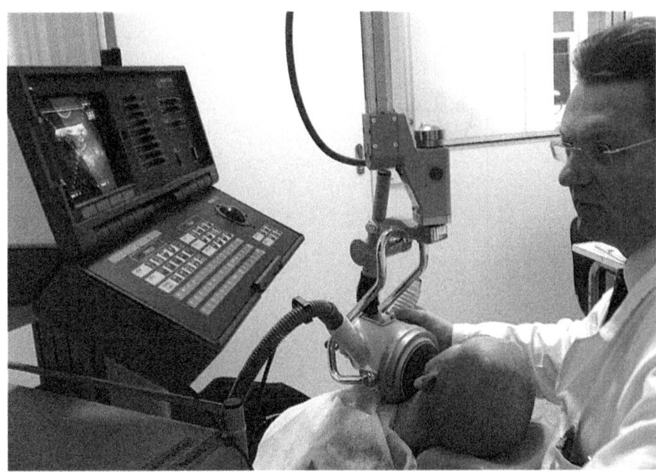

Fig. 5. Electromagnetic ESWL in a patient with a submandibular stone.

techniques (**Figs. 3** and **4**).[36] The contraindications for ESWL are complete distal duct stenosis, pregnancy, and the presence of a cardiac pacemaker. Relative contraindications include acute sialadenitis or other acute inflammatory processes of the head and neck; treatment should be postponed in these cases.[27,30,37]

With regard to the effectiveness of electromagnetic ESWL of salivary stones, it is difficult to compare the published results directly because of criteria differences used to define outcomes:[30] definition of complete or partial success ($\leq$2 and

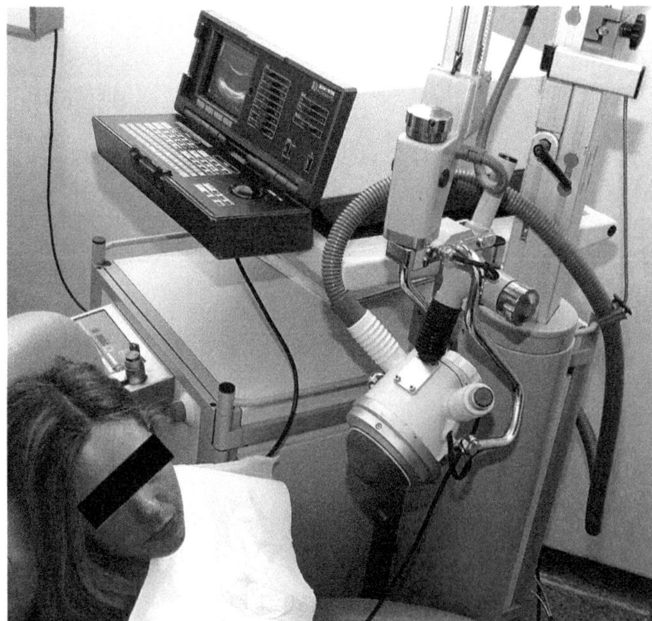

Fig. 6. Step-by-step procedure of ESWL.

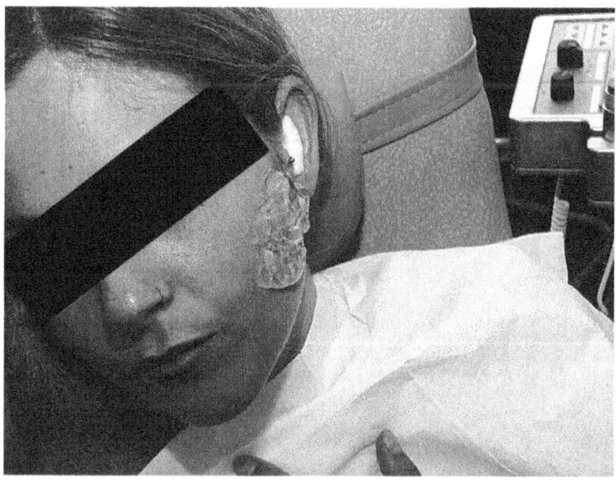

Fig. 7. Step-by-step procedure of ESWL.

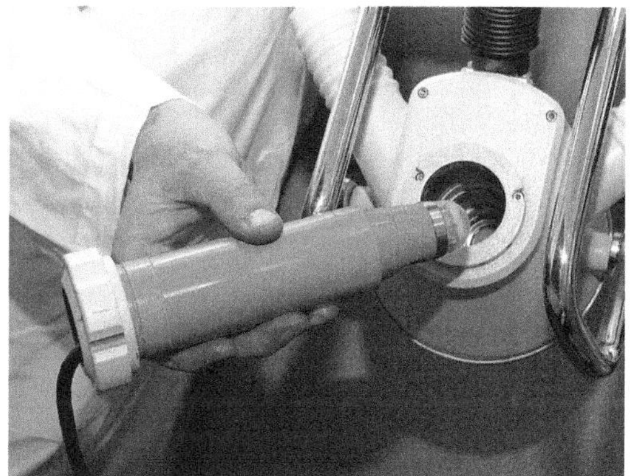

Fig. 8. Step-by-step procedure of ESWL.

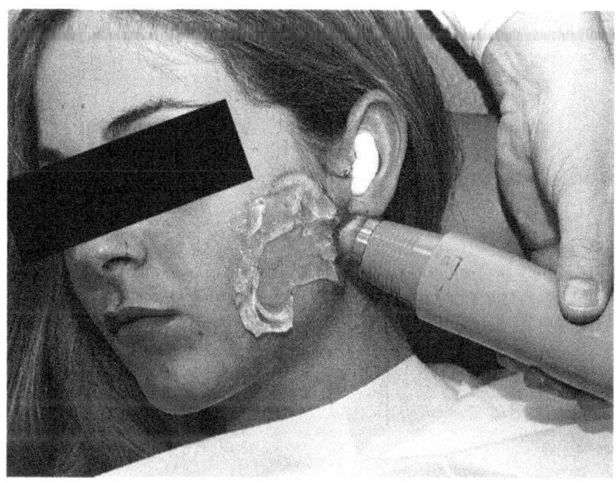

Fig. 9. Step-by-step procedure of ESWL.

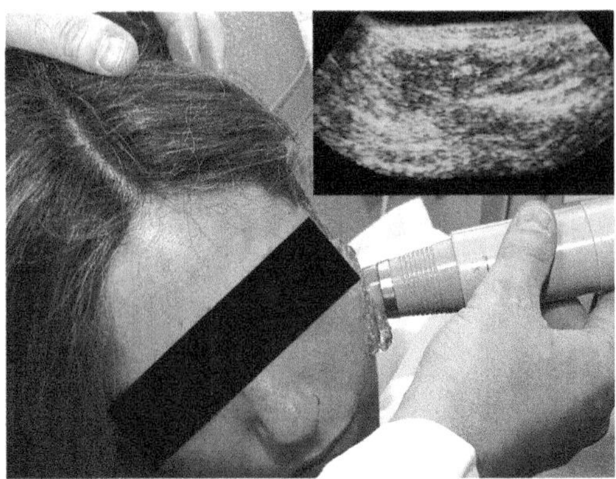

Fig. 10. Step-by-step procedure of ESWL.

>2 mm, respectively) or symptom status after lithotripsy.[14,27,28] On the basis of the published findings, the success rate is higher in the case of parotid than in the case of submandibular stones: complete stone clearance has been reported in 39% to 69% of parotid stones[9,15,16,26–30] but only 26% to 42% in submandibular stones (see **Table 1**)[9,15,16,26–30] treated electromagnetically, and, respectively, 33% to 81%[31–34] and 29% to –40%,[31,32,35] of those treated piezoelectrically (see **Table 2**).

ESWL is safe, and only minor and self-limiting untoward effects have generally been reported, including pain over the treated area, glandular swelling, ductal bleeding, and cutaneous petechiae (**Table 3**).[11,13–15,26,28–31,33,35,38–40]

PERSONAL EXPERIENCE

Population and Setting

Between December 1993 and December 2002, 322 consecutive patients (group A) with single or multiple symptomatic submandibular (234) or parotid (88) salivary stones were enrolled at the ear, nose, and throat department of University of Milan and underwent a complete cycle of extracorporeal lithotripsy ESWL.[28] The exclusion criteria

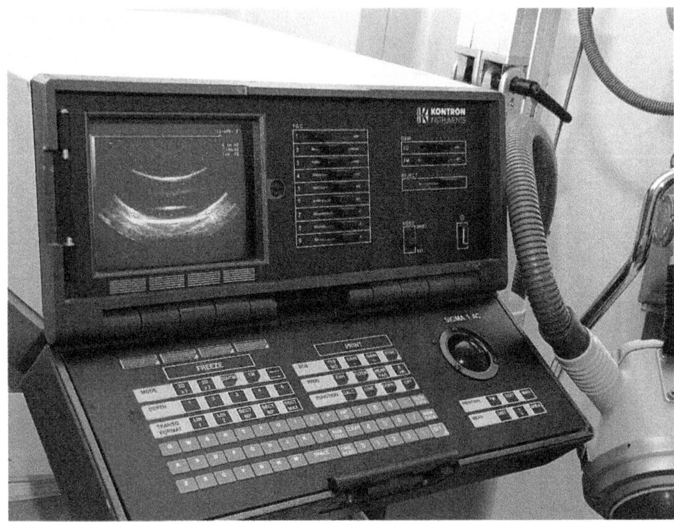

Fig. 11. Step-by-step procedure of ESWL.

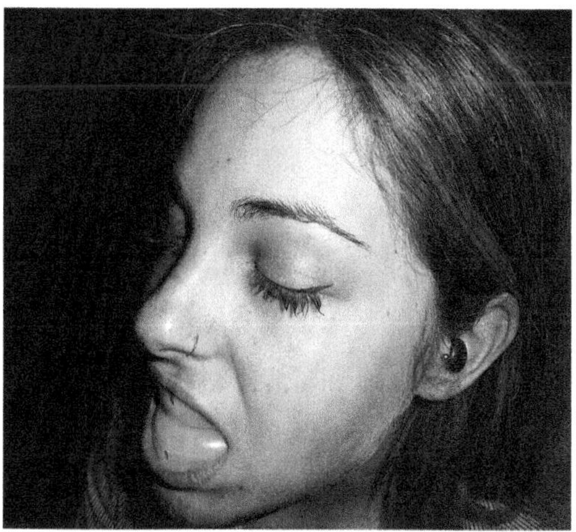

Fig. 12. Step-by-step procedure of ESWL.

were distal stones amenable to surgical duct dilatation and dissection or mobile intraductal stones that could be removed by means of a Dormia basket. Univariate and multivariate statistical analysis of this cohort showed that a favorable treatment result was significantly associated with parotid duct location and diameter of the stone (<7 mm). Based on the results of the previous study, between January 2004 and December 2008 a further 93 patients with parotid (48) or submandibular stones (45) with diameters of 3 to 7 mm were selectively recruited and treated with ESWL (group B). The demographic and clinical data of the two groups are compared in **Table 4**.

Intervention

For diagnostic purposes, all of the patients in both groups underwent US of the major salivary glands using a high-resolution small-parts US transducer (5- to 10-MHz broadband probe, Ultramark 9 HDI scanner, ATL Ultrasound, Bothell, Washington).

Step-by-Step Procedure for Extracorporeal Shock Wave Lithotripsy

Lithotripsy is performed using a dedicated extracorporeal electromagnetic device (Minilith SL1, Storz Medical, Kreuzlingen, Switzerland) with a mobile arm that is

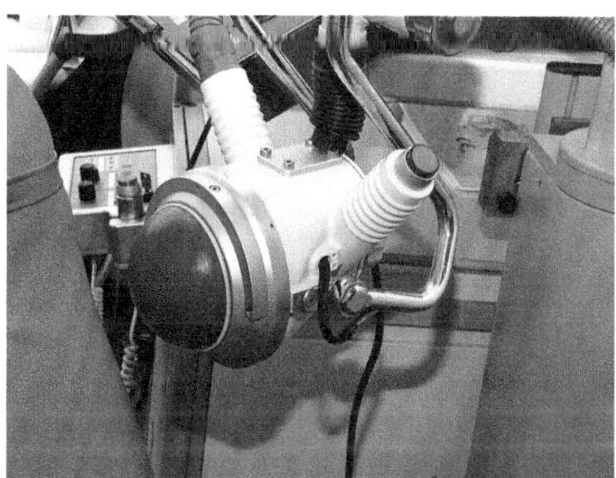

Fig. 13. Step-by-step procedure of ESWL.

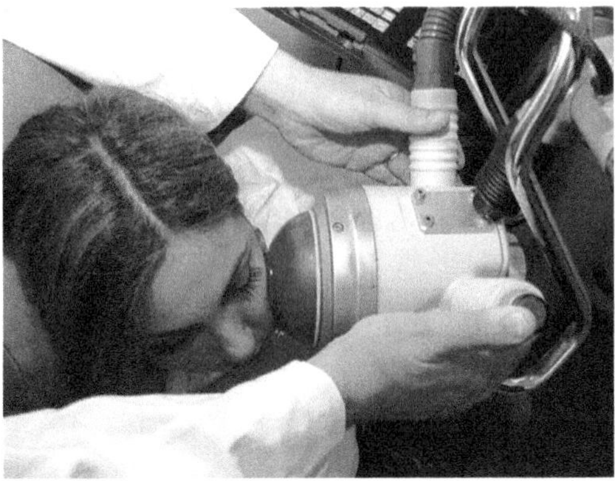

Fig. 14. Step-by-step procedure of ESWL.

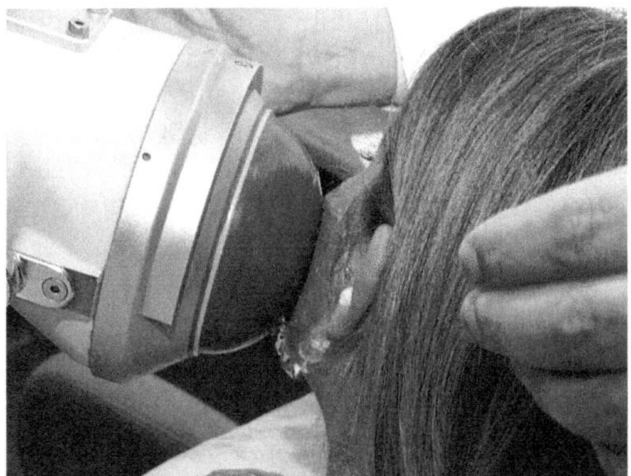

Fig. 15. Step-by-step procedure of ESWL.

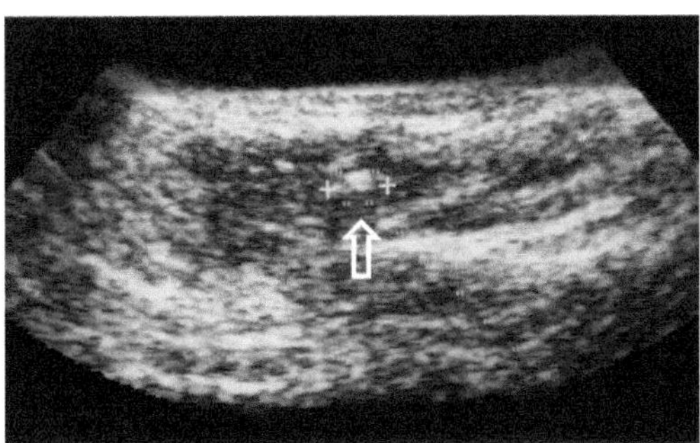

Fig. 16. Step-by-step procedure of ESWL.

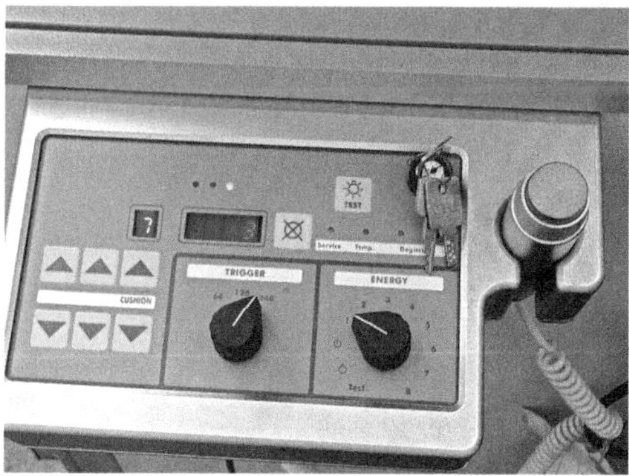

Fig. 17. Step-by-step procedure of ESWL.

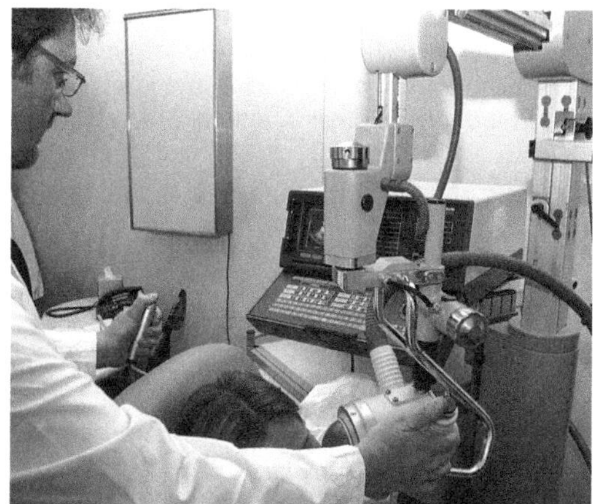

Fig. 18. Step-by-step procedure of ESWL.

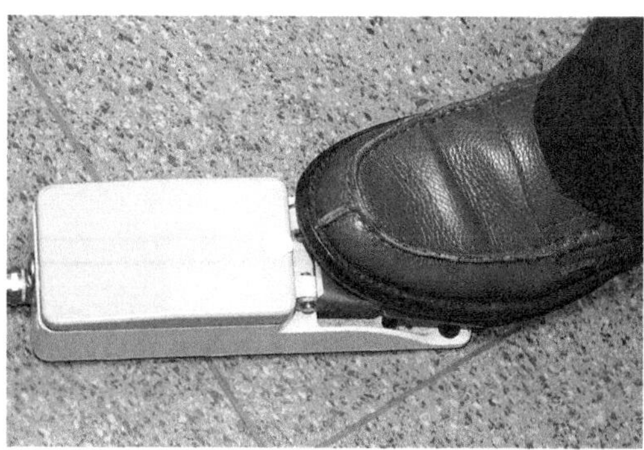

Fig. 19. Step-by-step procedure of ESWL.

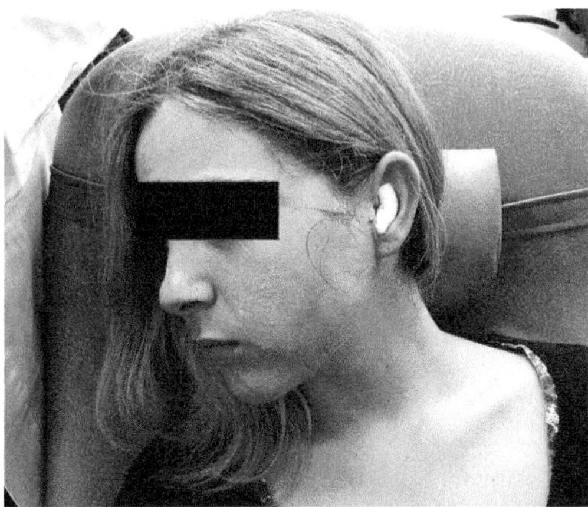

Fig. 20. Step-by-step procedure of ESWL.

maneuvered by the operator (Pasquale Capaccio) until the stone is positioned in the focus area (**Fig. 5**). The shock waves in this device are generated by a small-diameter cylindric electromagnetic source and focused on the target area by means of a parabolic reflector through a water cushion covered with a latex membrane. The patients are comfortably seated in a dentist's chair in a semireclined position (**Fig. 6**).

PHASE 1. ULTRASONOGRAPHIC INDIVIDUATION OF THE SALIVARY STONE

- US jelly is applied on the skin surface overlying the affected area (parotid or submandibular region) to allow conduction of US aiming beam and lithotripsy shock waves to the body (**Fig. 7**).
- The inline US scanner (7.5 MHz, Sigma 1-AC, Kontron Instruments, Everett, Massachusetts, USA), a high-resolution small-parts US transducer positioned along the longitudinal axis of the transducer, is extracted from the pressure-wave source (**Fig. 8**) and positioned over the jelly (**Fig. 9**). This system enables individuating the stone in the preoperative period (**Fig. 10**), positioning the salivary stone within

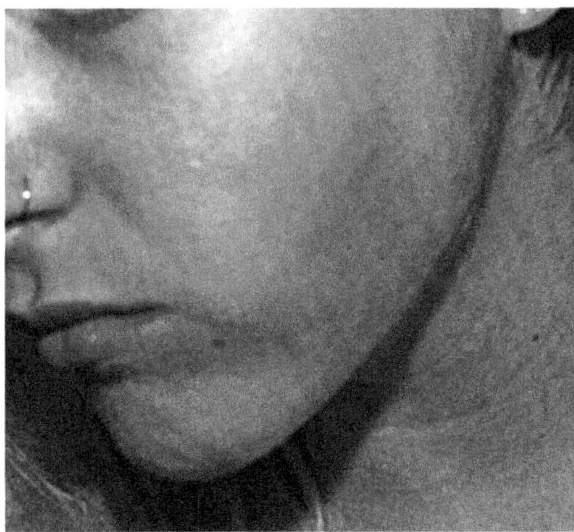

Fig. 21. Step-by-step procedure of ESWL.

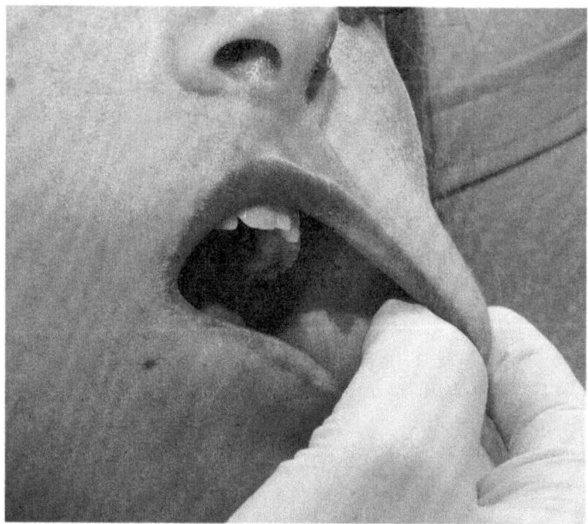

Fig. 22. Step-by-step procedure of ESWL.

the shock wave focus (2.4 mm of diameter; ie, all stones larger than this are amenable to treatment) before the procedure, and performing continuous sonographic monitoring during the operative session (**Fig. 11**).

- The inline scanner is reinserted in the pressure-wave source.

PHASE 2. OPERATIVE SESSION

- Ear and tooth guards are inserted on the treated side (**Fig. 12**).
- The shock waves are generated by a small-diameter cylindric electromagnetic source and focused on the target area by means of a parabolic reflector through a water cushion covered with a latex membrane (**Fig. 13**). Suspension of the pressure-wave source on a customized multijointed arm allows treatment comfort for patients and the physicians (**Figs. 14** and **15**).

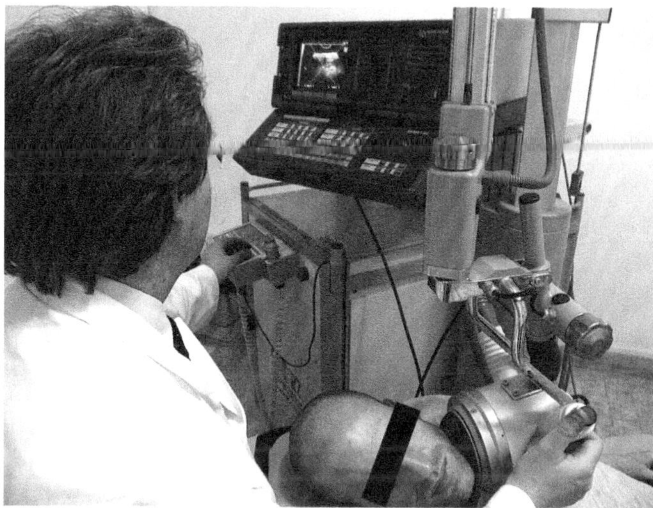

Fig. 23. Step-by-step procedure of ESWL.

- Additional US jelly is applied on the cutaneous surface.
- By means of a gentle movement of the mobile arm, it is possible to exactly target the stone within the shock wave focus (**Fig. 16**).
- Through the switch panel, it is possible to regulate the distance between the extremity of the inline scanner and the latex membrane by modifying the amount of water in the cushion (**Fig. 17**).
- Patients are invited to quit any unexpected movement and to raise an arm in case of necessity during the procedure.
- An operator is positioned behind the patient and may regulate, through the switch panel, the pulse frequency of the shock waves (0.5–2 Hz) and the increasing energy of the pulses (eight steps) (see **Fig. 17**).
- A typical session of ESWL requires a mean administration of 3000 shock waves and typically lasts approximately 30 minutes (range 20–37 minutes). The pulse frequency of the waves vary from 0.5 to 2 Hz, with the energy of the pulse gradually increased in six consecutive steps.
- The delivery of the shock waves is controlled by means of a button switch or a kick start (**Figs. 18** and **19**).

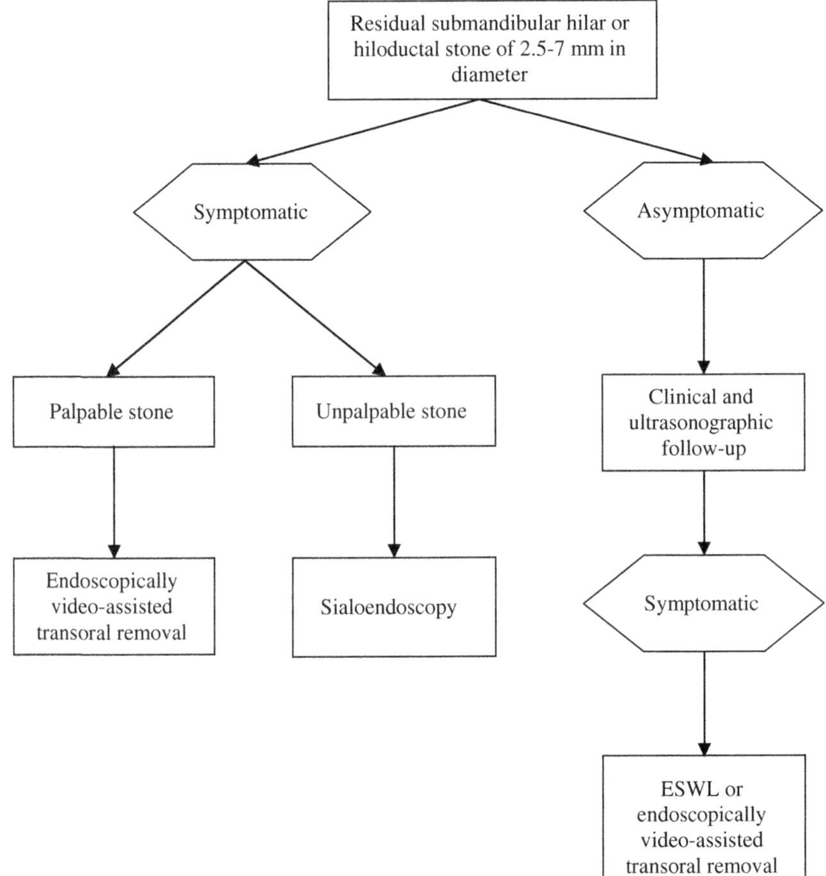

Fig. 24. Therapeutic algorithm for failure of ESWL for residual submandibular hilar or hiloductal stones.

PHASE 3. POSTOPERATIVE CARE

- After the procedure, the multijointed arm is moved from the operative position (**Fig. 20**).
- The occurrence of any untoward effects (cutaneous petecchiae or flushing, duct oral bleeding) is checked (**Figs. 21** and **22**). Intraoral examination and salivary gland bimanual palpation favor the immediate expulsion of microliths from the duct system.
- The procedure is repeated weekly unless the occurrence of acute sialadenitis requires a cycle of antibiotic and anti-inflammatory therapy.
- All the figures refer to the treatment of parotid stones (see **Figs. 6–22**); the same procedure is applied in the case of submandibular stones by locating the water cushion of the multijointed arm over the submandibular region (**Fig. 23**).

Further information about the treatment modality is given in **Table 4**.

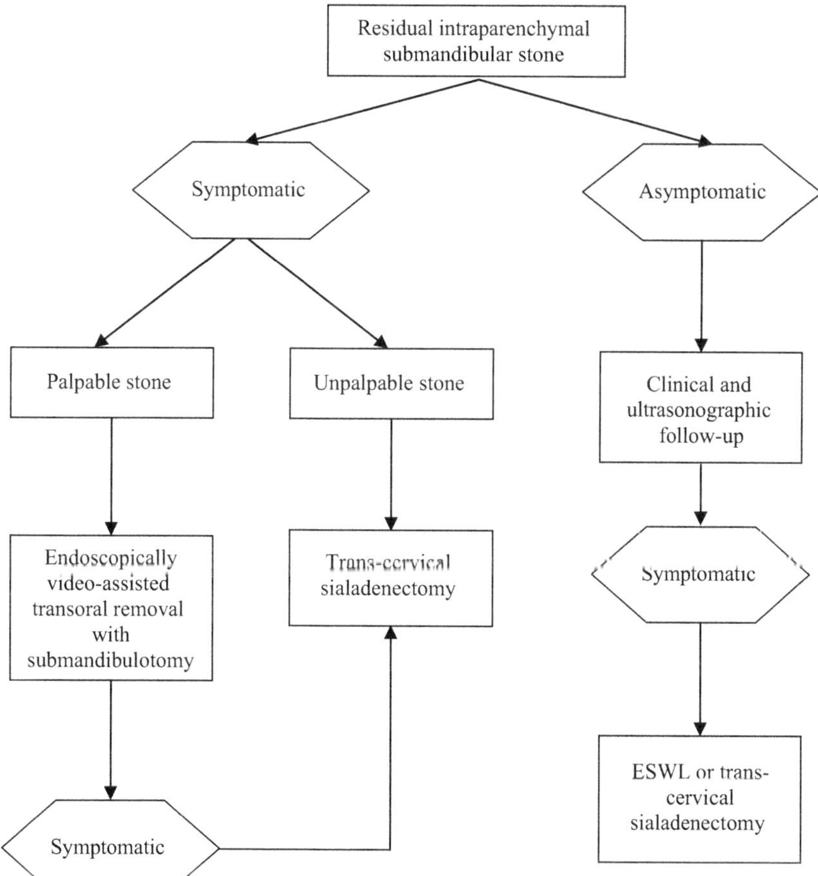

Fig. 25. Therapeutic algorithm for failure of ESWL for residual intraparenchymal submandibular stones.

RESULTS

The follow-up consisted of repeated US evaluations at 1 week, and then at 1, 3, 6, and 12 months post therapy. Outcomes were classified by means of three US features: complete stone clearance (the absence of any stone fragments), residual stone fragments less than or equal to 2 mm in diameter (the US detection of sandy material that could be flushed out by means of spontaneous or citric acid-induced salivation), or residual stone fragments more than 2 mm.

The therapeutic results in the two groups are shown in **Table 4**. Outcomes were generally better in group B, with the complete clearance of submandibular stones observed in 48.8% (vs 35.9% in group A) and complete clearance of parotid stones in 68.8% versus 69.3%. Residual submandibular and parotid stones of less than 2 mm were observed, respectively, in 27.3% and 27.3% of the patients in group A and 22.2% and 22.9% of those in group B with the corresponding results for residual stones of 2 mm or larger were 36.7% and 3.4% in group A and 29.8% and 8.3% in group B.

Tolerance and Further Therapeutic Measures

The procedure was well tolerated by all of the patients, and only mild and self-limiting untoward effects occurred, such as local pain, glandular swelling,

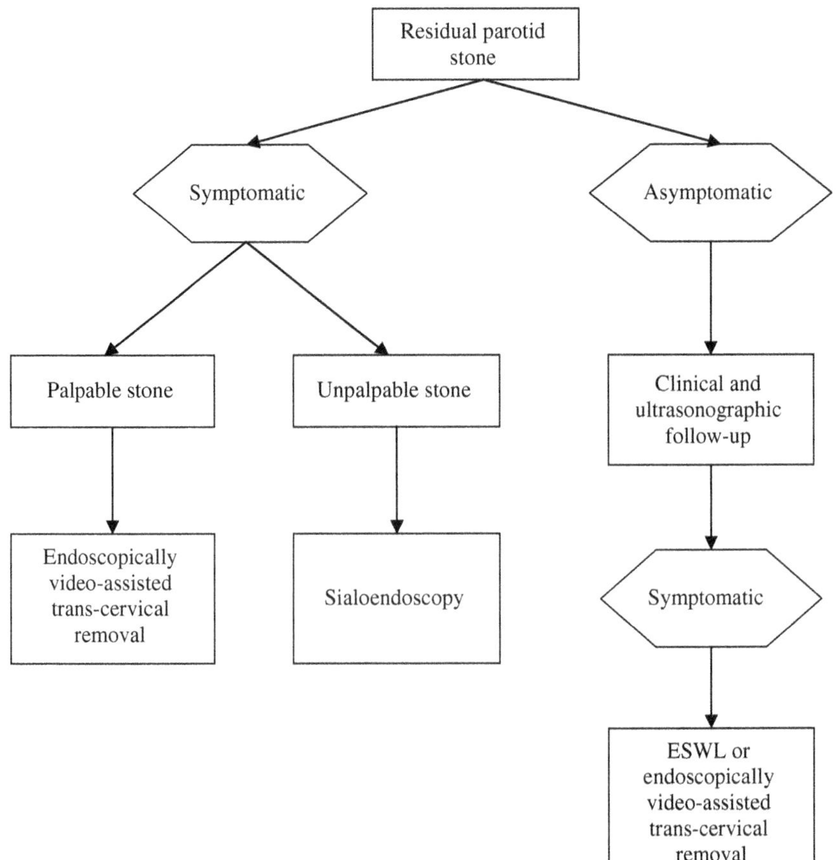

Fig. 26. Therapeutic options in the case of failure of ESWL for residual parotid stones.

self-limiting ductal hemorrhage, transient cutaneous petechiae, and temporary tinnitus (see **Table 4**).

A postlithotripsy papillotomy with submandibular stone retrieval was required in 26 group A patients (8.1%) and nine group B patients (9.7%), and, 10 patients of group A (3.1%) and one patient of group B underwent submandibular sialadenectomy. Operative sialoendoscopy was used in nine group B patients, and eight patients underwent the transoral removal of residual hilum-parenchymal submandibular stones. The recurrence of calculi in the treated gland was observed in four patients (1.25%) in group A after 10 to 58 months and two patients (1.94%) in group B after 8 to 36 months (see **Table 4**).

SUMMARY

Encouraged by increasingly frequent patient demands for minimally invasive and conservative therapies, ESWL is now used widely in dedicated centers in European and Eastern countries. Based on the authors' and others' experience, ESWL leads to good results, particularly for parotid stones, intraductal locations, and stones with a diameter of less than 7 mm.[14,15,24,28–34,36,37] Multivariate analysis of one of the authors' previous studies showed that favorable outcomes were significantly associated with a younger age (<46 years), parotid location (intraductal), stone diameter (<7 mm), and a lower number of therapeutic sessions.[28] Using US to carefully select patients for location and stone diameter, it is possible to obtain better therapeutic results, as can be seen from the success rate for submandibular stones increasing from 35.9% to 48.8% (**Fig. 24**).

Despite the use of specific indications for ESWL, US shows that a significant number of patients have residual fragments in the affected gland even though most of them are asymptomatic and do not require further procedures. The patients who remain symptomatic can be further treated by means of combined sialoendoscopy or the transoral removal of the residual stones (see **Figs. 24–26**).

Previous studies have shown that recurrent calculi are observed in few patients with US evidence of complete clearance after lithotripsy. US is a valid diagnostic tool when following ESWL patients, but it is not accurate in the case of stones with a diameter of less than 1.5 mm. Consequently, the undetectable microliths can act as a nidus for recurrence, which is why operative sialendoscopy should be performed after lithotripsy to clean the salivary duct system.

On the basis of the authors' experience of minimally invasive and conservative procedures over the past 15 years, it is possible to suggest specific indications based on size and site of the stones (parotid vs submandibular; intraductal vs hilum-parenchymal) (see **Figs. 24–26**).

Papillotomy followed by duct dissection remains the best therapeutic option for distal stones, whereas mobile duct stones can be successfully removed by means of endoscopically or radiologically controlled retrieval (see **Fig. 24**). ESWL is effective for all parotid stones and hilum-parenchymal submandibular stones with a diameter of 3 to 7 mm (see **Figs. 24** and **26**). Palpable and impacted stones in the proximal third of the duct or hilum-parenchymal submandibular region that measure more than 7 mm should undergo transoral removal (possibly endoscopically video assisted) under general anesthesia or sedation, and large palpable parotid stones (>10 mm) can be successfully retrieved by means of an endoscopically assisted transcervical procedure under general anesthesia (see **Figs. 25** and **26**).[11]

All of these procedures can be used singly or in combination with other conservative procedures to ensure the functional gland preservation. Although sometimes expensive and time consuming, the multimodal conservative approach can lead to an overall success rate of approximately 80%, reducing the indication for gland excision to 2% to 5% of cases.[11] In particular, single or combined ESWL is very much a part of the modern minimally invasive and functional management of salivary calculi.

REFERENCES

1. Epker BN. Obstructive and inflammatory diseases of the major salivary glands. Oral Surg Oral Med Oral Pathol 1972;33(1):2–27.
2. Marchal F, Dulguerov P, Becker M, et al. Specificity for parotid sialendoscopy. Laryngoscope 2001;111(2):264–71.
3. Rauch S, Gorlin RJ. Diseases of the salivary glands. In: Gorlin RJ, Goldman HM, editors. Thoma's oral pathology. St Louis (MO): Mosby; 1970. p. 997–1003.
4. Bodner L. Salivary gland calculi: diagnostic imaging and surgical management. Compendium 1993;14(5):572–86.
5. Capaccio P, Bottero A, Pompilio M, et al. Conservative transoral removal of hilar submandibular salivary calculi. Laryngoscope 2005;115(4):750–2.
6. Escudier MP. The current status and possible future for lithotripsy of salivary calculi. In: Haug RH, editor. Atlas of oral and maxillofacial surgery clinics of North America. Philadelphia: Saunders; 1998. p. 117–32.
7. Fodra C, Kaarmann H, Iro H. Sonographie und Röntgennativaufnahme in der Speichelsteindiagnostik—experimentelle Untersuchungen [Sonography and plain roentgen image in diagnosis of salivary calculi—experimental studies]. HNO 1992;40(7):25–8.
8. Traxler M, Schurawitzki H, Ulm C, et al. Sonography of nonneoplastic disorders of the salivary glands. Int J Oral Maxillofac Surg 1992;21(6):360–3.
9. Yoshimura Y, Inoue Y, Odagawa T. Sonographic examination of sialolithiasis. J Oral Maxillofac Surg 1989;47(9):907–12.
10. Hald J, Andreassen UK. Submandibular gland excision: short- and long-term complications. ORL J Otorhinolaryngol Relat Spec 1994;56(2):87–91.
11. Capaccio P, Torretta S, Ottaviani F, et al. Modern management of obstructive salivary diseases. Acta Otorhinolaryngol Ital 2007;27(4):161–72.
12. Iro H, Schneider T, Nitsche N, et al. Extracorporeal piezoelectric lithotripsy of salivary calculi: initial clinical experiences. HNO 1990;38(7):251–5.
13. Wehrmann T, Kater W, Marlinghaus EH, et al. Shock wave treatment of salivary duct stones: substantial progress with a minilithotripter. Clin Investig 1994; 72(8):604–8.
14. Ottaviani F, Capaccio P, Campi M, et al. Extracorporeal electromagnetic shock-wave lithotripsy for salivary gland stones. Laryngoscope 1996;106(6):761–4.
15. Escudier MP, Brown JE, Drage NA, et al. Extracorporeal shockwave lithotripsy in the management of salivary calculi. Br J Surg 2003;90(4):482–5.
16. Konigsberger R, Freyh J, Goetz A, et al. Endoscopically-controlled electrohydraulic intracorporeal shock wave lithotripsy (EISL) of salivary stones. J Otolaryngol 1993;22(1):12–3.
17. Iro H, Benzel W, Gode U, et al. Pneumatic intracorporeal lithotripsy of salivary stones: an in vitro and in vivo animal investigation. HNO 1995;43(3):172–6.
18. Arzoz E, Santiago A, Esnal F, et al. Endoscopic intracorporeal lithotripsy for sialolithiasis. J Oral Maxillofac Surg 1996;54(7):847–50.
19. McGurk M, Prince MJ, Jang ZX, et al. Laser lithotripsy: a preliminary study on its application for sialolithiasis. Br J Oral Maxillofac Surg 1994;32(4):218–21.

20. Ito H, Baba S. Pulsed dye laser lithotripsy of submandibular gland salivary calculus. J Laryngol Otol 1996;110(10):218–21.
21. Chaussy C, Brendel W, Schmiedt E. Extracorporeally induced destruction of kidney stones by shock waves. Lancet 1980;2(8207):1265–8.
22. Ell C, Kerzel W, Schneider HT, et al. Piezoelectric lithotripsy: stone disintegration and follow-up results in patients with symptomatic gallbladder stones. Gastroenterology 1990;99(5):1439–44.
23. Ashby RA, deBurgh Norman JE, Iro H, et al. Salivary calculi and obstructive sialadenitis. In: deburgh Norman JE, McGurk M, editors. Color atlas and text of the salivaryglands diseases, disorders and surgery. Barcelona (Spain): Mosby-Wolfe; 1995. p. 243–66.
24. Iro H, Meier J, Nitsche N, et al. Extracorporeal piezoelectric lithotripsy of salivary calculi. In vitro studies. HNO 1989;37(9):365–8.
25. Iro H, Nitsche N, Schneider HT. Extracorporeal shockwave lithotripsy of salivary gland stones. Lancet 1989;2(8654):115.
26. Kater W, Meyer WW, Wehrmann T, et al. Efficacy, risks, and limits of extracorporeal shock wave lithotripsy for salivary gland stones. J Endourol 1994;8(1):21–4.
27. Ottaviani F, Capaccio P, Rivolta R, et al. Salivary gland stones: US evaluation in shock wave lithotripsy. Radiology 1997;204(2):437–41.
28. Capaccio P, Ottaviani F, Manzo R, et al. Extracorporeal lithotripsy for salivary calculi: a long-term clinical experience. Laryngoscope 2004;114(6):1069–73.
29. McGurk M, Escudier MP, Brown JE. Modern management of salivary calculi. Br J Surg 2005;92(1):107–12.
30. Schmitz S, Zengel P, Alvir I. Long-term evaluation of extracorporeal shock wave lithotripsy in the treatment of salivary stones. J Laryngol Otol 2008;122(1):65–71.
31. Iro H, Schneider HT, Födra C, et al. Shockwave lithotripsy of salivary duct stones. Lancet 1992;339(8805):1333–6.
32. Aïdan P, De Kerviler E, LeDuc A, et al. Treatment of salivary stones by extracorporeal lithotripsy. Am J Otol 1996;17(4):246–50.
33. Iro H, Zenk J, Waldfahrer F, et al. Extracorporeal shock wave lithotripsy of parotid stones. Results of a prospective clinical trial. Ann Otol Rhinol Laryngol 1998;107(10):860–4.
34. Külkens C, Quetz JU, Lippert BM. Ultrasound-guided piezoelectric extracorporeal shock wave lithotripsy of parotid gland calculi. J Clin Ultrasound 2001;29(7):389–94.
35. Zenk J, Bozzato A, Winter M, et al. Extracorporeal shock wave lithotripsy of submandibular stones: evaluation after 10 years. Ann Otol Rhinol Laryngol 2004;113(5):378–83.
36. Lustmann T, Regev E, Melamed Y. Sialolithiasis; a survey of 245 patients and review of the literature. Int J Oral Maxillofac Surg 1990;19(3):135–8.
37. Eggers G, Chilla R. Ultrasound guided lithotripsy of salivary calculi using an electromagnetic lithotriptor. J Oral Maxillofac Surg 2005;34(8):890–4.
38. Yoshizaki T, Maruyama Y, Motoi I, et al. Clinical evaluation of extracorporeal shock wave lithotripsy for salivary stones. Ann Otol Rhinol Laryngol 1996;105(1):63–7.
39. Katz P, Fritsch MH. Salivary stones: innovative techniques in diagnosis and treatment. Curr Opin Otolaryngol Head Neck Surg 2003;11(3):173–8.
40. Fritsch MH. A new sialendoscopy teaching model of the duct and gland. J Oral Maxillofac Surg 2008;66(11):2409–11.

The Role of Adenectomy for Salivary Gland Obstructions in the Era of Sialendoscopy and Lithotripsy

Pasquale Capaccio, MD*, Sara Torretta, MD, Lorenzo Pignataro, MD

KEYWORDS

• Parotid • Submandibular • Sialadenitis
• Lithotripsy • Sialendoscopy

Obstructive sialadenitis is the major cause of salivary gland disorders, and accounts for approximately 50% of all benign disease.[1] Patients typically present with the so called "meal-time syndrome."[2] Recurrent and painful periprandial glandular swelling is typical and may be complicated by bacterial superinfection indicated by a purulent papillary discharge.[3,4]

Salivary gland obstruction may be caused by the presence of sialolithiasis, stenosis or anatomic variations in the ductal system, intraductal fibromucinous plugs, polyps, or foreign bodies, all of which impair physiologic salivary down-flow and lead to stasis. Sialolithiasis is still the main cause of salivary obstruction, and is detectable in more than 65% of cases.[5] Between 80% and 90% of all cases of sialolithiasis affect the submandibulary gland, probably because of the intrinsic features of its secretion.[2,6] The parotid gland is involved in only 5% to 10% of cases.[6]

The second most frequent cause of salivary obstruction is duct disorders, mainly strictures and kinks that prevalently involve the parotid duct system (75% of cases), although other reported disorders include accessory ducts, sphincteric-like structures, pelvis-like formations, and intraductal evaginations.[7–13] Salivary obstruction may also be related to the presence of intraductal mucous plugs, foreign bodies or polyps, sialodochitis, *ab estrinseco* compression from neoplastic masses or reactive

Department of Specialist Surgical Sciences, Fondazione I.R.C.C.S. Ospedale Maggiore Policlinico, Mangiagalli e Regina Elena, University of Milan, Via F. Sforza 35, Milano 20122, Italy
* Corresponding author.
E-mail address: pasquale.capaccio@unimi.it (P. Capaccio).

Otolaryngol Clin N Am 42 (2009) 1161–1171
doi:10.1016/j.otc.2009.08.013
0030-6665/09/$ – see front matter
oto.theclinics.com

intraparenchymal lymph nodes, or the granulation tissue associated with immunologic disorders (ie, Sjögren's syndrome), but radioiodine therapy and *ab estrinseco* ostial compression by dentures (in the case of the parotid gland) have been also reported.[1,8,11]

Invasive adenectomy has sometimes been favored because distinguishing the cause of mechanical obstruction based on a clinical assessment and traditional radiography, ultrasonography, conventional sialography, or CT is not simple and sometimes cannot be done.

Invasive surgery has also been justified based on a mistaken belief that the salivary gland obstruction is associated with an irreversible parenchymal inflammation that impairs salivary function, but this has been recently denied by scintigraphic and histopathologic findings of the secretory function recovery and histologic normalization after stone removal.[14–17]

The introduction of new diagnostic tools has substantially improved diagnosis, with the incidence of idiopathic obstruction reduced to only 5% to 10% of cases.[11] Ultrasonography is considered a valuable diagnostic technique, especially in the case of stones, but it has the limitation of being an operator-dependent procedure. Sialoendoscopy has recently partially filled a diagnostic gap because it allows direct visualisation.[9,14] Dynamic MR sialography has also been proposed as a useful diagnostic procedure for salivary duct disorders and the preoperative evaluation of patients undergoing sialoendoscopy.[18,19]

These modern diagnostic tools now make it possible to plan appropriate therapy based on the site and specific cause of the obstruction. Over the past 20 years, new and minimally invasive conservative therapies have been proposed, particularly for sialolithiasis, including extracorporeal shock wave lithotripsy (ESWL), operative sialoendoscopy, interventional radiology, the transoral removal of submandibular stones, and endoscopically video-assisted transcervical or transoral removal of parotid and submandibular stones.

Conservative treatment using sialoballoon dilatation under sialoendoscopic or radiologic fluoroscopic guidance is another useful technique.[20] Minimally invasive gland preservation for salivary gland obstruction has greatly reduced the need for sialadenectomy. Conservative therapeutic options, alone or in combination, can preserve a functional gland in situ in 97% of cases.[21] The published success rates of each of these techniques over the past 10 years are shown in **Tables 1** and **2**.[5,21–40]

Botulinum toxin therapy can be proposed in patients who have recurrent sialadenitis with no radiologic or sialoendoscopic cause of obstruction.[41]

With this background, the residual indications for parotid and submandibular sialadenectomy for salivary gland obstruction in the era of ESWL and operative sialoendoscopy can be better assessed.

IS THERE A RESIDUAL INDICATION FOR SIALADENECTOMY FOR SALIVARY GLAND OBSTRUCTION?

Until the 1950s, parotid gland excision for benign and inflammatory disorders was not considered a standard procedure.[42] The following years saw a more aggressive approach, with total or near-total parotidectomy being advocated for treating chronic parotid sialadenitis.[43] However, because total parotidectomy was associated with a significant rate of facial nerve injury, some authors[44] suggested the use of superficial parotidectomy. In 1978, Casterline and Jaques[43] reported that "near total parotidectomy with removal of the parotid duct can be performed

Table 1
Overall results in patients undergoing minimally invasive and gland preserving techniques for obstructive stones

Author	No. of Patients	Site	Procedure	Success Rate	Residual Obstruction Rate	Sialadenectomy
Zenk et al[22]	231	SM	Hilar transoral removal	91%	6%	2%
Nahlieli et al[23]	12	P	Endoscopically assisted removal	75%	25%	—
Marchal et al[24]	129	SM	Sialoendoscopy	85%	—	—
Escudier et al[25]	122	P and SM	ESWL	33%	Asymptomatic obstruction, 35% Symptomatic obstruction, 32%	2%
Capaccio et al[26]	322	P and SM	ESWL	45%	Fragments smaller than 2 mm, 27% Fragments bigger than 2 mm, 28%	3%
Makdissi et al[14]	43	SM	Hilar transoral removal	97%	5%	2%
Zenk et al[27]	191	P and SM	ESWL	50%	50%	—
Katz[28]	1773	P and SM	ESWL Sialoendoscopy	63% 96%	—	3%
McGurk et al[29]	455	P and SM	ESWL Transoral removal Interventional radiology	39% 96% 75%	15%	2%
Eggers and Chilla[30]	38	P and SM	ESWL	55%	—	—
Zenk et al[31]	683	SM	Transoral removal	86%	14%	—
Nahlieli et al[32]	172	SM	Sialoendoscopy	94%	4%	3%
Iro et al[21]	4691	P and SM	ESWL Sialoendoscopy Interventional radiology Transoral removal	81%	17%	3%

Abbreviations: ESWL, extracorporeal shock wave lithotripsy; P, parotid; SM, submandibular.

safely and should be the procedure of choice in patients with chronic, relapsing parotid sialadenitis."

More recently, Bates and colleagues[45] suggested the usefulness of total or near-total gland resection as an effective and low-morbidity procedure in the case of

Table 2
Overall results in patients undergoing minimally invasive and gland preserving techniques for all obstructive causes

Author	No. of Patients	Site	Procedure	Success Rate	Residual Obstruction Rate	Sialadenectomy
Nahlieli et al[33]	236	P and SM	Sialoendoscopy	88%	6%	4%
Marchal et al[5]	55	P	Sialoendoscopy	85%	15%	1%
Ziegler et al[34]	72	P and SM	Sialoendoscopy	87%	11%	8%
McGurk et al[35]	8	P	Endoscopically assisted removal	100%	—	—
Brown[36]	348	P and SM	Interventional radiology	Stones, 75% Strictures, 72%	16% 10%	—
Koch et al[37]	39	P	Sialoendoscopy	76%	—	5%
Yu et al[38]	68	P and SM	Intraoral removal Sialoendoscopy	87% 81%	—	—
Papadaki et al[39]	94	P and SM	Sialoendoscopy	85%	11%	5%
Walvekar et al[40]	56	P and SM	Sialoendoscopy	74%	21%	2%

Abbreviations: P, parotid; SM, submandibular.

parotid and submandibular sialadenitis. In 1998, Bhatty and colleagues[46] stated that superficial parotidectomy was the preferred treatment in selected cases of severe and recurrent chronic parotitis, despite the frequent risk for postoperative facial nerve weakness caused by the frequent adhesion of the facial nerve to glandular tissue. Traditionally, sialadenectomy has been indicated for not only chronic aspecific sialadenitis but also intraparenchymal stones.[47,48]

Based on this historical background, the traditional management of salivary gland obstruction seems to consist of superficial parotidectomy and traditional transcervical submandibular removal in the case of hilum–parenchymal obstructions; transoral surgical procedures such as sialolithectomy for distal duct stones; and sialodochoplasty for distal duct strictures.[49–51] Even though sialadenectomy is a relatively standard procedure, it is not devoid of postoperative complications, such as neurologic sequelae which, in the case of parotidectomy, may include transient (2%–76%)[43,46,52–56] or permanent (1%–3%)[45,52,55,56] facial nerve injury; sensory loss of the greater auricular nerve (2%–100%)[52–54]; or Frey's syndrome (8%–33%).[46,52–54,56] In the case of submandibular extirpation, these complications may include temporary (1%–23%)[57–60] or permanent (1%–8%)[45,57,59] marginalis mandibulae nerve injury; temporary (1%–2%)[57,59] or permanent (3%)[57] hypoglossal nerve palsy; or temporary (2%–6%)[41–60] or permanent (2%)[57] lingual nerve lesions. Other complications include aesthetic sequelae, such as hematomas (parotid gland, 2%–9%; submandibular gland, 2%–4%)[45,52–57,60]; salivary fistulas (parotid gland, 2%–18%; submandibular gland, 1%)[45,52,53,55,56] or sialoceles (parotid gland, 5%–11%; submandibular gland, 1%–3%)[52–54,59]; wound infections (parotid gland, 5%–6%; submandibular gland,

3%–8%)[46,54,56,57,59,60]; hypertrophic scars (parotid gland, 3%–6%; submandibular gland, 2%–5%)[52–54,56,57,59]; and inflammation caused by residual stone in the salivary duct (parotid gland, 2–14; submandibular gland, 2%–8%)[43,45,52–55,57–59]

Tables 3 and **4** provide detailed descriptions of the frequency of postoperative sequelae after parotid and submandibular gland excision for chronic and obstructive inflammatory disorders of salivary glands.

Specific treatment indications for each type of obstructive ductal disorder can be outlined, and each treatment technique may be used alone or in combination (**Tables 1** and **2**).

Given the high success rates and low morbidity of minimally invasive and conservative procedures, gland extirpation should only be considered when the modern management of salivary obstruction fails, but fortunately this is unlikely because the different options can be combined in a multimodal approach.

However, despite these encouraging results, the most powerful published studies are based on relatively short follow-up periods, and stable remissions should be evaluated over time. Nevertheless, available clinical evidence supports minimally invasive gland preservation because it significantly reduces the use of invasive sialadenectomy, which is still associated with well-known functional and neurologic sequelae. In this regard, transoral submandibular sialadenectomy was recently proposed to reduce the number of these sequelae, but the paucity of treated patients means that no final conclusion can yet be made.

Minimally invasive procedures and ESWL have contraindications and exclusion criteria, such as the presence of atresia or diffuse stenosis of the main salivary duct (diagnosed with MR–sialography or x-ray sialography), and the inability to adequately open the mouth for all transoral procedures. These situations may lead directly to sialadenectomy.

Sialadenectomy for obstructive salivary disorders may be also indicated in the case of failure or intraoperative complication after minimally invasive procedures. Some examples of further residual indications for sialadenectomy include

- Patients previously submitted to multiple stricture dilatations with endoscopic balloon treatments on recurrence of the stricture
- Multiple and massive unilateral or bilateral intraparenchymal stones with symptomatic and recurrent sialadenitis
- Complications during intraoperative sialendoscopic procedures (ie, hilar entrapping of the basket transorally unremovable)
- Failure to remove a hilo-parenchymal submandibular or parotid stone during transoral or transcervical video-assisted removal techniques
- Persistent symptomatic sialadenitis in patients who have Sjögren's syndrome not responding to systemic or local video-endoscopic steroid lavage
- Persistent symptomatic sialadenitis in patients previously treated with ^{131}I whose condition does not respond to systemic therapy or duct rehabilitation

Patient treatment has progressed to new algorithms, which have resulted in more physiologic outcomes. Gland and duct repair and preservation are the primary goal. Single or multimodal treatment has resulted in success rate near 100%. Nevertheless, failures or contraindications to minimally invasive procedures and ESWL exist. In these cases, adenectomy is the final common pathway and also the best treatment option.

Table 3
Overall results in patients undergoing parotidectomy for chronic and obstructive salivary disease

Author	No. of Glands Removed	Type of Obstruction	Surgery	Facial Nerve Injury	Greater Auricular Nerve Injury	Greater Auricular Neuroma	Frey's Syndrome	Hematoma	Wound Infection	Seroma	Fistula	Sialocele	Hypertrophic Keloid	Recurrences
Casterline and Jaques[43]	26	Chronic parotitis, 100%	SP, 35% NTP, 65%	CTP or PTP, 69%	—	—	—	—	—	4%	—	—	—	4%
Bhatty et al[46]	17	Stones, 58%[a] Strictures, 32%[a] Sialectasis, 10%[a]	SP	PTP, 76%	—	5%	15%	—	5%	—	—	—	—	—
Bates et al[45]	47	Chronic parotitis, 66% Chronic parotitis and stones, 26% Chronic atrophic parotitis, 8%	SP, 30% NTP, 70%	CTP or PTP, 25% PP, 2%	—	—	—	4%	—	—	2%	—	—	2%

Moody et al[52]	39	Chronic parotitis, 100%	SP, 51% SP + duct ligation, 46% TP, 3%	CTP, 49% PTP, 3%–10%[d]	3%	—	8%	3%	—	—	5%	10%	5%	8%
Moody et al[53]	44	Chronic parotitis, 89% Parotitis and stones, 9% Strictures, 2%	SP, 49% SP + duct ligation, 49% TP, 2%	CTP, 47% PTP, 2%–8%[b]	2%	—	11%	2%	—	—	6%	11%	6%	11%
Amin et al[54]	21	Chronic parotitis 100%	SP	CTP, 9% PTP, 62%[c]	100%	14%	33%	5%	5%			5%	5%	14%
Patel et al[55]	78	Acute and chronic parotitis, 55% Chronic parotitis and stones, 23% Benign lymphoepithelial lesions, 17% Atrophic parotitis, 5%	SP, 22% NTP, 78%	CTP or PTP, 33% PP, 1%	—	—	—	4%	—	1%	3%	—	—	3%
Nouraei et al[56]	34	Parotitis, 85% Parotitis and sialectasis, 15%	SP TP	CTP, 41% PTP, 21%–38%[e] PP, 3%	—	3%	21%	9%	6%	—	18%	—	3%	—

Abbreviations: CTP, complete temporal palsy; NTP, near-total parotidectomy; PP, permanent palsy, PTP, partial temporal palsy; SP, superficial parotidectomy; TP, total parotidectomy.

[a] Computed on 19 patients, including 2 conservatively treated.

[b] Marginalis mandibulae branch 8%; temporal branch 2%; zygomatic branch 2%.

[c] Buccal and/or marginalis mandibulae branch.

[d] Marginalis mandibulae branch 10%; temporal branch 3%; zygomatic branch 3%.

[e] Marginalis mandibulae branch 26%; temporal branch 32%; zygomatic branch 21%; buccal branch 38%; cervical branch 18%.

Table 4
Overall results in patients undergoing submandibular adenectomy for chronic and obstructive salivary disease

Author	N of Gland Removed	Type of Obstruction	Facial Nerve Injury	LingualNerve Injury	Hypoglossal Nerve Injury	Hemorrhage	Wound Infection	Fistula	Sialocele	Xerostomia	Hypertrophic Keloid	Recurrences
Berini-Aytes and Gay-Escoda[57]	124	Stones, 100%	TP, 4% PP, 8%	PP, 2%	PP, 3% TP, 1%	4%	7%	—	—	—	5%	7%
Ellies et al[58]	171	Sialadenitis, 64% Sialadenitis and stones, 34% Stones, 2%	TP, 1%	TP, 6%	—	—	—	—	—	—	—	8%
Bates et al[45]	41	Sialadenitis and stones, 73% Sialadenitis and sialectasis, 27%	PP, 1%	—	—	—	—	—	—	—	—	—
Gallo et al[59]	119	Stones, 40% Chronic sialadenitis, 29% Chronic and fibrotic sialadenitis, 31%	TP, 4% PP, 3%	TP, 2%	TP, 1%	—	5%	—	3%	2%	2%	2%
Christie et al*	128	Chronic sialadenitis and stones, 64% Chronic sialadenitis, 36%	TP, 23% PP, 1%	TP, 5%	TP, 2%	—	8%	1%	1%	4%	5%	5%
Preuss et al[60]	207	Sialadenitis, 43% Stones, 57%	TP, 6%	TP, 3%	—	2%	3%	—	—	—	—	—

Abbreviations: TP, temporal palsy; PP, permanent palsy.
* Taken from Gallo et al.[59]

REFERENCES

1. Capaccio P, Minetti AM, Manzo R, et al. The role of the sialoendoscopy in the evaluation of obstructive salivary disease. Int J Maxillo Odontostomatol 2003; 2(1):9–12.
2. Escudier MP. The current status and possible future for lithotripsy of salivary calculi. In: Saunders WB, editor. Atlas of oral and maxillofacial surgery clinics of North America. Philadelphia: Saunders; 1998. p. 117–32.
3. Brown AL, Shepherd D, Buckenham TM. Per oral balloon sialoplasty: results in the treatment of salivary duct stenosis. Cardiovasc Intervent Radiol 1997;20(5): 337–42.
4. Marchal F, Kurt AM, Dulguerov P, et al. Retrograde theory in sialolithiasis formation. Arch Otolaryngol Head Neck Surg 2001;127(1):66–8.
5. Marchal F, Dulguerov P, Becker M, et al. Specificity for parotid sialendoscopy. Laryngoscope 2001;111(2):264–71.
6. Bodner L. Salivary gland calculi: diagnostic imaging and surgical management. Compendium 1993;14(5):572–86.
7. Nahlieli O, Bar T, Shacham R, et al. Management of chronic recurrent parotitis: current therapy. J Oral Maxillofac Surg 2004;62(9):1150–5.
8. Ngu RK, Brown JE, Whaites EJ, et al. Salivary duct strictures-nature and incidence in benign salivary obstruction. Dentomaxillofac Radiol 2007;36(2):63–7.
9. Koch M, Zenk J, Bozzato A, et al. Sialoscopy in case of unclear swelling of the major salivary glands. Otolaryngol Head Neck Surg 2005;133(6):863–8.
10. Nahlieli O, Hecht-Nakar L, Nazarian Y, et al. Sialoendoscopy: a new approach to salivary gland obstruction pathology. J Am Dent Assoc 2006;137(10):1394–400.
11. Nahlieli O. Endoscopic techniques for diagnosis and treatment of salivary gland diseases. Tuttlingen (Germany): Endo-Press; 2005.
12. Rose SS. A clinical and radiological survey of 192 cases of recurrent swellings of the salivary glands. Ann R Coll Surg Engl 1954;15(6):370–401.
13. Nahlieli O, Nazarian Y. Sialadenitis following radioiodine therapy-a new diagnostic and treatment modality. Oral Dis 2006;12(5):476–81.
14. Makdissi J, Escudier MP, Brown JE, et al. Glandular function after intraoral removal of salivary calculi from the hilum of the submandibular gland. Br J Oral Maxillofac Surg 2004;42(6):538–41.
15. Yoshimura Y, Morishita T, Sugihara T. Salivary gland function after sialolithiasis: scintigraphic examination of submandibular glands with 99m Tc-pertechnetate. J Oral Maxillofac Surg 1989;47(7):704–10.
16. Marchal F, Kurt AM, Dulguerov P, et al. Histopathology of submandibular glands removed for sialolithiasis. Ann Otol Rhinol Laryngol 2001;110(5):464–9.
17. Nahlieli O, Shacham R, Yoffe B, et al. Diagnosis and treatment of strictures and kinks in salivary gland ducts. J Oral Maxillofac Surg 2001;59(5):484–90.
18. Morimoto Y, Ono K, Tanaka T, et al. The functional evaluation of salivary glands using dynamic MR sialography following citric acid stimulation: a preliminary study. Oral Surg Oral Med Oral Pathol Oral Radiol Endod 2005;100(3):357–64.
19. Capaccio P, Cuccarini V, Ottaviani F, et al. Comparative ultrasonographic, magnetic resonance sialographic, and videoendoscopic assessment of salivary duct disorders. Ann Otol Rhinol Laryngol 2008;117(4):245–52.
20. Capaccio P, Torretta S, Ottaviani F, et al. Modern management of obstructive salivary diseases. Acta Otorhinolaryngol Ital 2007;27(4):161–72.
21. Iro H, Zenk J, Escudier MP, et al. Outcome of minimally invasive management of salivary calculi in 4,691 patients. Laryngoscope 2009;119(2):263–8.

22. Zenk J, Constantinidis J, Al-Kadah B, et al. Transoral removal of submandibular stone. Arch Otolaryngol Head Neck Surg 2001;127(4):432–6.
23. Nahlieli O, London D, Zagury A, et al. Combined approach to impacted parotid stones. J Oral Maxillofac Surg 2002;60(12):1418–23.
24. Marchal F, Dulguerov P, Becker M, et al. Submandibular diagnostic and interventional sialendoscopy: new procedure for ductal disorders. Ann Otol Rhinol Laryngol 2002;111(1):27–35.
25. Escudier MP, Brown JE, Drage NA, et al. Extracorporeal shockwave lithotripsy in the management of salivary calculi. Br J Surg 2003;90(4):482–5.
26. Capaccio P, Ottaviani F, Manzo R, et al. Extracorporeal lithotripsy for salivary calculi: a long-term clinical experience. Laryngoscope 2004;114(6):1069–73.
27. Zenk J, Koch M, Bozzato A, et al. Sialoscopy: initial experience with a new endoscope. Br J Oral Maxillofac Surg 2004;42(4):293–8.
28. Katz P. New techniques for the treatment of salivary lithiasis: sialoendoscopy and extracorporal lithotripsy: 1773 cases. Ann Otolaryngol Chir Cervicofac 2004; 121(3):123–32.
29. McGurk M, Escudier MP, Brown JE. Modern management of salivary calculi. Br J Surg 2005;92(1):107–12.
30. Eggers G, Chilla R. Ultrasound guided lithotripsy of salivary calculi using an electromagnetic lithotriptor. J Oral Maxillofac Surg 2005;34(8):890–4.
31. Zenk J, Gottwald F, Bozzato A, et al. Submandibular sialoliths. Stone removal with organ preservation. HNO 2005;53(3):243–9.
32. Nahlieli O, Shacham R, Zagury A, et al. The ductal stretching technique: an endoscopic-assisted technique for removal of submandibular stones. Laryngoscope 2007;117(6):1031–5.
33. Nahlieli O, Baruchin AM. Long-term experience with endoscopic diagnosis and treatment of salivary gland inflammatory diseases. Laryngoscope 2000;110(6):988–93.
34. Ziegler CM, Steveling H, Seubert M, et al. Endoscopy: a minimally invasive procedure for diagnosis and treatment of diseases of the salivary glands. Six years of practical experience. Br J Oral Maxillofac Surg 2004;42(1):1–7.
35. McGurk M, Makdissi J, Brown JE. Intra-oral removal of stones from the hilum of the submandibular gland: report of technique and morbidity. Int J Oral Maxillofac Surg 2004;33(7):683–6.
36. Brown JE. Interventional sialography and minimally invasive techniques in benign salivary gland obstruction. Semin Ultrasound CT MR 2006;27(6):465–75.
37. Koch M, Iro H, Zenk J. Role of sialoscopy in the treatment of Stensen's duct strictures. Ann Otol Rhinol Laryngol 2008;117(4):271–8.
38. Yu CQ, Yang C, Zheng LY, et al. Selective management of obstructive submandibular sialadenitis. Br J Oral Maxillofac Surg 2008;46(1):46–9.
39. Papadaki ME, McCain JP, Kim K, et al. Interventional sialoendoscopy: early clinical results. J Oral Maxillofac Surg 2008;66(5):954–62.
40. Walvekar RR, Razfar A, Carrau RL, et al. Sialendoscopy and associated complications: a preliminary experience. Laryngoscope 2008;118(5):776–9.
41. Capaccio P, Torretta S, Osio M, et al. Botulinum toxin therapy: a tempting tool in the management of salivary secretory disorders. Am J Otol 2008;29(5):333–8.
42. Gerry RG, Seigman EL. Chronic sialadenitis and sialography. Oral Surg Oral Med Oral Pathol 1955;8(5):453–78.
43. Casterline PF, Jaques DA. The surgical management of recurrent parotitis. Surg Gynecol Obstet 1978;146(3):419–22.
44. Beahrs OH, Devine KD, Woolner LB. Parotidectomy in the treatment of chronic sialadenitis. Am J Surg 1961;102:760–4.

45. Bates D, O'Brien CJ, Tikaram K, et al. Parotid and submandibular sialadenitis treated by salivary gland excision. Aust N Z J Surg 1998;68(2):120–4.
46. Bhatty MA, Piggot TA, Soames JV, et al. Chronic non-specific parotid sialadenitis. Br J Plast Surg 1998;51(7):517–21.
47. Rallis G, Mourouzis C, Zachariades N. A study of 55 submandibular salivary gland excisions. Gen Dent 2004;52(5):420–3.
48. Goh YH, Sethi DS. Submandibular gland excision: a five-year review. J Laryngol Otol 1998;112(3):269–73.
49. Baurmash HD. Chronic recurrent parotitis: a closer look at its origin, diagnosis, and management. J Oral Maxillofac Surg 2004;62(8):1010–8.
50. Motamed M, Laugharne D, Bradley PJ. Management of chronic parotitis: a review. J Laryngol Otol 2003;117(7):521–6.
51. Cohen D, Gatt N, Olschwang D, et al. Surgery for prolonged parotid duct obstruction: a case report. Otolaryngol Head Neck Surg 2003;128(5):753–4.
52. Moody AB, Avery CM, Taylor J, et al. A comparison of one hundred and fifty consecutive parotidectomies for tumors and inflammatory disease. Int J Oral Maxillofac Surg 1999;28(3):211–5.
53. Moody AB, Avery CM, Walsh S, et al. Surgical management of chronic parotid disease. Br J Oral Maxillofac Surg 2000;38(6):620–2.
54. Amin MA, Bailey BMW, Patel SR. Clinical and radiological evidence to support superficial parotidectomy as the treatment of choice for chronic parotid sialadenitis: a retrospective study. Br J Oral Maxillofac Surg 2001;39(5): 348–52.
55. Patel RS, Low TH, Gao K, et al. Clinical outcome after surgery for 75 patients with parotid sialadenitis. Laryngoscope 2007;117(4):644–7.
56. Nouraei SA, Ismail Y, Ferguson MS, et al. Analysis of complications following surgical treatment of benign parotid disease. ANZ J Surg 2008;78(3):134–8.
57. Berini-Aytes L, Gay-Escoda C. Morbidity associated with removal of the submandibular gland. J Craniomaxillofac Surg 1992;20(5):216–9.
58. Ellies M, Laskawi R, Araglebe C, et al. Surgical management of nonneoplastic diseases of the submandibular gland. A follow-up study. Int J Oral Maxillofac Surg 1996;25(4):285–9.
59. Gallo O, Berloco P, Bruschini L, et al. Treatment for non-neoplastic disease of the submandibular gland. In: McGurk M, Renehan AG, editors. Controversies in the management of salivary gland disease. Oxford (UK): Oxford University Press; 2001. p. 297–310.
60. Preuss SF, Klussmann JP, Wittekindt C, et al. Submandibular gland excision: 15 years of experience. J Oral Maxillofac Surg 2007;65(5):953–7.

Algorithms for Treatment of Salivary Gland Obstructions

Michael Koch, MD*, Johannes Zenk, MD, Heinrich Iro, MD

KEYWORDS

- Salivary glands • Obstruction of salivary glands
- Treatment of salivary glands • Stenosis • Sialolithiasis
- Sialendoscopy • Minimally invasive

Chronic sialadenitis is commonly associated with an acute chronic inflammation and obstruction of the excretory duct. The differentiation between chronic sialadenitis and obstruction of the excretory duct is difficult. The main causes of obstructive disorders are stones in about 60% to 70%, stenosis in about 15% to 25%, inflammation of the duct (sialodochitis) in about 5% to 10%, and other obstructions, such as anatomic variations or foreign bodies, in about 1% to 3%.[1–3]

Until just a few years ago, the operative removal of the glands was recommended as the therapeutic method of choice in as many as 40% of all cases after unsuccessful conservative treatment.[4–8] The development of a variety of minimally invasive techniques has led to a fundamental change in therapeutic perspectives.[9–16] Various forms of therapy for obstructive disorders are meanwhile reported in the literature: interventional sialography and other radiologically controlled methods, such as ultrasound-guided techniques,[3,16,17]and sialendoscopy.[9,15] Sialendoscopy has received broad acceptance in the diagnostic examination and management of obstructive disorders of the salivary glands because of its direct visualization of findings without the use of contrast medium and with the lack of exposure to radiation, combined with a high success rate.[2,14,18–23] Other gland-preserving techniques, such as transoral duct slitting[11,16,21,24–31] or transcutaneous stone retrieval,[30,32–34] have found their way into the therapeutic spectrum for obstructive sialadenitis.

The aim of this article is to present algorithms for the treatment of obstructive diseases of the salivary glands. Experience gained by the authors' study group and the results gleaned from a thorough research and analysis of the literature form the basis for these algorithms.

Department of Otorhinolaryngology, Head and Neck Surgery, Friedrich Alexander University of Erlangen-Nuremberg, Waldstrasse 1, 91054 Erlangen, Germany
* Corresponding author.
E-mail address: Michael.Koch@uk-erlangen.de (M. Koch).

Otolaryngol Clin N Am 42 (2009) 1173–1192
doi:10.1016/j.otc.2009.08.002
oto.theclinics.com
0030-6665/09/$ – see front matter

PRETHERAPEUTIC DIAGNOSTIC EXAMINATIONS

Ultrasound and sialendoscopy are the authors' methods of choice for diagnosing sialadenitis. In the absence of ultrasound, sialography is still regarded as a standard technique. Ultrasound allows a presumptive diagnosis to be made quickly, safely, cost effectively, and with great precision. Sialendoscopy serves to provide a direct demonstration of the obstruction and thus allows confirmation of the diagnosis. Furthermore, it can also lead to endoscopy-controlled treatment (interventional sialendoscopy) during the same session.[3,9,13,19,21,35,36]

ALGORITHM FOR THE TREATMENT OF SIALOLITHIASIS

With an incidence of approximately 60% to 70%, stones are the most common cause of all salivary-duct obstructions; their prevalence in the general population is approximately 1%.[3,37,38] Conservative measures of treatment like massage of the gland, sialgogues, antiinflammatories, and where indicated, antibiotic medication should precede more invasive measures.

Decisive parameters for the further management are size, location (distal duct, hilar region, intraparenchymal ductal system), number and positional relationship of the stones to the surrounding tissue (adhesive, impacted, mobile). Stone impaction may, for example, be suspected sonographically (**Fig. 1**) but can only be demonstrated with certainty by sialendoscopy (**Fig. 2**).

Small (≤5 mm) and mobile stones located in the main excretory duct as far as the hilar region, and possibly even as far as first- and second-order ducts, can be extracted primarily by endoscopically controlled means, in the submandibular and in the parotid gland, with a success rate of 70% to 90% (**Fig. 3**, Video 1). Video 1 of a sialendoscopic extraction is found online at http://www.oto.theclinics.com.[21,31,36,39–43]

Stones of soft consistency with a size of up to 5 to 7 mm may initially be fragmented within the ducts during interventional sialendoscopy and the fragments then retrieved by endoscopically controlled means. Fragmentation may alternatively be accomplished using microinstruments (**Fig. 4**, Video 2 [Video 2 of intraductal sialendoscopically

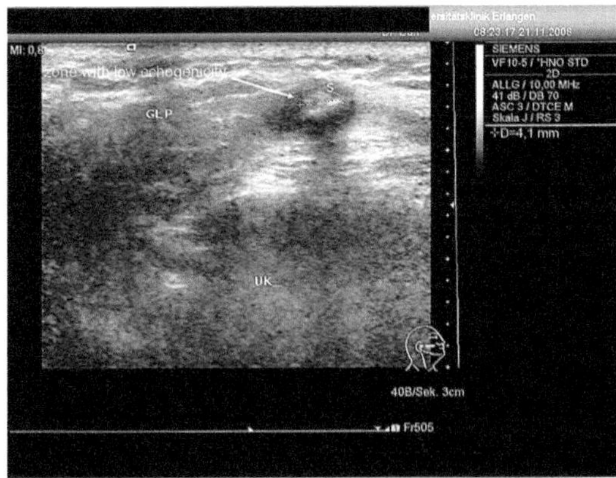

Fig. 1. High-resolution ultrasonography: small stone (4.5 mm) in the proximal segment of the Stensens duct. The arrow indicates the hypoechoic marginal zone of the stone as a sign of impaction. The glandular parenchyma is altered and appears hypoechoic. GLP, parotid gland: S, stone; UK, mandible.

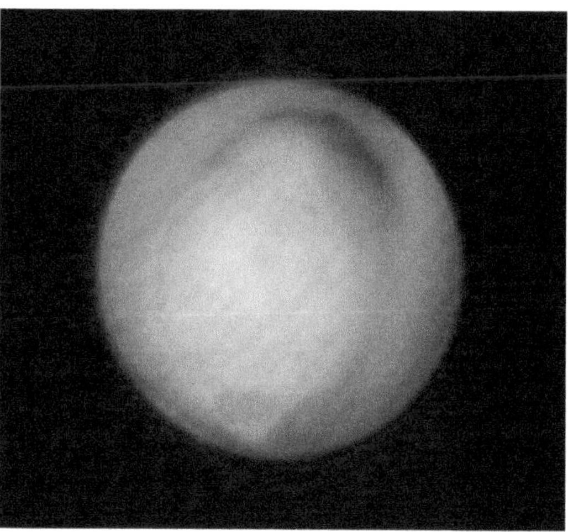

Fig. 2. Sialendoscopic image of a larger, impacted stone in the parotid gland: this is an indication for extracorporeal shock-wave lithotripsy (ESWL).

controlled instrumental fragmentation is found online at http://www.oto.theclinics.com])[21,41,43] or laser technique (**Fig. 5**).[18,39,44–46]

Radiologically controlled or fluoroscopic methods are performed with a success rate of up to 80%.[25,47] Stones that are not accessible using the sialendoscope, those that are impacted, and intraparenchymal stones are disintegrated and fragmented using extracorporeal shock-wave lithotripsy (ESWL). ESWL represents the therapeutic alternative of first choice in many cases of stones of the parotid gland.[19,21,22,31,35,41–43] The mobile fragments can then once again be extracted in an endoscopically controlled manner.[21]

Intractable stones of the papilla and the distal ductal system of the parotid gland can be retrieved by way of an extended papillotomy or distal duct slitting. The majority of

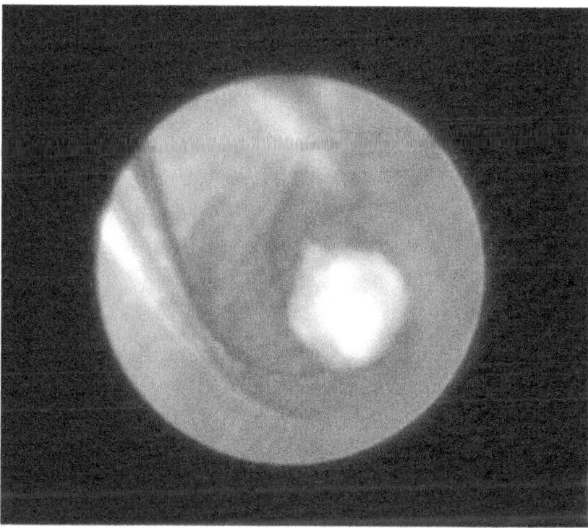

Fig. 3. Sialendoscopic image of a smaller, mobile stone of the submandibular gland, There is the indication here for primary sialendoscopic extraction.

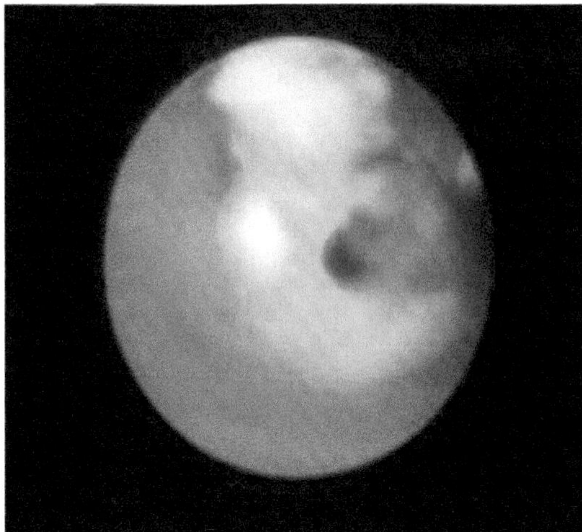

Fig. 4. Sialendoscopic image of a marginally large, mobile stone in the parotid gland, which is too large for primary sialendoscopic extraction. Treatment is therefore by intraductal endoscopically controlled instrumental fragmentation (micro-drill). The fragments can be retrieved by sialendoscopy.

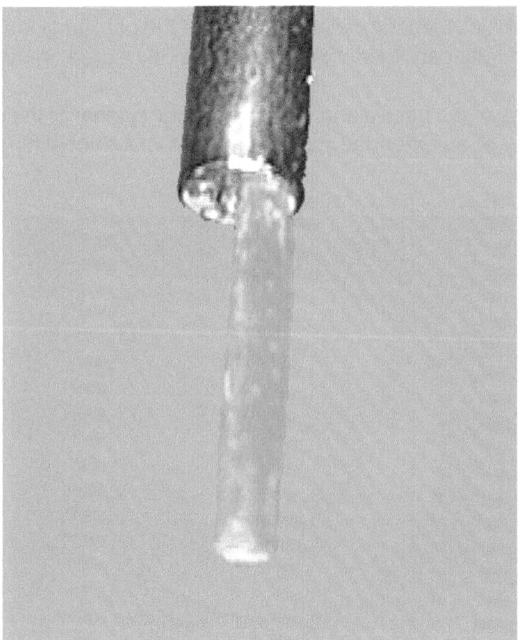

Fig. 5. Terminal part of the sialendoscope with laser fibers in the working channel. Intracorporeal laser fragmentation is the alternative for stones that are too large for primary sialendoscopic extraction. Residual fragments can be removed by sialendoscopy.

these cases require the implantation of a stent to prevent the development of a stenosis.[7,8,21,48,49] For the submandibular duct, the various modifications of transoral duct slitting are the methods of choice for larger or impacted stones; the success rate amounts to more than 90%. The incision can be done beyond the hilar region as far as intraparenchymal areas.[11,16,21,24–31]

The combined endoscopic-transcutaneous stone retrieval was developed for therapy-resistant stones of the parotid gland and carries a success rate of as high as 90%.[30,33,34] As an alternative to the removal of the gland, repeat injections of botulinum toxin may be administered as the therapy of last choice.[50]

Therapeutic Strategy for Stones of the Submandibular Gland

Only approximately 10% of all stones have an intraparenchymal location (**Fig. 6**). As a rule, conservative measures are sufficient for stones without symptoms.

Distal Stones and Those in the Main Excretory Duct

Small mobile stones ($\leq$5 mm) are retrieved primarily by interventional sialendoscopy or other interventional methods (sialography, ultrasound-controlled). Concomitant papillotomy may be necessary.

Transoral duct slitting is the treatment of first choice for impacted stones and stones with a size of more than 5 mm. Endoscopic mobilization or fragmentation may be considered for a stone size of 5 to 7 mm, but this is regarded as treatment of second choice.

If several stones are present, they are treated similarly according to their size and may need to undergo a combined form of management.

Stones in the Hilar Region

Small mobile stones ($\leq$5 mm) may be retrieved by interventional techniques. Stones of borderline sizes (5–7 mm) may undergo attempts at endoscopic mobilization and fragmentation, followed by fragment extraction. Transoral-duct slitting is primarily indicated for larger stones or impacted stones (**Fig. 7**).

Sonographic localization is very helpful for planning the management of smaller impacted stones located deep in the hilar region (from a sialendoscopic view, ducts of the first order) (**Figs. 8–10**). If the stone can be visualized during sialendoscopy and is palpable, then transoral duct slitting is performed (**Fig. 11**). ESWL is indicated in visible and impacted stones in the duct system from first order, which are not palpable (in most cases calculi of 5 mm or less in size, Video 3), or if the stone is

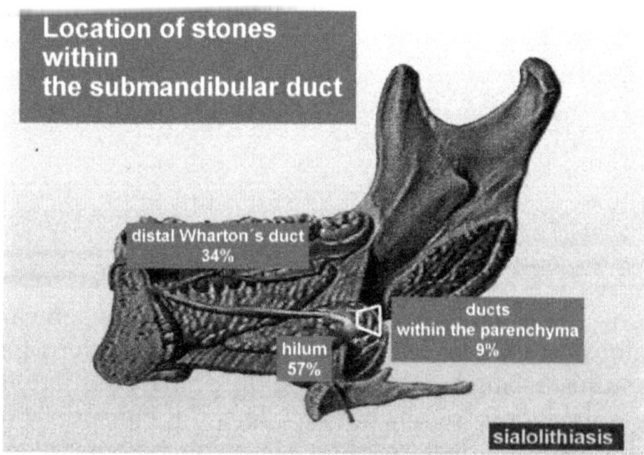

Fig. 6. Location and frequency of stones in the submandibular gland.

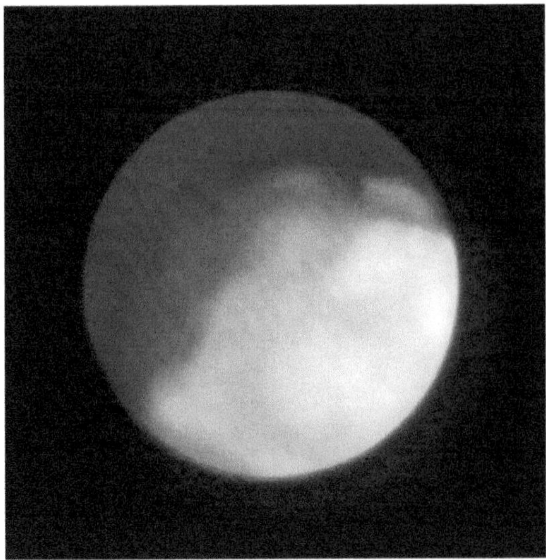

Fig. 7. Sialendoscopic image of a large, impacted stone in the hilum of the submandibular gland, which is an indication to transoral duct slitting.

not visible during sialendoscopy. Video 3 of an impacted stone in hilum is found online at http://www.oto.theclinics.com. The indication for ESWL is for impacted, nonpalpable stones in a duct of the first order (usually smaller calculi up to 5 mm in size) or for stones which cannot be visualized during sialendoscopy. If several stones are present, they are treated similarly and may need to undergo a combined form of management. Residual fragments may be retrieved using interventional means.

Intraparenchymal Stones

If the calculi can be visualized during endoscopy, an attempt may be made to extract small mobile stones by endoscopy, mobilization, or fragmentation. Transoral duct

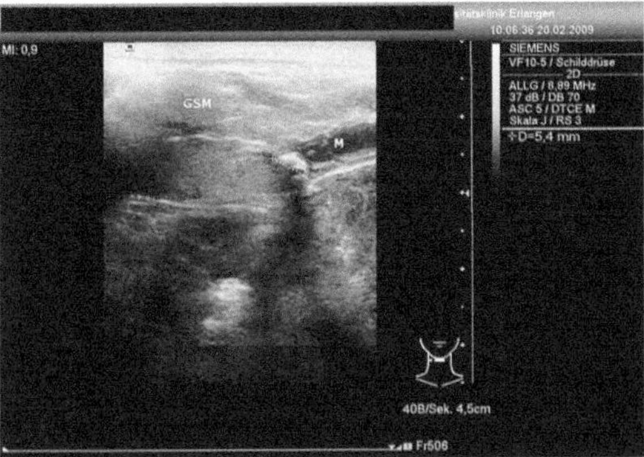

Fig. 8. High-resolution ultrasonography of smaller stones of the submandibular gland for the purpose of demonstrating the subsequent therapeutic options based on the sonographic finding. The stone (5.4 mm) in the hilar region, primary indication for interventional therapy. If the stone is sialendoscopically not mobile and is bimanually well palpable, then this is an indication for transoral duct slitting. GSM, submandibular gland; MM, mylohyoid muscle; Stone with the size of 5.4 mm is marked (+).

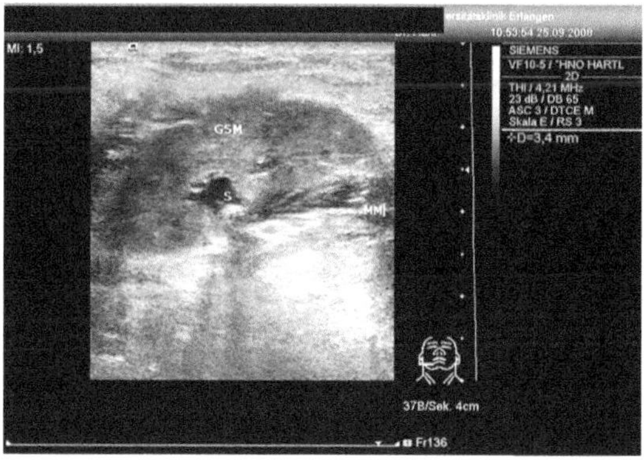

Fig. 9. Stone (3.4 mm) located deep in the hilar region, almost intraparenchymal: indication for primary interventional sialendoscopy. Should this not be possible, then there would be the indication for transoral duct slitting (stone is endoscopically visible and palpable) or for ESWL (stone not visualized at endoscopy). GSM, submandibular gland; MM, mylohyoid muscle; S, stone.

slitting with opening of the gland is indicated for large stones, which are palpable from inside the mouth.

If a small stone cannot be visualized endoscopically or cannot be removed endoscopically, then ESWL is indicated. The success rate is significantly reduced with stones larger than 10 mm in size.

Removal of the gland should be undertaken as a therapeutic option if at least three ESWL sessions were unsuccessful or for stones larger than 10 mm in size that cannot be retrieved by the transoral route or for several intraparenchymal stones. **Diagram 1** illustrates the algorithm for the management of submandibular stones.

Therapeutic Strategy for Stones of the Parotid Gland

Twenty percent to twenty-five percent of all stones have an intraparenchymal location (**Fig. 12**). The stones are more commonly impacted (see **Fig. 2**).

Conservative measures may be sufficient for stones with no symptoms (see earlier discussion).

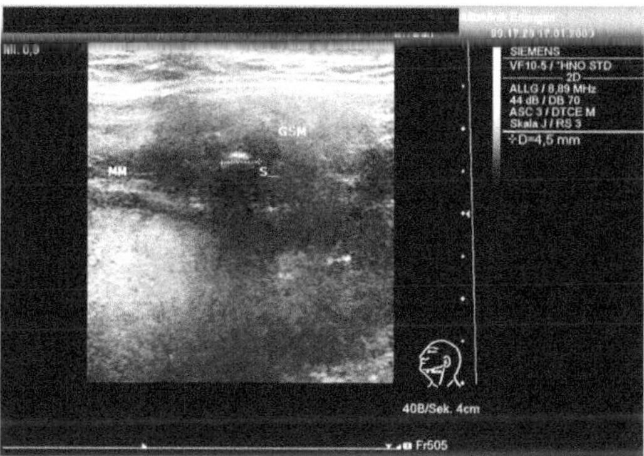

Fig. 10. Stone (4.5 mm) intraparenchymal: indication for ESWL. GSM, submandibular gland; MM, mylohyoid muscle; S, stone.

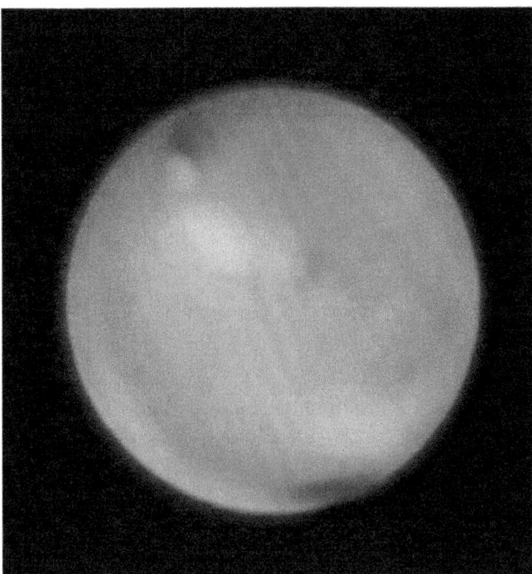

Fig. 11. Sialendoscopic image of a smaller, impacted stone in the hilum of the submandibular gland (upper duct system after division of the main duct). Interventional sialendoscopy not indicated. If the stone is palpable, then transoral duct slitting is the therapy of choice if the stone is palpable. In this case the stone was not palpable, therefore ESWL was indicated. The situation corresponds to that of the sonographic finding in **Fig. 9**.

Stones in the Papilla and the Distal Excretory Duct

For visible small stones in the papilla, spontaneous passage may be provoked with the aid of bougienage. Small mobile stones (≤5 mm) are retrieved by interventional sialendoscopy or other interventional methods (sialography, ultrasound controlled). Endoscopic mobilization or fragmentation may be considered for a stone size between 5 to7 mm. Major operative manipulations to the papilla are obsolete as a primary therapeutic measure, as they frequently result in stenosis. A mini-papillotomy may be performed without the risk of creating a stenosis for stones/fragments that have been grasped by various instruments during interventional sialendoscopy, but have proved to be too large for passage through the papilla. A mini-papillotomy consists of a superficial incision in the papilla, not involving the duct epithelium and extending maximally 3 to 4 mm (**Fig. 13**).[21]

Regardless of the stone location, ESWL is the therapy of choice for impacted stones or stones with a size greater than 5 mm that are not retrievable even by interventional means. Extraction using interventional sialendoscopy is indicated for persistent fragments in the ductal system. If ESWL is not available, stone retrieval may be achieved by a combined endoscopic and transcutaneous approach in the distal excretory duct. If several stones are present, they are treated similarly according to their size and may need to undergo a combined form of management.

Stones in the Middle, Proximal Duct, and Hilar Region

Small mobile stones (≤5 mm) are primarily treated using available interventional methods (sialendoscopy, sialography, or ultrasound controlled) while preserving the

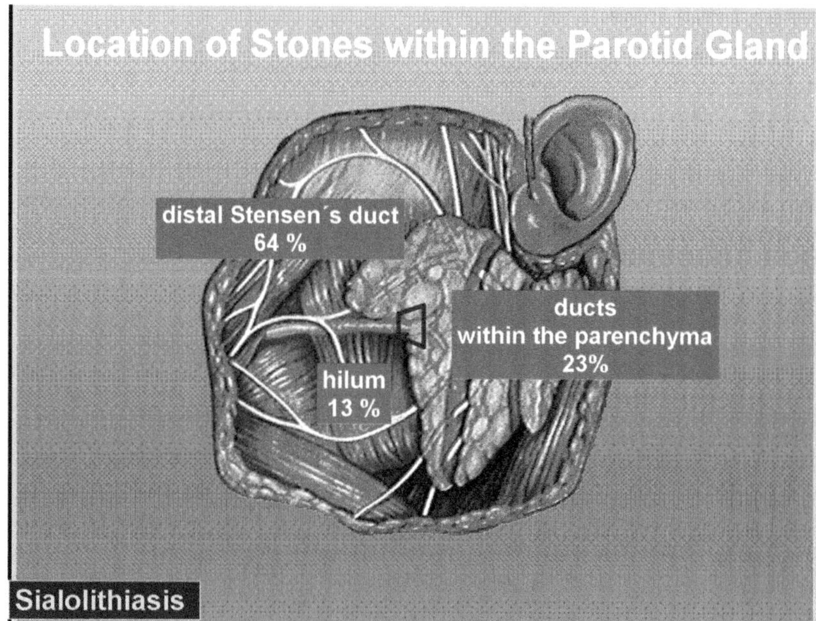

Fig. 12. Location and frequency of stones in the parotid gland.

gland. ESWL is primarily indicated for small stones that are not amenable to sialendoscopy or for impacted stones. Residual fragments, on the other hand, may be extracted by interventional means.

Patients who have therapy-resistant calculi or a contraindication to ESWL (cardiac pacemaker) are treated by a combined endoscopic-transcutaneous approach. The prerequisite for this is the endoscopic accessibility of the stone.

If several stones are present, they are treated similarly and may need to undergo a combined form of management.

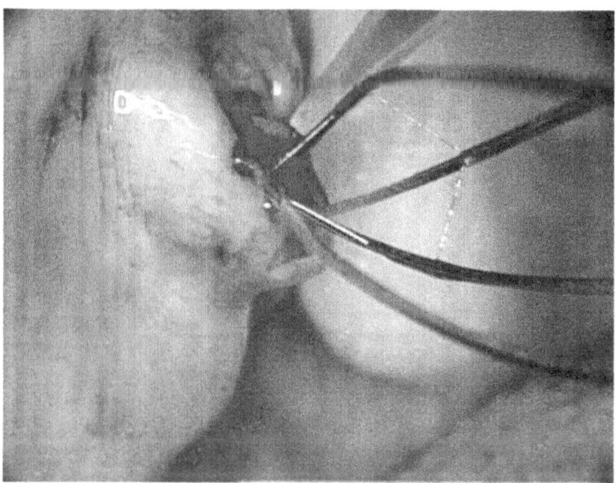

Fig. 13. Situation during mini-papillotomy, which is necessary for the extraction of a stone to facilitate its passage through the papilla of the parotid gland.

Intraparenchymal Stones

If the calculi can be visualized during endoscopy, an attempt may also be made to extract small mobile stones by endoscopy, mobilization, or fragmentation (see earlier discussion). Alternatively, and in all other cases in which a small stone cannot be visualized during endoscopy, ESWL is performed. Residual fragments, on the other hand, may be retrieved by a combined use of interventional means. Therapy-resistant stones, or patients who have a contraindication to ESWL, are indications for the combined endoscopic-transcutaneous approach. The prerequisite for this is the endoscopic accessibility of the stone.

Parotidectomy is indicated when minimally invasive measures, including ESWL, have not been successful after at least three sessions or several intraparenchymal stones are present (n >3). **Diagram 2** illustrates the current therapeutic strategy.

ALGORITHM FOR THE MANAGEMENT OF STENOSES

An impression of the characteristics of the stenosis may be gained using ultrasound or sialography, but especially with the aid of sialendoscopy.[2,51] The decisive factors for therapy, however, are location, the number of stenoses, their length, the degree of obstruction, and the character of the tissue in the region of the stenosis.

Sialendoscopy has the advantage of direct assessment, allowing an inflammatory stenosis to be differentiated from a fibrous stenosis. The majority of the former may be successfully treated conservatively (irrigation and intraductal steroid instillation), whereas the latter can usually only be managed by an additional endoscopically controlled instrumental dilatation.[49] The intraductal administration of drugs has already been performed in the treatment of chronic parotitis with varying degrees of success.[52–54] Intraductal administration of steroids, during sialendoscopic irrigation and after the intervention, has proved to be an important part of the therapy.[49,55]

Interventional sialendoscopy is the operative treatment of first choice for any stenosis, with a success rate of 70% to 90% (**Fig. 14**, Video 4).[2,18,22,35,49,55] Video 4 of sialendoscopic dilatation of stenosis is found online at http://www.oto.theclinics.

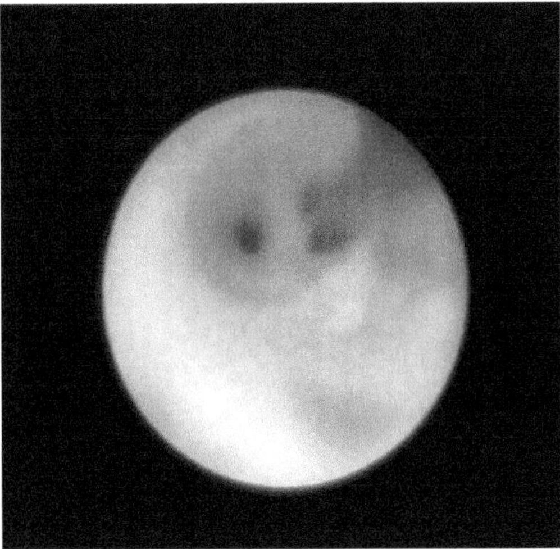

Fig. 14. Fibrous filiform stenosis of the Stensen's duct before instrumental dilatation with the mini-drill.

com. Alternatively, dilatation by interventional sialography may also be performed; the success rates are comparable and amount to 80%.[3,16,56] Operative interventions on the papilla may be successfully conducted for a complete obstruction in this region. Apart from papillotomy and distal duct slitting, resection of the affected segment of duct and repair by suturing into the buccal mucosa promise success.[7,8,21,48,49] Opening the duct using a combined endoscopic-transcutaneous approach and performing plastic-surgical repair with the insertion of a vein patch (sialodochoplasty) has been suggested for stenoses located further proximally.[34] Stent implantation is an important measure for preventing recurrent stenosis.[49,55] Ligation of the duct is an option and avoids parotidectomy, should the other forms of treatment fail. It is, however, viewed with varying degrees of acceptance with regard to its value and long-term effect; the success rates only amount to maximally 50%.[7,8,13,30,34] As an additional treatment option, repeat intraglandular application of botulinum toxin may also be attempted as an alternative to removal of the gland.[50]

Therapeutic Strategy for Stenosis of the Submandibular Gland

Symptom-free stenoses, especially if there is an associated recognizable atrophy of the gland, require no, or an exclusively conservative, form of treatment (as described above in algorithm for the treatment of sialolithiasis). The basic treatment rule applies for symptomatic stenoses: inflammatory stenoses are treated primarily conservatively, whereas fibrous stenoses are operated on.

Papillary Stenosis or Distal Ductal Stenosis

Transoral papillotomy or duct slitting is the treatment of first choice, being completely adequate in nearly all cases.

Stenosis of the Proximal Ductal System and Hilar Region

Localized (inflammatory and fibrous) stenoses are an indication for sialendoscopic, or alternatively, sialographically controlled dilatation in the presence of a corresponding narrowing of the lumen. Diffuse stenoses are generally first treated conservatively, whereas diffuse fibrous stenoses undergo transoral duct slitting, and if necessary, by extending the duct slitting beyond the hilum into the gland parenchyma (submandibulotomy). If scar formation extends far into the parenchyma, removal of the gland is indicated, if there are appropriate symptoms.

Stenoses of the Intraparenchymal Ductal System

Interventional sialendoscopy is indicated for a localized stenosis that can be visualized at sialendoscopy. If the stenosis cannot be visualized at endoscopy or is diffuse in nature, then conservative means of treatment are initiated. Removal of the gland is indicated in individual cases if relevant symptoms are present and the parenchyma of the gland lacks any tendency to atrophy. Alternatively, repeat injection of botulinum toxin into the gland parenchyma may arrest the symptoms, if surgery cannot be performed. **Diagram 3** illustrates the current therapeutic strategy.

Therapeutic Strategy for Stenosis of the Parotid Gland

The majority of stenoses occur in the parotid gland duct, with a differentiation between inflammatory (**Fig. 15**) and fibrous stenosis (see **Fig. 14**) being frequently possible. Symptom-free stenoses, especially if there is an associated recognizable atrophy of the gland, require no, or an exclusively conservative, form of treatment (as described above in algorithm for the treatment of sialolithiasis). Sialendoscopy-based conservative treatment is indicated in cases with inflammatory stenoses and in all cases with

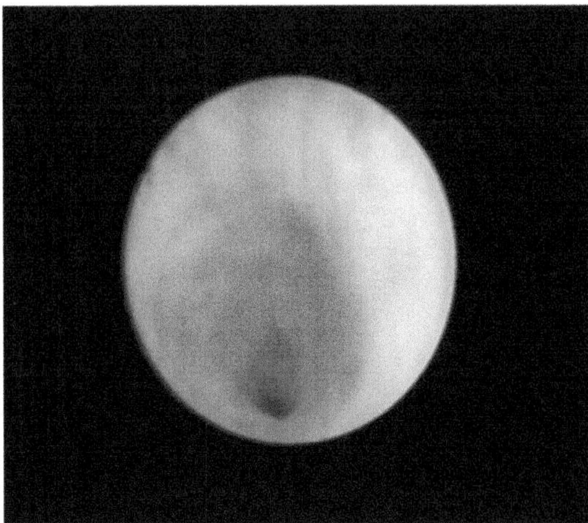

Fig. 15. Inflammatory stenosis of the Stensen's duct.

diffuse stenoses as a primary therapy, but also in all cases after performing an interventional sialendoscopy. It consists of irrigation of the duct system (eg, Ringer solution and cortisone) while performing sialendoscopy and in postinterventional weekly intraductal applications of cortisone for 4 to 8 weeks.[21,49]

Papillary Stenosis or Distal Ductal Stenosis

Conservative and sialendoscopy-based management is primarily indicated for the majority of cases with inflammatory stenosis. Interventional sialendoscopically, or alternatively, sialographically controlled dilatation is primarily the treatment of first choice for all fibrous stenoses or for high-grade or therapy-resistant inflammatory stenoses. Transoral surgery of the papilla or the distal ductal system is performed for therapy-resistant cases. Modifications of this approach include papillotomy, distal duct slitting, and resection of the stenosed segment of the duct with distal duct reinsertion into the buccal mucosa and creation of a neo-ostium. The majority of cases will

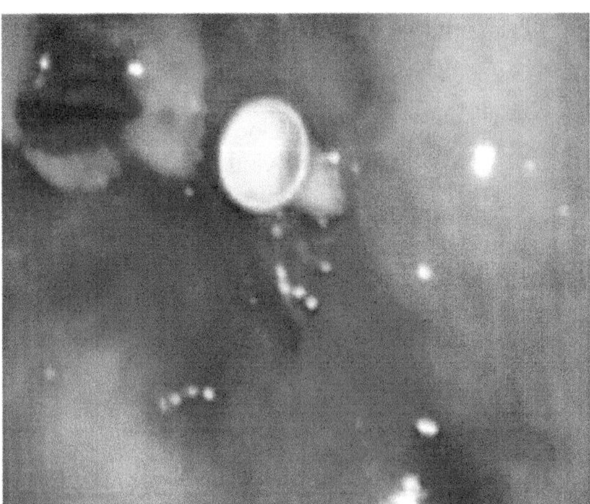

Fig. 16. Appearance after extended papillotomy for combined stenosis and stone in the papilla of the parotid gland with the insertion of a stent as a prophylaxis against the development of a recurrent stenosis.

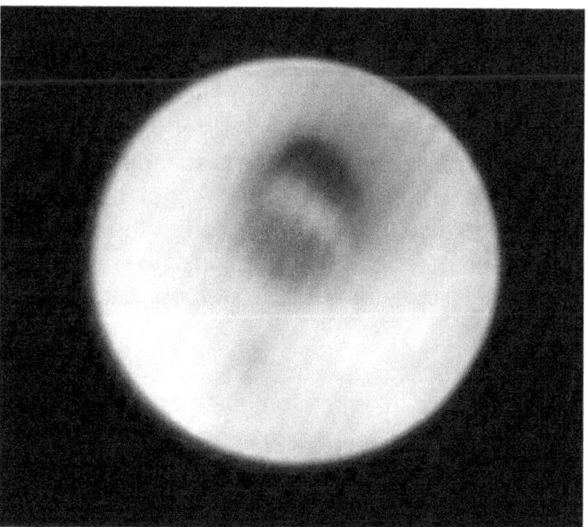

Fig. 17. Fibrinoid plaque, which had resulted in obstruction of the excretory duct of the parotid gland, before its endoscopically controlled extraction.

require the endoscopically controlled implantation of a stent to prevent the development of a stenosis (**Fig. 16**).

Stenosis of the Middle, Proximal Ductal System and Hilar Region

Conservative and sialendoscopy-based management is primarily indicated for localized or diffuse inflammatory, and for diffuse fibrous stenoses. Interventional management is indicated for localized fibrous stenosis, and less frequently, inflammatory stenoses in the presence of a corresponding narrowing of the lumen. The option of opening the stenosis using a combined transcutaneous-endoscopic operation is available for therapy-resistant cases. If parts of the duct wall require resection, an augmentation patch-plasty using a vein graft may be performed. If conservative management of diffuse stenoses including the injection of botolinum toxin fails, ligation of the excretory duct may avoid the complications that are possible following resection of the gland. Gland resection is the treatment of last choice.

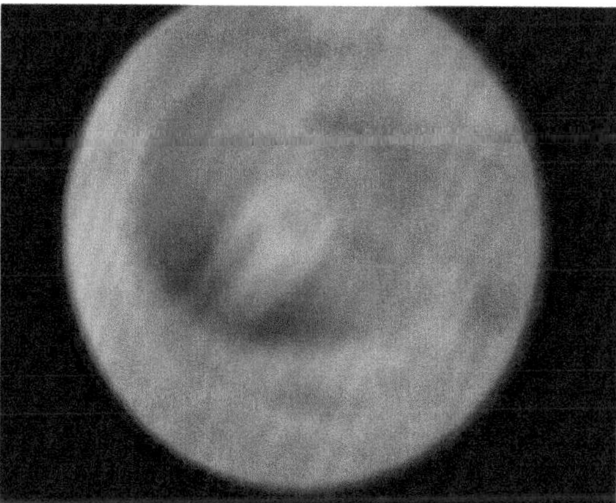

Fig. 18. Foreign body in the hilar region of the parotid gland (indwelling venous catheter, which had previously been inserted into the papilla as a stent), resulting in obstruction of the excretory duct of the parotid gland before its endoscopically controlled extraction.

Intraparenchymal Ductal System

Conservative and sialendoscopy-based management is primarily indicated for localized or diffuse inflammatory, and for diffuse fibrous, stenoses. Interventional sialendoscopy is indicated for localized stenoses that can be visualized at sialendoscopy, although the combined transcutaneous-endoscopic operation is suitable for therapy-resistant cases. Conservative therapeutic measures are undertaken for stenoses that cannot be visualized endoscopically or are diffuse in nature. Ligation of the duct or repeat injection of botulinum toxin into the gland parenchyma or ligation of the duct may help to avoid excision of the gland. **Diagram 4** illustrates the current therapeutic strategy.

Sialodochitis

Sialodochitis is characterized by inflammation, edematous thickening of the duct wall, and obstruction by mucous or fibrous plaques (**Fig. 17**). In the majority of cases, it is observed in the parotid gland.[2,57,58] The intraductal steroid administration while performing irrigation during sialendoscopy and after the intervention has emerged as an important component of its management.[49,55]

Therapeutic Strategy for Sialodochitis

The treatment of choice is the endoscopically controlled irrigation of the ductal system and intraductal steroid administration. This treatment should be continued for 4 to 8 weeks. Obstructing plaques are removed using interventional sialendoscopy (**Diagram 5**).

Special Situations

Rare causes of swelling of a salivary gland include anatomic variations, such as significant convolutions, kinking, web-like retractions in the ductal system, polyps of the

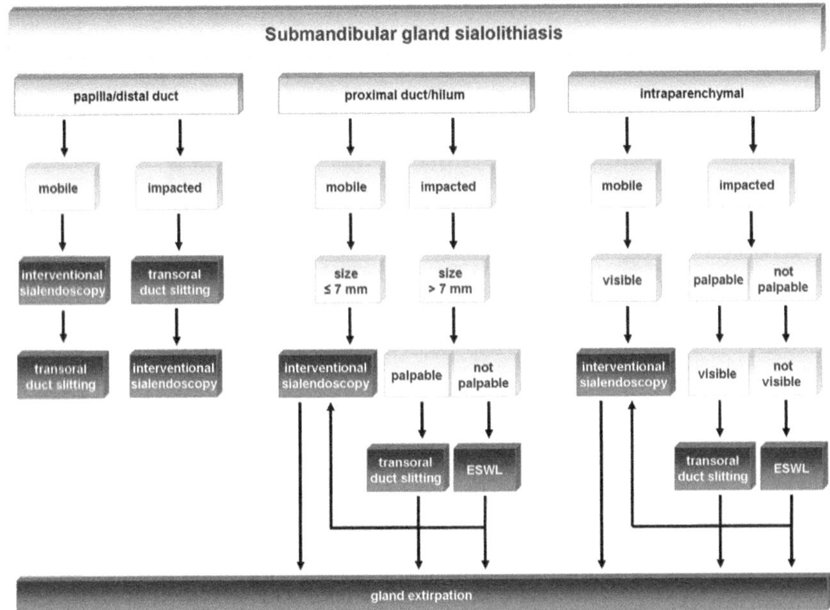

Diagram 1. Treatment algorithm for sialolithiasis of the submandibular gland.

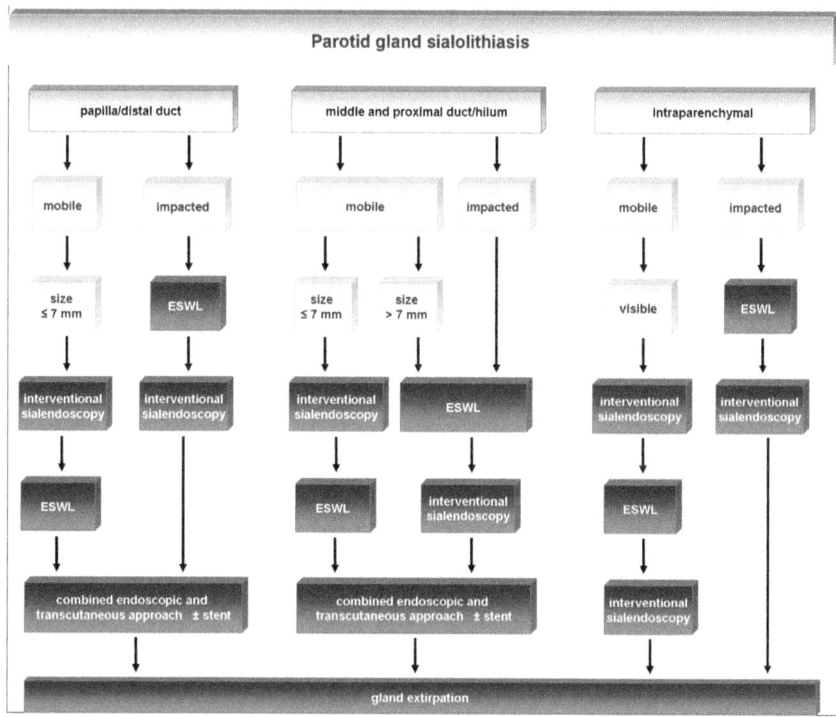

Diagram 2. Treatment algorithm for sialolithiasis of the parotid gland.

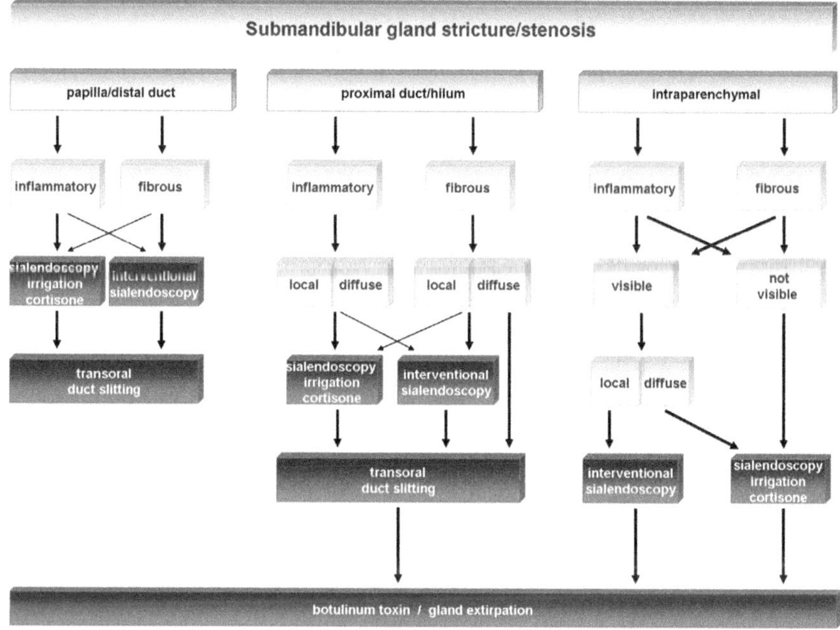

Diagram 3. Treatment algorithm for stricture/stenosis of the submandibular gland.

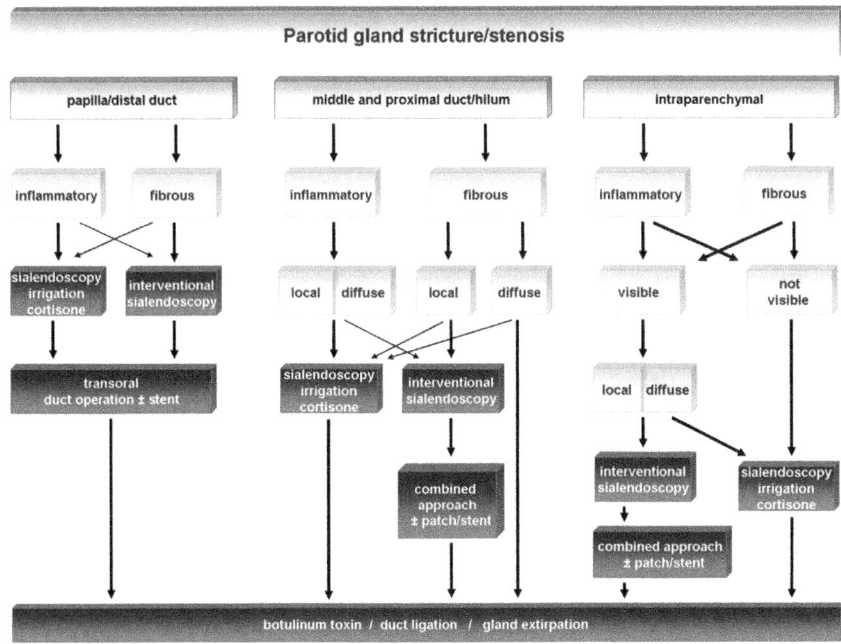

Diagram 4. Treatment algorithm for stricture/stenosis of the parotid gland.

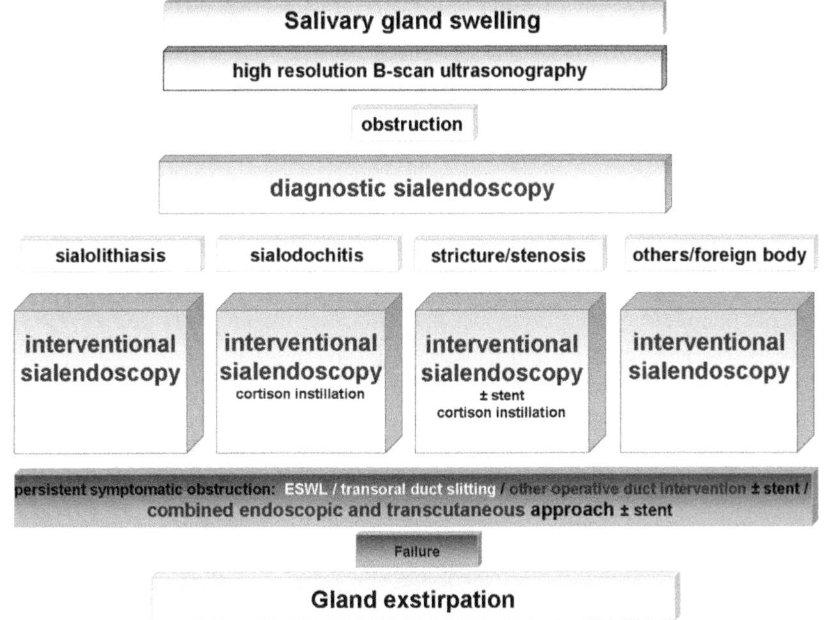

Diagram 5. Overview of the treatment plan and therapeutic strategy for obstructive salivary gland diseases.

duct wall, and foreign bodies.[2,15,19] These variations can only be diagnosed and treated sialendoscopically [2,19,21] Marked convolutions and kinking of the Wharton duct that still give rise to symptoms, despite conservative or endoscopically controlled treatment, may undergo techniques of transoral-duct slitting or modifications, such as the duct-stretching technique.[11,24,26,27,29,30]

Therapeutic Strategy for Rare, Special Situations That Result in Obstruction

Interventional sialendoscopy is the treatment of first choice. During this procedure, for example, obstructing webs can be divided, polyps removed, or a foreign body extracted (**Fig. 18**, Video 5). Video 5 of sialendoscopic extraction of a foreign body is found online at http://www.oto.theclinics.com.

Transoral operations of the ductal system are an alternative if the pathologic lesion of the submandibular gland can be demonstrated by sialendoscopy (see **Diagram 5**).

SUMMARY

The treatment of obstructive diseases of the major salivary glands has undergone a fundamental transformation over the past 10 to 15 years. The rate of gland removal has been significantly reduced to below 5%. The disadvantage of the more recent therapeutic procedures is that the use of these techniques in a daily clinical routine is linked to the availability of the instruments and equipment. Temporal, staffing, and organizational requirements for the hospital are sometimes increased. The treatment is sometimes associated with a financial burden and time stress for patients because of the possible need for several sessions. Acceptance by patients, however, is high because glandular function is maintained without invasive operative measures. Sialendoscopically based procedures, in particular, play a central role in the minimally invasive therapeutic concept shown here. However, analysis of large patient groups shows that it is not one individual therapeutic modality that provides maximal therapeutic results but rather the combination of various methods.[16,21,28,31,43] This statement is reflected in the treatment algorithms described in the present article (**Diagrams 1–5**).

APPENDIX: VIDEOS ONLINE

Supplementary videos can be found in the online version of this article at Salivary Gland Obstruction Treatment Videos.

REFERENCES

1. Rice DH. Non-inflammatory, non-neoplastic disorders of the salivary glands. Otolaryngol Clin North Am 1999;32:835–43.
2. Koch M, Zenk J, Bozzato A, et al. Sialoscopy in cases of unclear swelling of the major salivary glands. Otolaryngol Head Neck Surg 2005;133:863–8.
3. Brown JE. Interventional sialography and minimally invasive techniques in benign salivary gland obstruction. Semin Ultrasound CT MR 2006;27:465–75.
4. O'Brien CJ, Murrant NJ. Surgical management of chronic parotitis. Head Neck 1993;15:445–9.
5. Sadeghi N, Black MJ, Frenkiel S. Parotidectomy for the treatment of chronic recurrent parotitis. J Otolaryngol 1996;25:305–7.
6. Amin MA, Bailey BM, Patel SR. Clinical and radiological evidence to support superficial parotidectomy as the treatment of choice for chronic parotid sialadenitis: a retrospective study. Br J Oral Maxillofac Surg 2001;39:348–52.

7. Moody AB, Avery CM, Walsh S, et al. Surgical management of chronic parotid disease. Br J Oral Maxillofac Surg 2000;38:620–2.
8. Motamed M, Laugharne D, Bradley PJ. Management of chronic parotitis: a review. J Laryngol Otol 2003;117:521–6.
9. Katz P. [New method of examination of the salivary glands: the fiberscope]. Inf Dent 1990;72:785–6 [in French].
10. Iro H, Schneider HT, Fodra C, et al. Shockwave lithotripsy of salivary duct stones. Lancet 1992;339:1333–6.
11. Zenk J, Constantinidis J, Al-Kadah B, et al. Transoral removal of submandibular stones. Arch Otolaryngol Head Neck Surg 2001;127:432–6.
12. Nahlieli O, Sacham R, Yoffe B, et al. Superficial parotidectomy for chronic recurrent parotitis? J Oral Maxillofac Surg 2002;60:970, author reply 970.
13. Baurmash HD. Chronic recurrent parotitis: a closer look at its origin, diagnosis, and management. J Oral Maxillofac Surg 2004;62:1010–8.
14. Nahlieli O, Bar T, Shacham R, et al. Management of chronic recurrent parotitis: current therapy. J Oral Maxillofac Surg 2004;62:1150–5.
15. Nahlieli O, Nakar LH, Nazarian Y, et al. Sialoendoscopy: a new approach to salivary gland obstructive pathology. J Am Dent Assoc 2006;137:1394–400.
16. McGurk M, Escudier MP, Thomas BL, et al. A revolution in the management of obstructive salivary gland disease. Dent Update 2006;33:28–30, 33–26.
17. Geisthoff UW, Lehnert BK, Verse T. Ultrasound-guided mechanical intraductal stone fragmentation and removal for sialolithiasis: a new technique. Surg Endosc 2006;20:690–4.
18. Marchal F, Becker M, Dulguerov P, et al. Interventional sialendoscopy. Laryngoscope 2000;110:318–20.
19. Nahlieli O, Baruchin AM. Long-term experience with endoscopic diagnosis and treatment of salivary gland inflammatory diseases. Laryngoscope 2000;110:988–93.
20. Katz P, Fritsch MH. Salivary stones: innovative techniques in diagnosis and treatment. Curr Opin Otolaryngol Head Neck Surg 2003;11:173–8.
21. Koch M, Zenk J, Iro H. [Diagnostic and interventional sialoscopy in obstructive diseases of the salivary glands]. HNO 2008;56:139–44 [in German].
22. Papadaki ME, McCain JP, Kim K, et al. Interventional sialoendoscopy: early clinical results. J Oral Maxillofac Surg 2008;66:954–62.
23. Walvekar RR, Razfar A, Carrau RL, et al. Sialendoscopy and associated complications: a preliminary experience. Laryngoscope 2008;118:776–9.
24. Baurmash HD. Submandibular salivary stones: current management modalities. J Oral Maxillofac Surg 2004;62:369–78.
25. McGurk M, Escudier MP, Brown JE. Modern management of salivary calculi. Br J Surg 2005;92:107–12.
26. Zenk J, Gottwald F, Bozzato A, et al. [Submandibular sialoliths. Stone removal with organ preservation]. HNO 2005;53:243–9 [in German].
27. McGurk M. Surgical release of a stone from the hilum of the submandibular gland: a technique note. Int J Oral Maxillofac Surg 2005;34:208–10.
28. Iro H, Dlugaiczyk J, Zenk J. Current concepts in diagnosis and treatment of sialolithiasis. Br J Hosp Med (Lond) 2006;67:24–8.
29. Nahlieli O, Shacham R, Zagury A, et al. The ductal stretching technique: an endoscopic-assisted technique for removal of submandibular stones. Laryngoscope 2007;117:1031–5.
30. McGurk M, MacBean A, Fan KF, et al. Conservative management of salivary stones and benign parotid tumours: a description of the surgical technique involved. Ann Roy Australia Coll Dent Surg. 2004;17:41–4.

31. Iro H, Zenk J, Escudier MP, et al. Outcome of minimally invasive management of salivary calculi in 4,691 patients. Laryngoscope 2009;119:263–8.
32. Baurmash H, Dechiara SC. Extraoral parotid sialolithotomy. J Oral Maxillofac Surg 1991;49:127–32.
33. Nahlieli O, London D, Zagury A, et al. Combined approach to impacted parotid stones. J Oral Maxillofac Surg 2002;60:1418–23.
34. Marchal F. A combined endoscopic and external approach for extraction of large stones with preservation of parotid and submandibular glands. Laryngoscope 2007;117:373–7.
35. Marchal F, Dulguerov P, Becker M, et al. Specificity of parotid sialendoscopy. Laryngoscope 2001;111:264–71.
36. Marchal F, Dulguerov P, Becker M, et al. Submandibular diagnostic and interventional sialendoscopy: new procedure for ductal disorders. Ann Otol Rhinol Laryngol 2002;111:27–35.
37. Rauch S. [Diseases of the Salivary Glands]. Wien Med Wochenschr 1965;115: 261–5 [in German].
38. Escudier MP, McGurk M. Symptomatic sialoadenitis and sialolithiasis in the English population, an estimate of the cost of hospital treatment. Braz Dent J 1999;186:463–6.
39. Ito H, Baba S. Pulsed dye laser lithotripsy of submandibular gland salivary calculus. J Laryngol Otol 1996;110:942–6.
40. Chu DW, Chow TL, Lim BH, et al. Endoscopic management of submandibular sialolithiasis. Surg Endosc 2003;17:876–9.
41. Nahlieli O, Shacham R, Bar T, et al. Endoscopic mechanical retrieval of sialoliths. Oral Surg Oral Med Oral Pathol Oral Radiol Endod 2003;95:396–402.
42. Marchal F, Dulguerov P. Sialolithiasis management: the state of the art. Arch Otolaryngol Head Neck Surg 2003;129:951–6.
43. Katz P. [New techniques for the treatment of salivary lithiasis: sialoendoscopy and extracorporal lithotripsy: 1773 cases]. Ann Otolaryngol Chir Cervicofac 2004;121: 123–32 [in French].
44. Iro H, Zenk J, Benzel W. Laser lithotripsy of salivary duct stones. Adv Otorhinolaryngol 1995;49:148–52.
45. Arzoz E, Santiago A, Esnal F, et al. Endoscopic intracorporeal lithotripsy for sialolithiasis. J Oral Maxillofac Surg 1996;54:847–50 [discussion: 851–84].
46. Raif J, Vardi M, Nahlieli O, et al. An Er:YAG laser endoscopic fiber delivery system for lithotripsy of salivary stones. Lasers Surg Med 2006;38:580–7.
47. Brown JE, Drage NA, Escudier MP, et al. Minimally invasive radiologically guided intervention for the treatment of salivary calculi. Cardiovasc Intervent Radiol 2002; 25:352–5.
48. Cohen D, Gatt N, Olschwang D, et al. Surgery for prolonged parotid duct obstruction: a case report. Otolaryngol Head Neck Surg 2003;128:753–4.
49. Koch M, Iro H, Zenk J. Role of sialoscopy in the treatment of Stensen's duct strictures. Ann Otol Rhinol Laryngol 2008;117:271–8.
50. Ellies M, Gottstein U, Rohrbach-Volland S, et al. Reduction of salivary flow with botulinum toxin: extended report on 33 patients with drooling, salivary fistulas, and sialadenitis. Laryngoscope 2004;114:1856–60.
51. Ngu RK, Brown JE, Whaites EJ, et al. Salivary duct strictures: nature and incidence in benign salivary obstruction. Dentomaxillofac Radiol 2007;36:63–7.
52. Galili D, Marmary Y. Juvenile recurrent parotitis: clinicoradiologic follow-up study and the beneficial effect of sialography. Oral Surg Oral Med Oral Pathol 1986;61: 550–6.

53. Bowling DM, Ferry G, Rauch SD, et al. Intraductal tetracycline therapy for the treatment of chronic recurrent parotitis. Ear Nose Throat J 1994;73:262–74.
54. Antoniades D, Harrison JD, Epivatianos A, et al. Treatment of chronic sialadenitis by intraductal penicillin or saline. J Oral Maxillofac Surg 2004;62:431–4.
55. Nahlieli O, Shacham R, Yoffe B, et al. Diagnosis and treatment of strictures and kinks in salivary gland ducts. J Oral Maxillofac Surg 2001;59:484–90 [discussion: 490–2].
56. Brown JE. Minimally invasive techniques for the treatment of benign salivary gland obstruction. Cardiovasc Intervent Radiol 2002;25:345–51.
57. Qi S, Liu X, Wang S. Sialoendoscopic and irrigation findings in chronic obstructive parotitis. Laryngoscope 2005;115:541–5.
58. Chikamatsu K, Shino M, Fukuda Y, et al. Recurring bilateral parotid gland swelling: two cases of sialodochitis fibrinosa. J Laryngol Otol 2006;120:330–3.

Algorithms for Treatment of Salivary Gland Obstructions *Without* Access to Extracorporeal Lithotripsy

Michael H. Fritsch, MD, FACS

KEYWORDS

• Salivary • Endoscopy • Stone • Stenosis • Duct

TREATMENT OF SALIVARY OBSTRUCTIONS

For the North American continent, the extracorporeal shockwave lithotriptor designed for salivary glands is not yet available for use in treating patients. The reasons are multiple, but mainly hinge on the costs associated with the Food and Drug Administration (FDA) approval application. The process must be initiated by an applicant company. In the case of lithotriptors, the company must weigh recouping the costs of FDA filing against the number of anticipated customers for an instrument approaching half a million dollars in cost. It is uncertain when such a lithotriptor device will become available. Also, renal lithotriptors are not appropriate for use on salivary stones and can lead to major complications. Until salivary lithotriptors become available, physicians in North America will continue to see patients with obstructive salivary duct stones; they will need to proceed with treatments without extracorporeal shockwave lithotripsy (ESWL).

Standard North American treatment for salivary duct and gland obstructions remains the sialadenectomy of either the parotid or submandibular glands. On removal of the gland and the duct containing the stone, no further obstructive symptoms will occur; however, the gland's function is lost to the patient and can affect well-being. In a young patient, the other glands may compensate for the loss. With age, however, the remaining salivary glands may fall into decline for any one of many reasons. The missing excised gland could have made a significant percentage contribution to function and rendered the patient asymptomatic. Additionally, there is always the possibility of a gland resection complication, especially of nerve deficiencies.

Department of Otolaryngology–Head and Neck Surgery, Indiana University Medical Center, 702 Barnhill Drive, Suite 0860, Indianapolis, IN 46202, USA
E-mail address: mfritsch@iupui.edu

Otolaryngol Clin N Am 42 (2009) 1193–1197
doi:10.1016/j.otc.2009.08.001 oto.theclinics.com
0030-6665/09/$ – see front matter

In patients with salivary stones and strictures, without access to ESWL, the salivary endoscope with endoscopic instruments is the major tool for accomplishing a minimally-invasive, gland-preserving procedure. Without a lithotriptor, endoscope use becomes expanded to bridge the difference between a large stone, preferably treated with ESWL, and a stone requiring open resection. By expanding endoscope use, new and challenging situations arise requiring skill at manipulation of the endoscopic instrumentation. As a stone increases in size, it changes in character. A small stone will float within the duct and can be grasped with forceps or wire basket for removal. As the stone enlarges, it begins to dilate the duct and thin the duct wall. The inflammatory nature of the stone, the sequestered saliva, the stone pressure on the mucosa, and the bacterial challenges cause the duct lining to change. A normally smooth duct becomes waffled and may even form granulation tissue or polyps. The duct is expanded and the periphery of the stone is quite distant from the duct axis, which has implications for visualization during endoscopy. A thick adhesive stone "rind" may form at the interface between the stone and the duct mucosa. Multiple stones in a row may be present. The sialendoscopic physician's skills must be used to address all of these issues, which would otherwise be mastered through the use of ESWL. For these reasons, there are differences in the stone treatment algorithms used by physicians who have access to ESWL and those who do not.

PAROTID GLAND STONES

For parotid stones (**Fig. 1**) in the mid to proximal duct, sized 2.0 mm or smaller, removal by endoscopic forceps or basket is usually possible. If the stone is between 2.0 and 8.0 mm, endoscopic holmium laser lithotripsy with a 200 μm (or smaller) laser fiber followed by instrument removal is used, sometimes with a papillotomy. C-arm

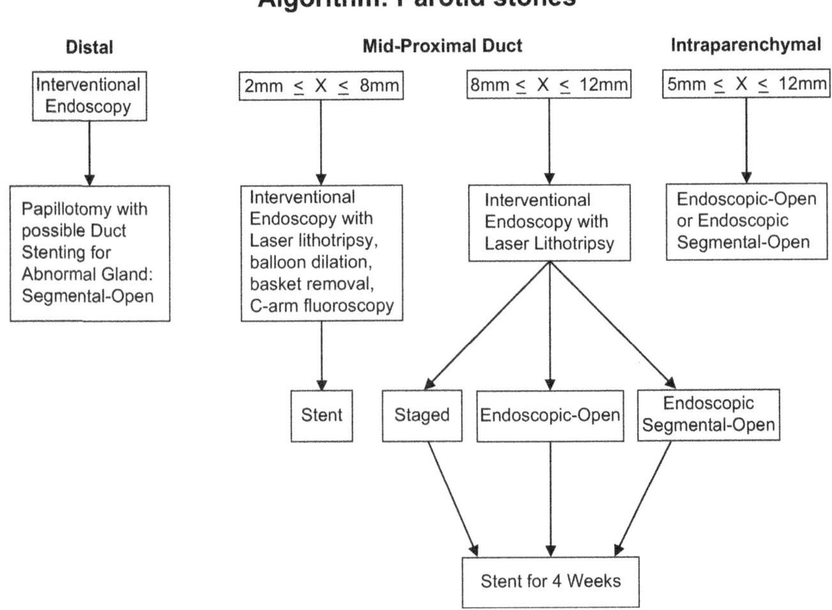

Fig. 1. Algorithm: parotid stones.

fluoroscopy with balloon dilation of the duct, followed by wire basket extraction, can also be used on these stones. For stones between 8.0 and 12.0 mm, a similar strategy is used as for the 2.0 to 8.0 mm group, recognizing that a progression to a staged endoscopic or an endoscopic-open approach will probably be needed.

For sialendoscopic removal of very large stones solely by endoscopic means, without external incisions, several steps are required. The challenge is that a good portion of the stone may lie outside of the duct axis and field of view.

The laser is first used to drill tunnels into and through the central parts of the stone. This achieves a decompression of the gland. It also begins the fragmentation process. To increase the lithoclastic laser shockwave, the laser power can be temporarily increased to produce greater fracturing.

Next, more peripheral tunnels are created. As the peripheral tunnels are created, cracks in the stone appear and the stone starts collapsing toward its center. A wire basket and forceps are used intermittently to retrieve fragments. The laser process continues.

When the greater portion of the stone has been removed, a stone "rind" usually adheres to the duct wall. By maneuvering the endoscope and using external digital compression, the endoscope or laser fiber can be used to dissect and separate the stone from the duct wall. The loosened rind pieces can then be fragmented with the laser. Mini-forceps are used only to retrieve fragments; they are not strong enough to crush stones.

The duct wall of the parotid is stretched by the stone, and after stone removal there is a combination of edema, de-epithelialization, redundant mucosa, and laser damaged areas. The inside of the duct needs time to heal properly and re-epithelialize. The duct inevitably scars and becomes stenosed after such trauma. For this reason, it is of paramount importance to use a stent, sometimes for up to 4 weeks. Usually, a 4F hollow stent is used. The stent must be placed into the empty "socket" where the stone was once positioned. A guidewire is placed into the socket through the endoscope under direct vision. Measurement of the endoscope before and after its withdrawal allows for precise stent length determination and placement depth. The stent is placed over the guidewire, and then the guidewire is slowly withdrawn. It is sewn into position with two 5-0 silk sutures through the stent.

If, during the course of endoscopic removal, the stone rind is seen to be too adherent to dislodge and remove, then further endoscopic work becomes fruitless. An Endoscopic-Open or Endoscopic-Staged approach may be chosen instead. If a staged procedure is chosen, fractures in the stone decompress the salivary pressure and make the gland temporarily asymptomatic between stages.

For stones in the secondary, tertiary, and quaternary ducts, the endoscope and laser together can usually remove them. If the stone is large and expands the thin ducts, tissue-expander-like, into the parenchyma (ie, "intraparenchymal stone"), then an endoscopic-open preauricular approach can be selected. The Endoscopic-Open approach only raises a parotid flap and dissects directly down to the stone to remove it. If the gland drainage-basin proximal to the duct obstruction is heavily diseased with ectasias or multiple stenoses, then the Endoscopic-Open procedure should be expanded to an Endoscopic Segmental-Open approach whereby the wedge-shaped diseased gland tissue is also resected.

PAROTID GLAND STENOSES OR STRICTURES

For parotid stenoses or strictures (**Fig. 2**) from the punctum to the hilum, 2 issues must be considered: the size of the stenotic opening and the degree of fibrosis.

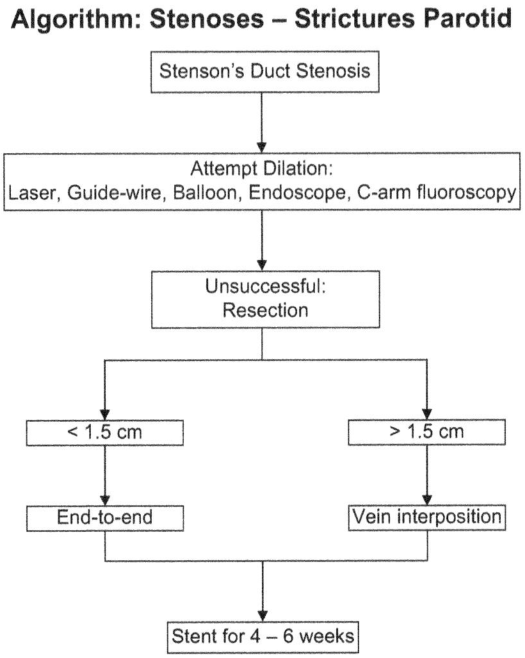

Algorithm: Stenoses – Strictures Parotid

Stenson's Duct Stenosis

Attempt Dilation:
Laser, Guide-wire, Balloon, Endoscope, C-arm fluoroscopy

Unsuccessful:
Resection

< 1.5 cm

> 1.5 cm

End-to-end

Vein interposition

Stent for 4 – 6 weeks

Fig. 2. Algorithm: parotid gland stenoses or strictures.

The opening size at the entry to the stenosis is important because the dilating balloons, whether soft or high-pressure, or the endoscope (itself used for dilation) must first enter the stenosis before dilation. It is possible that the balloons or endoscope are too wide to enter the stenotic opening. This can happen despite attempts to dilate the opening with a laser, with saline pressure, or with a guidewire that is used to guide the forceful advancement of the endoscope or an interventional radiology high-pressure balloon.

The consistency of the stenosis is important because a soft balloon will not be able to dilate a fibrotic "hard stenosis." Indeed, the balloon may rupture during inflation and even leave a large plastic foreign-body shard in the duct. Also, with a hard stenosis more than 2.0 to 3.0 mm long, it is technically difficult to lyse with a laser because of the curved nature of the duct versus the straight laser fiber. A blunt-tipped endoscope or interventional radiology balloon may also not gain entry. In these unusual cases, a stenotic segment resection with end-to-end or vein interposition graft should be considered. For duct defects of 1.5 cm or less, an end-to-end anastomosis can be achieved. For a deficit greater than 1.5 cm of missing duct, a vein graft interposition will be required. Either a dorsal hand vein or a saphenous malleolar ankle branch is useable; the saphenous graft will generally be more robust. In all cases, a stent is used for 4 to 6 weeks.

SUBMANDIBULAR GLAND STONES AND STRICTURES

For submandibular gland stones (**Fig. 3**) without access to ESWL, a major factor contributing to successful removal is that the Wharton duct is wider than the Stensen duct. The difference between the two ducts is considering ease of use for the endoscope with instrumentation. Larger stones can be successfully removed more often

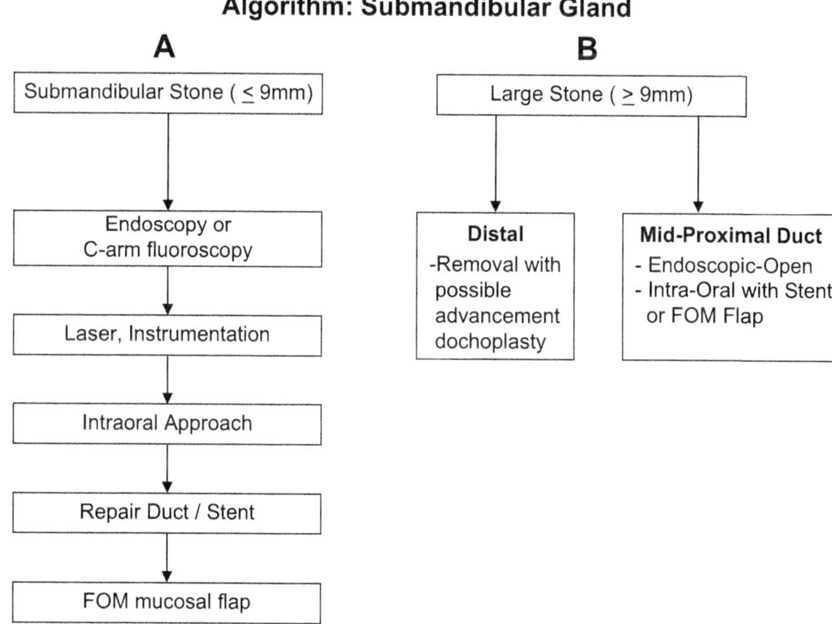

Fig. 3. Algorithm: submandibular gland.

from the submandibular gland duct with the endoscope than from Stensen duct. If attempts with the endoscope or with C-arm fluoroscopy are not successful, then an open intraoral approach is useful. Direct repair of the duct after stone removal, followed by stent placement, is best. If this cannot be achieved, then an advancement dochoplasty or a Sialo Drain (Sialo Technology, Ashkelon, Israel) is useful. If no duct can be ascertained, then a Floor-Of-Mouth (FOM) flap is sewn into the wall of the empty socket to create a mucosal-lined fistula to the FOM.

Incisionless Otoplasty

Michael H. Fritsch, MD, FACS

KEYWORDS

• Otoplasty • Incisionless • Cosmetic • Surgery
• Lop-ear • Surgical procedures

A typically used open-surgical otoplasty operation is the Mustarde procedure.[1] This procedure can give rise to difficulties in the postoperative period. Specifically, the wide incisions and the undermining of the skin and subcutaneous tissues create a dead space with the potential for hematomas, abscess formation, and perichondritis. The retention sutures are under cartilage-spring tension until scarring partially anchors the correction. Excision of excess skin on the posterior pinna is a widely variable and subjective maneuver that can lead to tenting or bridging. To achieve a successful result, considerable postoperative bandaging and maintenance efforts are required for the patient and physician.

The Incisionless Otoplasty techniques arose from a desire to achieve excellent cosmetic effects with a limitation of complications. Incisionless Otoplasty, Version 1.0, was published in 1995 and used a new method of placing percutaneous otoplasty retention sutures.[2] It completely removed the need for incisions and wide tissue undermining. The 2.0 version appeared in the literature in 2004 and added a new percutaneous technique for scoring and breaking the inherent pinna cartilage spring.[3] This served to remove any bow-string–like strain on the retention sutures caused by the cartilage spring. The 3.0 version is a further development of the 2.0 version. It streamlines the retention suture application for the antihelix and broadens the anatomic possibilities for suture application extending to the conchal bowl, the lobule, and to a combined antihelical and conchal bowl correction.

SURGICAL TECHNIQUE OF INCISIONLESS OTOPLASTY 3.0

Antihelical Correction

A 30-gauge needle and a tuberculin syringe are used to deliver nondistorting amounts of vasoconstrictive local anesthetic agent on the anterior and posterior surfaces of the pinna. A circum-auricular injection addresses the superficial temporal and postauricular artery contributions to help achieve tissue blanching. In children, a general anesthetic is used in addition to the local agent. For surgical draping, bilateral, plastic stick-on otologic drapes are applied so that both ears are simultaneously visible for comparison. For awake patients, the otologic drapes are scrolled together

Department of Otolaryngology-Head and Neck Surgery, Indiana University Medical Center, 702 Barnhill Drive, Suite 0860, Indianapolis, In 46202, USA
E-mail address: mfritsch@iupui.edu

Otolaryngol Clin N Am 42 (2009) 1199–1208
doi:10.1016/j.otc.2009.09.003
0030-6665/09/$ – see front matter

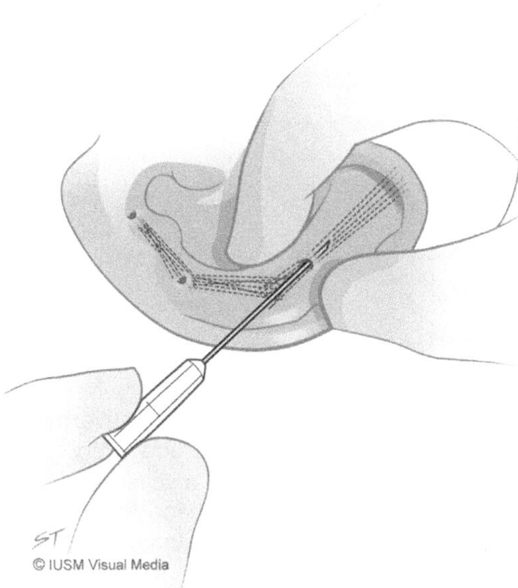

Fig. 1. As the first step in Version 3.0, a percutaneous 20-gauge needle thoroughly scores and punctures the cartilage along the planned antihelical fold. This maneuver breaks the inherent cartilage spring and renders the cartilage pliable. The area connecting the antihelical fold to the antitragus, and the area of the most superior antihelical fold under the helical rim are particularly important. This cartilage spring weakening is performed before any other areas or steps are undertaken. This is to prevent cutting already placed sutures with the needle.

above and below the face, so that the face is freely exposed. With general anesthesia, the otologic drapes are scrolled together covering the face.

Incisionless Otoplasty: step one cartilage scoring

The first surgical step is to precisely break the cartilage spring along the envisioned neoantihelical fold. A 20-gauge phlebotomy needle is used to score percutaneously the anterior cartilage surface and to create full thickness tunnels through the cartilage

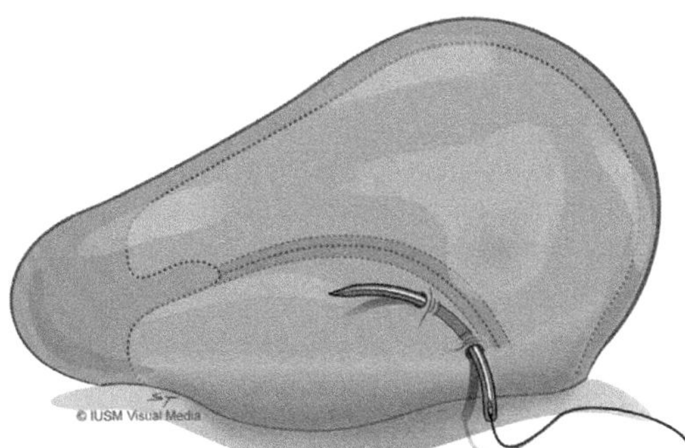

Fig. 2. Step two of Version 3.0 begins with the first short limb of the loop. It enters and exits the skin from the posterior surface. The needle completely penetrates the cartilage, but stays below the anterior skin.

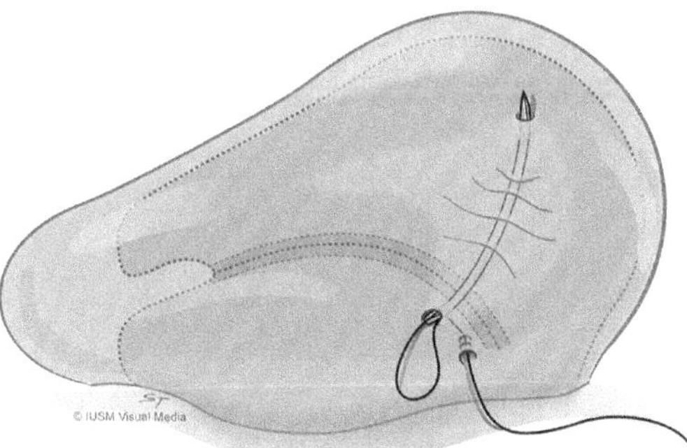

Fig. 3. The first long posterior limb of the suture loop brings the same needle to a point where the second short limb will take place.

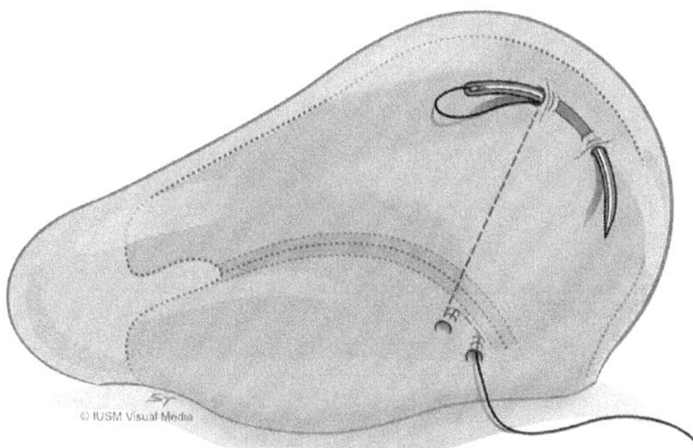

Fig. 4. The second short limb of the suture loop. Note that the needle always enters and exits the skin layer at 90 degrees to allow settling of the suture on the cartilage.

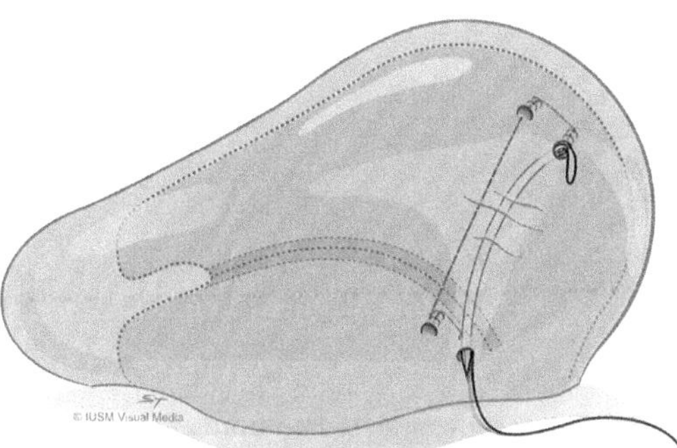

Fig. 5. The second long limb of the suture loop exits the skin through the original entry point of the loop.

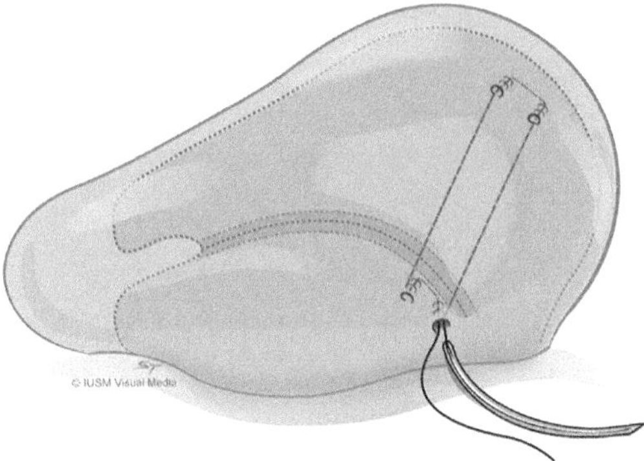

Fig. 6. A completed sutured loop contains two short limbs on the anterior cartilage surface, and two long limbs on the posterior cartilage surface.

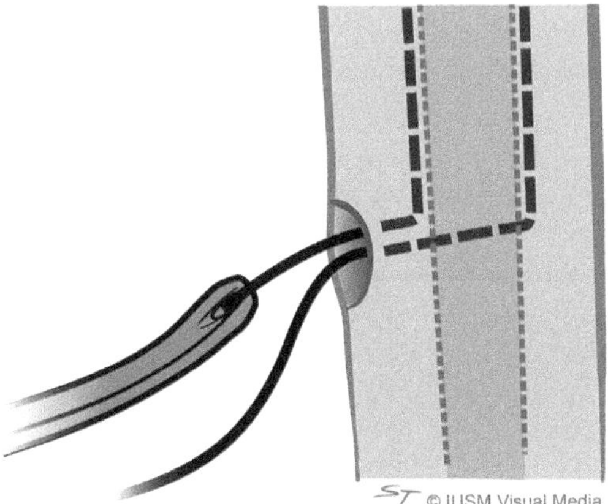

Fig. 7. The suture stays close to, or into, the perichondrium. Ninety-degree needle skin entries and exits are used. Exact tracing through the previous needle tract is performed. These aspects are especially important at the point where a knot will be placed, so that the knot is able to slip through the skin layer and down to the cartilage without becoming tethered in the superficial skin layers. It also prevents skin dimpling.

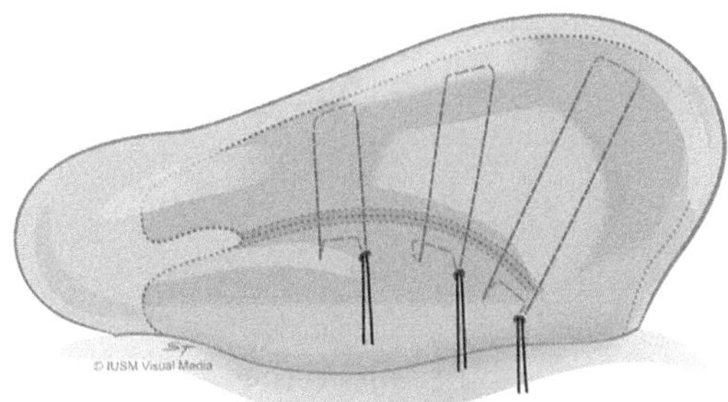

Fig. 8. A series of retention sutures is completed on both ears with two or three sutures per side maintaining the correction. Usually, one suture at the upper pole and one lateral to the ear canal suffice to hold the pliable cartilage in place. Bilateral slow, progressive tightening lowers the ear profile to the desired position; knots are placed.

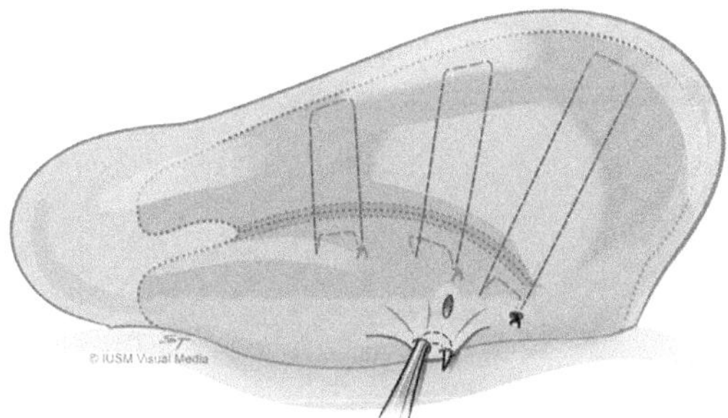

Fig. 9. In step three in Version 3.0, a single-prong hook pulls on the soft tissues adjacent to the suture loop knot. This action submerges the knot below the skin surface and allows it to rest on the cartilage as a final position.

(**Fig. 1**). By doing so, the cartilage spring is released and a palpably flaccid cartilage spring is noted. In this state, the neoantihelical fold can be retained in the desired aesthetic position without tension on the sutures. Additionally, the cartilage scores and tunnels will heal with scar tissue, further strengthening the correction.

Incisionless Otoplasty: step two suture placement

The second surgical step is to place percutaneous retention sutures to hold the neoantihelical fold in the new position.

The preferred suture is a braided, white, 3-0 polyester (Mersilene; Ethicon, Summersville, NJ, USA) with a cutting needle. The manufacturer's attached cutting needle is used. Marking-pen dots on the anterior pinna surface are useful for symmetrically planning the suture loops and as intraoperative targets for the surgeon.

The 3.0 version suture-retention loop starts on the posterior pinna, close to the postauricular sulcus (**Fig. 2**). The retention sutures are placed only from the posterior surface of the pinna and, unlike the 2.0 version, never emerge through the anterior side. The needle penetrates the cartilage and can be seen to burrow subcutaneously under the skin of the anterior conchal bowl for a short distance, before re-exiting on the posterior surface. A broad-based suture bite is used and the suture does not skim into the anterior skin, but stays buried next to the perichondrium to prevent any chance of skin erosion.

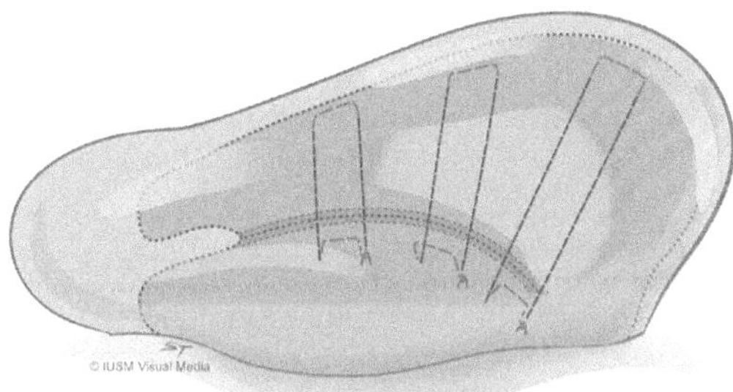

Fig. 10. A completed series of suture loops holding the neoantihelix in place. Any separate conchal bowl recession is performed before application of these antihelical retention sutures.

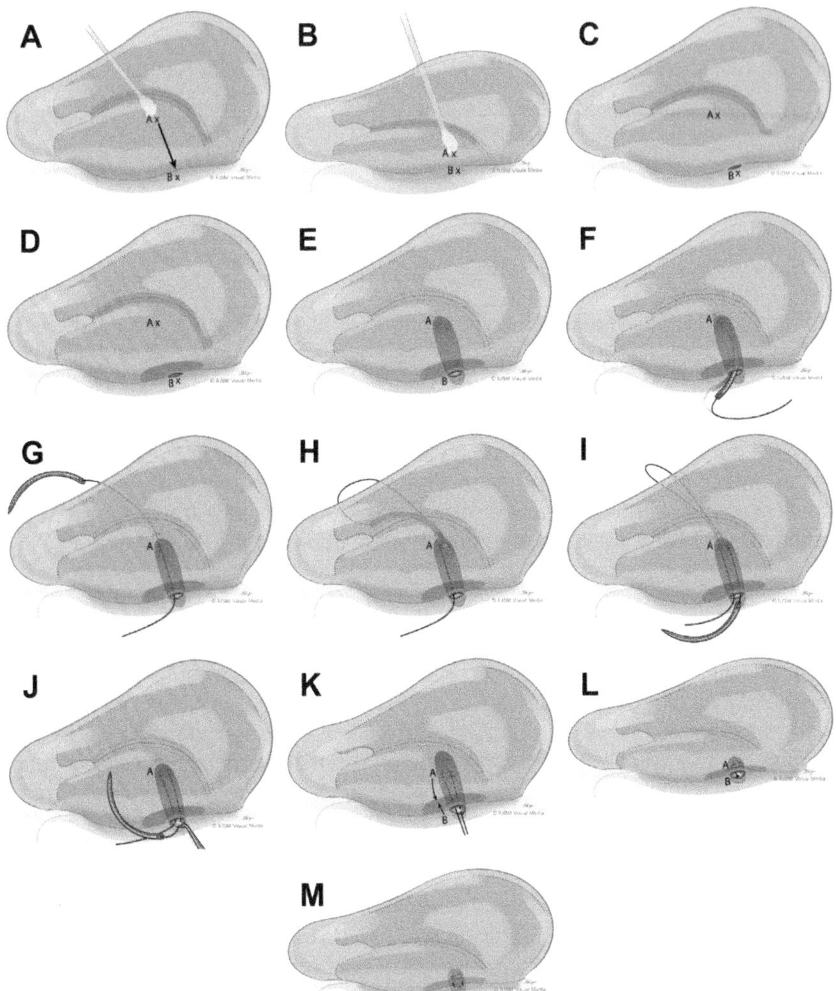

Fig. 11. (*A–M*) The Incisionless technique is used for the protuberant conchal bowl. Owing to the importance of removing soft tissue or bone between the conchal bowl and the mastoid bone, access is created through a small opening in the postauricular sulcus. A needle-tip monopolar cautery is useful for the soft tissue removal. The points of maximal effective correction (*A, B*) are the sites for suture anchoring. If antihelical work is needed, the antihelical cartilage spring scoring (step 1, 3.0 version) should be performed before placing any conchal bowl retention sutures. This prevents needle cuts of already placed conchal sutures.

Next, the needle is redirected for a longer distance, laterally on the postauricular side, toward the chosen spot for the next suture loop short limb (**Fig. 3**). The needle stays on the posterior surface of the cartilage, but it does enter into the perichondrium to keep the suture tacked close to the cartilage and prevent any chance of suture bridging. The process is progressively repeated until the entire loop is completed (**Figs. 4–6**). Conceptually, there are two short limbs of the suture loop on the anterior pinna cartilage surface, and two long limbs on the posterior surface of the cartilage.

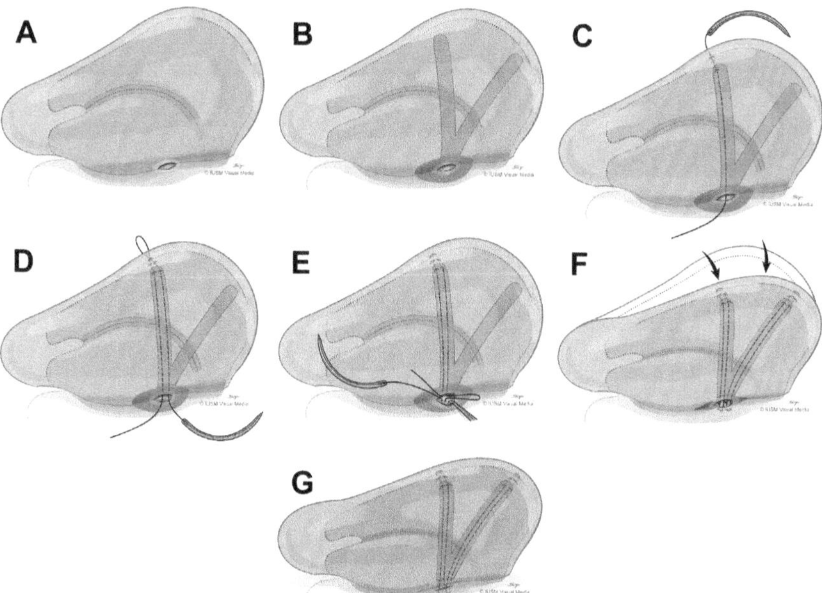

Fig. 12. (*A–G*) A Combined technique for correction of both the conchal bowl and antihelical fold can be used. The surgeon should palpate the ears to determine exactly where the maximum effectiveness for the retention sutures lays. Soft-tissue or bone removal between the conchal bowl and the mastoid is performed. Narrow tunnels on the postauricular cartilage create a scar band to augment the retention sutures and attach to the conchal bowl correction.

The 3.0 version is intraoperatively compatible with the 2.0 version and the two may be used in combination. Sometimes, it is easier to use a 2.0 version stitch for part of the suture loop if difficult angles or thick cartilage are encountered.

Exit and precise re-entry of the needle into exactly the same needle hole prevents epithelial inclusion cyst formation.[2] Skin entry and exit at a 90 degree angle to the skin surface into and out from the previous needle tract prevents dimpling of the skin and also allows the final suture knot to settle on the cartilage. This concept of following in the same needle tract is most important to achieving a successful result (**Fig. 7**).

The number of retention sutures placed for most ears is usually two or, sometimes, three (**Fig. 8**). Though some ears are asymmetric and will bend slightly differently, the sutures in the two ears should usually be placed in very similar positions to achieve the best results. Uncommonly, asymmetric application of the sutures is needed. According to individual needs, the final pinna measurements for the upper pole rim are usually 12 mm and for the midauricle rim at the top of the ear canal are usually 15 mm. These measurements may seem tight, but they help to assure long-term excellent results and give confidence to the patient that a complete correction was achieved.

Once the complete series of suture loops has been placed bilaterally, the loops are progressively tightened. This is done by gentle manual squeezing of the neoantihelix and simultaneous pulling on the individual suture ends. A metal ruler and the surgeon's visual assessment are used to assure adequate tightening, adjustments, and bilateral symmetry. Repetitive tightening and loosening are discouraged as the cartilage may be cut. It is preferable to slowly tighten bilaterally until final symmetry is achieved.

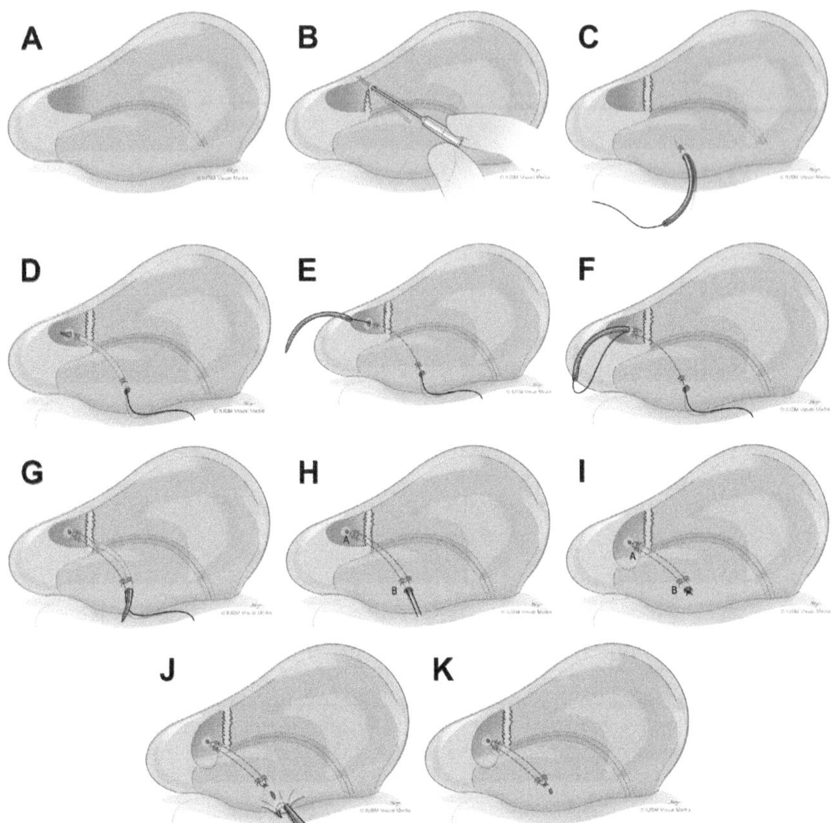

Fig. 13. (*A–K*) Correction of the lobule begins with separation of the cauda helicis from the pinna cartilage. The flail cauda helicis can be grasped with the needle from behind or with a stitch penetrating to the anterior cauda helicis surface. After tightening the suture and pulling the lobule posteriorly, a knot is placed. It is submerged under the skin using a single-prong hook.

Incisionless Otoplasty: step three knot submersion

The third step places the suture knots into a subcutaneous position. After tightening the sutures, the knots are thrown. After completing the knots, they are exterior to the skin. To submerge the knots under the skin and into their final subcutaneous positions on the cartilage, a single-prong hook is used. It is hooked into the skin adjacent to the knot (**Fig. 9**). The hook pulls the skin so that the inelastic suture with knot submerges below the skin (**Fig. 10**). A review of the three key surgical steps by video is useful.[4]

Postoperative mastoidectomy-type dressings can be used for the first night to assure protection against digital contamination of the ears and a bruise-free result. Actual ecchymoses are rare. Bacitracin ointment application, water precautions, and oral antibiotics continue for 1 week. The ears are painful for the first day after surgery and there may be some soreness of the ears for up to 7 days.

Incisionless Otoplasy: Conchal Bowl, Lobule, and 2.0 Techniques

The conchal bowl may contribute to ear protrusion and is corrected using the Conchal Recession Incisionless technique. Only after the antihelical cartilage spring has been

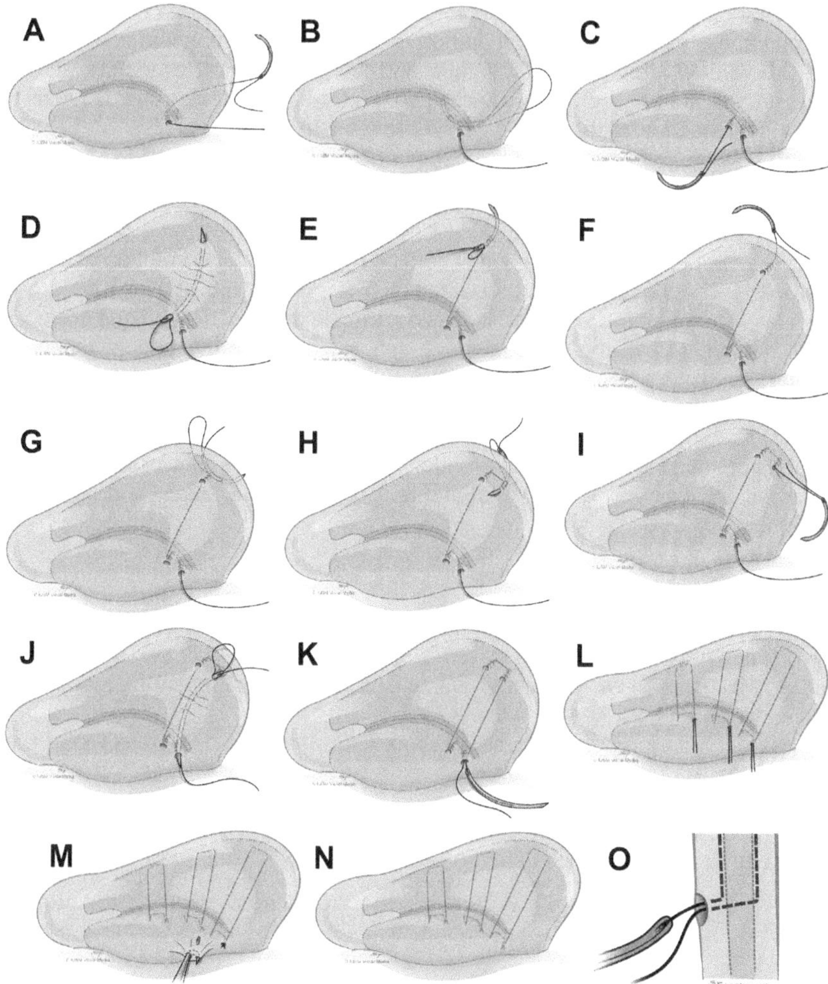

Fig. 14. (*A–O*) Incisionless Otoplasty 2.0 version correction of the antihelical fold is technically easier to perform than the 3.0. The individual steps are more straightforward. The need to enter and exit the skin at a 90-degree angle and stay within the previously created needle tracts is crucial. The knots will glide through the skin to rest on the cartilage and there will be no dimpling of the skin (see **Fig. 7**). Small ink dots on the anterior surface demarcating the short limbs can help the surgeon to precisely place the needle steps.

weakened, (step one, 3.0), so as not to later cut any conchal bowl sutures, is attention turned to the conchal bowl. The conchal bowl may be recessed by itself as a single procedure apart from the antihelix, or completed before the antihelical retention sutures are placed (**Fig. 11**).[3] Alternately, the conchal bowl and antihelical fold may be corrected simultaneously with the same set of retention sutures using the Combined Incisionless technique (**Fig. 12**).

The lobule may also be protuberant. Even if the rest of the otoplasty procedure is performed well, lack of attention to the lobule can decrease aesthetic results. Key to lobule correction is to palpate and identify the cauda helicis. It is separated from the pinna by transcutaneous needle dissection or by a 3.0 mm incision. The Incisionless technique is used to pin the cauda helicis to the posterior conchal bowl (**Fig. 13**).

The 2.0 version is an easier technique and lends itself well to accumulating an operative understanding of Incisionless techniques. The 2.0 is easier because the complex single action of the 3.0 version is broken into separate smaller steps. Work is performed from the posterior and anterior sides of the auricle (see **Fig. 14**).

SUMMARY

Incisionless Otoplasty 3.0 techniques should be considered for correction of the antihelical fold and conchal bowl protuberances. The present 3.0 applications are the Antihelical Correction, the Conchal Recession, the Simultaneous technique correction of both the antihelical and conchal bowl deficiencies, and the Lobule technique. Compared with Versions 1.0 and 2.0, the 3.0 retention suture placement is more streamlined. The surgeon can combine and interchange parts of Versions 2.0 and 3.0 within the same operation and with other open procedures. Owing to the noninvasive nature of the operation, there is a markedly decreased potential for complications. Incisionless Otoplasty in all its variations is a safe, reliable, exact and repeatable operation.

REFERENCES

1. Mustarde JC. The correction of prominent ears by buried mattress sutures: a ten-year survey. Plast Reconstr Surg 1967;39(4):382–6.
2. Fritsch MH. Incisionless Otoplasty. [Version 1.0: early technique without address of the cartilage spring]. Laryngoscope 1995;105:1–11.
3. Fritsch MH. Incisionless Otoplasty. [Version 2.0: percutaneous breakage of cartilage spring added to 1.0 version]. Facial Plast Surg 2004;20(4):267–70.
4. Incisionless Otoplasty surgery video. Available at: http://othn.iu.edu/incisionlessotoplasty/ or, Google: "Michael H Fritsch, MD, FACS", and scroll to "Incisionless Otoplasty".

Endoscopy of the Inner Ear

Michael H. Fritsch, MD, FACS

KEYWORDS

• Endoscopy • Otic • Otology • Inner ear • Stem cells

Surgery of the inner ear remains an elusive goal. Intervention usually means loss of function. Even procedures that superficially invade the labyrinth may give rise to hearing loss. Nevertheless, successful procedures, such as stapedectomy and canal plugging, are performed, and function is preserved. Even with naturally occurring pathologies that destroy the otic capsule, such as cholesteatoma, function can be spared. However, the possibilities of traumatic hearing loss, tinnitus, and vertigo remain obstacles to progress towards more direct inner ear surgery.

Presently there are some patients with a relatively circumscribed otologic lesion, such as an erosive cholesteatoma or intralabyrinthine schwannoma, who nevertheless undergo a surgically destructive procedure of the entire inner ear. Currently methods of surgery were devised using the operating microscope as the enabling tool, which may limit preservation surgery. In addition, there is an ingrained belief in surgeons that opening of the labyrinth immediately leads to disabling or loss of all acoustic and vestibular function. Rather than chance a chronically debilitated ear as the surgical result, ablation surgery is chosen by the surgeon.

Recent advances in endoscopic technology have allowed for small diameter endoscope designs suitable for inner ear surgery. These endoscopes are narrow enough to fit through small openings into the otic capsule. They have optical and working channels and are the prototype surgical instruments for atraumatic entry into the inner ear. Completion of surgical goals without destroying the remaining anatomic content of the inner ear may be possible using micro-endoscopes.

Entry of endoscopes into the inner ear has already taken place. Endoscopic work has taken place as part of cochlear implant research.[1–3] Microscopic endoscopes to research hair cell physiology are also in use.[4] Research into stem cells for inner ear cell regeneration is progressing.[5] These early attempts point towards a goal of directly operating on the inner ear to structurally remediate a patient's medical problem.

Before reliable inner ear endoscopy outcomes can be expected in the future, much groundwork needs to be achieved. Understanding how to enter the inner ear with

Department of Otolaryngology-Head and Neck Surgery, Indiana University Medical Center, 702 Barnhill Drive, Suite 0860, Indianapolis, IN 46202, USA
E-mail address: mfritsch@iupui.edu

Otolaryngol Clin N Am 42 (2009) 1209–1222
doi:10.1016/j.otc.2009.08.018
oto.theclinics.com

minimal or no anatomic inner ear trauma is one part of the groundwork. There are other aspects, such as degree of trauma induced, recovery from trauma, and so forth. In this article, temporal bone (TB) laboratory studies together with clinical experiences of endoscopes contribute to early understanding of surgical entry into the inner ear using the endoscope.

MATERIALS AND PROCEDURES

TB Laboratory

Multiple sites of entry into the human inner ear were explored. Cadaver TBs, which were either dry or bare, or formaldehyde fixed with attached tissue, were used. Specific endoscopic entry sites for the otic capsule were divided into 3 areas: cochlea, vestibule, and the semi-circular canals (SCC). These multiple sites were evaluated for their relative visual clarity, disruption to normal structures, realistic approach angle, and surgical work through simultaneous double-entry sites.

Multiple specialized instruments and surgical steps were used. Sialendoscopes (K. Storz Medical, Tuttlingen, Germany) with an outer diameter of 0.75 mm and 3000 pixels (model no. 11576) and a diameter of 1.1 mm and 6000 pixels (model no. 11573) were used; the angle for both endoscopes was 0°. The endoscopes are categorized by the manufacturer as semirigid for salivary cases and rigid for otology-type work. Forceps (K. Storz, model no. 11577ZJ) with 1.0 mm outer diameter and a 200-μm laser fiber (Lumenis Inc., Santa Clara, CA) were also tested. To simulate schwannoma tumors, small pieces of white modeling clay (Permaplast Clay, AMACO, Indianapolis, IN) were placed in the vestibule and then mock-resected using the endoscope, laser fiber, and forceps.

To achieve adequate surgical exposure, all cases required a canal wall down (CWD) mastoidectomy with removal of the incus and malleus bones. Next, routine microscope-assisted otologic drilling through the otic capsule bone with soft surgery technique was used as a preliminary step to gain access to the inner ear structures before endoscopy commenced.

For the endoscopic surgical techniques, the Oval Window (OW) approach uses either footplate removal or a stapedotomy opening to access the vestibule; the endoscopic Extended-Oval Window (E-OW) approach gains wide exposure of the posterior vestibule through the fossula post-fenestram. In the E-OW approach, removing the stapes pyramid and stapedius muscle are followed by soft surgery techniques and the CO_2 laser over the postfenestram endosteum in a technique similar to laser stapedotomy (**Fig. 1**A, B). The E-OW approach can be performed with or without prior removal of the stapes footplate. In the OW and E-OW approaches, perilymph was revealed and the endoscope entered the vestibular cistern under the footplate or fossula post fenestram.

The vestibular cistern fluid space was used to gain wide endoscopic visualization and access to all the vestibular structures in the OW and E-OW approaches. The vestibular cistern is a volume of vestibular perilymph space between the footplate area and the utriculosaccular structures. The saccule and utricle rest between 1 and 2 mm from the plane of the footplate.[6] Because of the cistern space, there is adequate distance between the otic capsule and membranous structures to allow endoscopic entry without disrupting structures.

The endoscope was also used in the cochlear basal turn to guide a 30-gauge hypodermic needle (Becton Dickinson PrecisionGlide, Franklin Lakes, NJ) into the modiolus. The basal turn was opened by drilling away the anterior lip of the round window using soft surgery techniques. Then, the needle tip was visually guided to

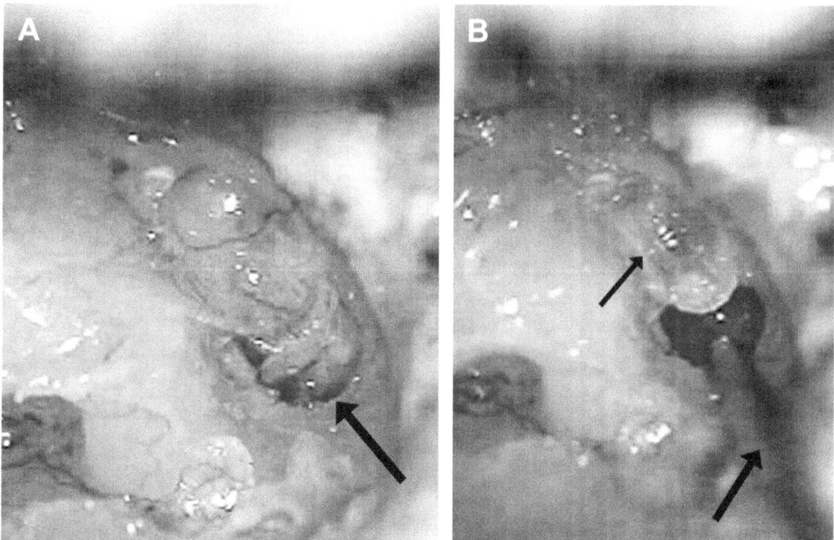

Fig. 1. Microscopic view of the left fixed cadaver TB OW revealing: (*A*) The area of the fossula post fenestram that has been "egg-shelled" (*arrow*) behind the footplate in preparation for an E-OW approach without footplate removal. (*B*) The 0.75-mm endoscope (*large arrow*) enters the left vestibule in preparation for vestibuloendoscopy using the E-OW approach. In this case, the surgical approach has not been enlarged to maximal size by excision of the stapes footplate (*small arrow*).

the modiolus using the endoscope. Fingertip pressure was sufficient to penetrate the bone with the needle into the desired modiolar position (**Fig. 2**). The middle turn is preferred.

The SCCs were approached by soft surgery drilling techniques. In the initial step, the otic capsule bone was drilled, then the endosteum was gently removed, followed by entry of the endoscope and advancing toward the vestibule. The SCCs and ampullae have different diameters and therefore different endoscopes were gently used in each SCC to visualize structures and instruments. To disrupt as little anatomy as possible, soft surgery techniques were used.

RESULTS

Table 1 provides an overview of the predicted surgical experience when using endoscopes to gain intralabyrinthine access directly into the cochlea and into the vestibule by OW/E-OW approaches. Each entry point is paired with the 2 endoscopic sizes tested. The technical and mechanical findings are listed, followed by the endoscopic visual findings to help the surgeon decide on a practical access point into the inner ear that visually targets the specific endolabyrinthine pathology at hand.

Table 2 provides an overview of the predicted surgical experience when using endoscopes to gain intralabyrinthine access through the semi-circular canals.

TB Laboratory

The dry- and wet-preserved TB study findings were consistent and their results are combined.

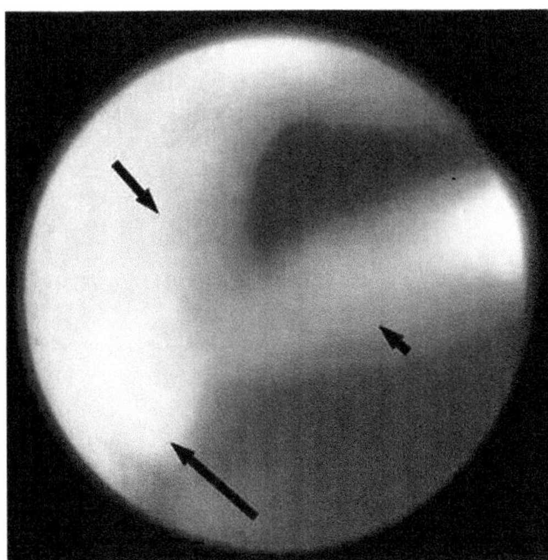

Fig. 2. Endoscopic view of left "wet" human TB scala tympani of the basal turn with a 30-gauge needle (*short arrow*) placed into the modiolus (*medium arrow*) or spiral ganglion in preparation for stem cell injection. The displaced bone and endosteum (*long arrow*) are seen inferior to the needle. With or without the endoscope, the middle turn is preferred in order to inject the central modiolar axis.

Cochlea

The basal and middle turns of the cochlea were accessible with both endoscope sizes, whereas the apical turn was too small for endoscopic entry (see **Table 1**).

In the basal turn, the 0.75-mm endoscope fitted both major scalae, but the 1.1-mm endoscope could be used only in the scala tympani. Simultaneous use of the endoscope and microforceps could only be performed in the basal turn and necessitated the use of both scalae with 1 instrument in each scala; patient use would be for a lesion straddling the 2 scalae. The laser fiber was useable simultaneously with both endoscope sizes within 1 scala. The major landmark structures of the cochlea, such as the stria vascularis, osseous spiral lamina, and modiolus, were clearly visualized (**Fig. 3**). The modiolus was in direct view and accessible for surgical entry. The maximal clear viewing distance along the basal turn was 3.5 mm beyond the endoscope tip. Alternately, the middle cranial fossa (MCF) approach to the basal turn provided visual clarity as good as the transmastoid middle ear approach; however, the morbidity of an MCF craniotomy would be incurred in patient use.

In the middle cochlear turn, the 0.75-mm endoscope fitted into the individual scalae. However, the endoscope was relatively large and was traumatic to the cochlear structures to a point that would cause bleeding in a patient. The 1.1-mm endoscope was too wide to insert into the individual middle turn scalae; however, if it was abutted against a cross section of both scalae, a clear viewing distance of 2 mm was achieved.

For the apical turn, exposure was achieved by first removing the overlaying tensor tympani muscle and tendon. Once the apical turn was opened using soft surgery with the drill, only the microscope was useable, as the endoscopes were too wide to enter.

Vestibule

Two entry sites were useful for endoscopy of the labyrinthine vestibule: the OW area and the horizontal semi-circular canal (H-SCC; discussed in the next section) (see **Tables 1** and **2**).

Table 1
Cochlear findings

Endoscopy Entry Point	Endoscope Size	Technical and Mechanical Findings	Visual Findings
Basal turn cochlea	0.75 mm	Entry possible into ST and SV	WB: wide views of basal turn structures, ST, SV, modiolus, basal membrane; view in anterior direction for 3.5 mm beyond endos tip in ST
	1.1 mm	Entry into ST	
	Other	Cochleostomy 1 mm anterior to RW; forceps size (1 mm) necessitates entry into separate scala from endos, laser fiber placement simultaneously in same scala as endos; CWD-TM or TM with anteriorization of soft tissue ear canal for approach; posterior direction viewing angle limited by anterior ear canal	
Middle turn cochlea	0.75 mm	Entry into ST both directions	WB: both directions viewable, tightly turned ST and SV allow only 1 mm view beyond endos; with 1.1-mm endos, structures only seen in cross section; MCF approach views like those in basal turn findings
	1.10 mm	Too wide for single scala, ST/SV viewed simultaneously in cross section	
	Other	Posterior viewing angle limited by anterior ear canal; Superior aspects of basal and middle turns viewable by MCF approach	
Apical turn cochlea	0.75 mm/1.10 mm	No endoscopic viewing without uncapping of entire apical turn by removing tensor tympani muscle and bone; apical turn destroyed by endoscopy attempts	Structures of uncovered apical turn fully visible; visualization during endos contact with structures is destructive; not of practical clinical application presently
	Other	Good approach angles from CWD-TM or TM with anteriorization of soft tissue ear canal	
OW/E-OW	0.75 mm/1.10 mm	Both endoscopes fit into OW/E-OW to enter vestibular cistern	WB: vestibular cistern gives wide views of entire V. Anterior view shows S, U, saccule-utricle interface, VA, anterior cochlear artery, S-SCC ampulla. Posterior view shows U, CC, P-SCC ampulla, H-SCC ampulla, P-SCC ampulla, posterior cochlear artery
	Other	Multiple good approach angles from CWD-TM or TM with anteriorization of soft tissue ear canal; transcanal approach limited by constricted angulation of endos; SS technique	

Abbreviations: CC, common crus; CWD, canal wall down; endos, endoscopes; E-OW, extended oval window approach; OW, oval window approach; RW, round window; S, saccule; SCC, semi-circular canal (H, horizontal; S, superior; P, posterior); SS, soft surgery; ST, scala tympani; SV, scala vestibuli; TM, tympanomastoidectomy; U, utricle; V, vestibule; VA, vestibular aquaduct; WB, wet temporal bone (vs dry bone no soft tissue).

Table 2
Vestibular findings

Endoscope Entry Point	Endoscope Size	Technical and Mechanical Findings	Endoscope Visual Findings
H-SCC Anterior limb	0.75 mm	Good entry into bony canal after drilling access with SS; membranous canal not passable without avulsion	DB: view encompasses area of S and U, S-SCC anterior limb; WB: 0.75 mm shows membranous canal in cross section or folded as endos advances and avulsion occurs with advance of endos; ampulla with cupula seen with both 0.75-, 1.10-mm endos
	1.10 mm	Entry into ampulla after removal of bony SCC	
	Other	Good approach angle from CWU-TM for both endos	
Posterior limb	0.75 mm	Entry as for H-SCC anterior limb	Endos angled toward medial wall of vestibule; WB: utricle; DB: U and S areas
	1.10 mm	Entry into posterior V after removal of bony canal	
	Other	Good approach angle from CWU-TM for both endos	
S-SCC Anterior limb	0.75 mm	Good entry into bony canal after drilling access with SS; membraneous canal not passable without avulsion	Ampulla with cupula seen with both 0.75- and 1.10-mm endos; WB: beyond ampulla into U; DB: view encompasses area of footplate, hook of cochlear duct, SV, VA
	1.10 mm	Entry into ampulla after removal of bony SCC	
	Other	MCF approach angle for both endoscopes	
CC/limb	0.75 mm	CC accessible through limb of S-SCC, membraneous canal avulsed with advance of endos	WB: visualization of membranous S-SCC DB: CC leads to view of posterior vestibule, OW
	1.10 mm	Not accessible through S-SCC limb until drilled to CC	
	Other	Extreme MCF approach angle for both endoscopes, not practically useful at present	
P-SCC Inferior limb	0.75 mm	Entry into bony canal after drilling access with SS	WB: Good view of ampulla with cupula
	1.10 mm	Accessible after P-SCC bony canal removed to ampulla	DB: cribriform area of nerve seen, posterior-most vestibule.
	Other	CWU-TM with good approach angle	
CC/limb	0.75 mm	CC accessible through limb of P-SCC	WB: P-SCC limb enters into CC with membranous SCC seen
	1.10 mm	Not accessible through superior limb until drilled to common crus	DB: CC view of posterior vestibule
	Other	MCF approach angle for both endoscopes	

Abbreviations: CC, common crus; CWU, canal wall up; DB, dry temporal bone; endos, endoscopes; E-OW, extended oval window approach; OW, oval window approach; S, saccule; SCC, semi-circular canal (H, horizontal; S, superior; P, posterior); SS, soft surgery; SV, scala vestibuli; TM, tympanomastoidectomy; U, utricle; V, vestibule; VA, vestibular aquaduct; WB, wet temporal bone (vs dry bone no soft tissue).

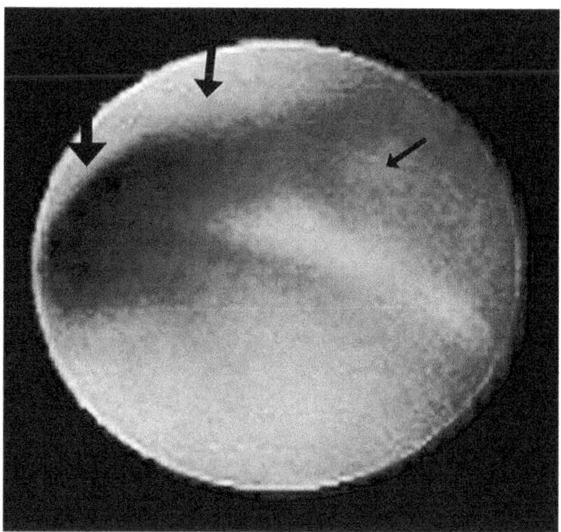

Fig. 3. Endoscopic view of the right cochlea basal turn using the 1.3-mm endoscope looking anteriomedially through a cochleostomy in the scala tympani. The modiolus (*large arrow*), osseous spiral lamina (*medium arrow*), and spiral ligament (*small arrow*) are landmarks shown in this fixed cadaver specimen.

For both approaches (OW and E-OW), the endoscopes fitted easily into the OW niche and into the openings created. Simultaneous instrumentation, with the endoscope and instruments in separate openings, was possible using both approaches.

Both approaches were used to visualize the vestibule. With the OW approach, the anterior and middle portions of the vestibule were easily seen and revealed light reflections on the saccule, utricle, the vestibular aqueduct, the canal openings of the H-SCC, and the superior semi-circular canal (S-SCC) (**Fig. 4**). The OW approach gave a wider view of the vestibule when enlarged in a posterior direction into the fossula post fenestram as an E-OW technique. The E-OW approach without removal of the footplate (ie, postfenestram only) allowed for endoscopic visualization and surgical work on the entire posterior vestibule (**Figs. 5** and **6**).

SCC

In the SCCs, the canals have a different diameter than the ampullae. For this reason, different endoscopes were used in different areas of the SCC to gain different inner ear perspectives (see **Table 2**).

In all SCCs, the 0.75 mm endoscope could not pass the canal's membranous structures without trauma, the structures could not be marginalized within the canal, and they were disrupted when the endoscope was advanced. The 1.1-mm endoscope was only useable if bone removal proceeded up to an ampulla. Direct endoscopic visualization of the entire anterior and mid vestibule was made through the anterior limbs of the H-SCC and S-SCC. Endoscopy through the posterior limb of the H-SCC visualized the posterior vestibule. The bony confines of the posterior limb of the H-SCC only accommodated passage of the 0.75-mm endoscope and the laser fiber. The inferior limb of the posterior canal gave only a circumscribed view of the ampulla and just 1.0 mm beyond it. Endoscopy through the common crus gave a broad view of the posterior and inferior vestibule. The common crus and anterior SCC approach using a rigid endoscope is not practical for patients, since entry through

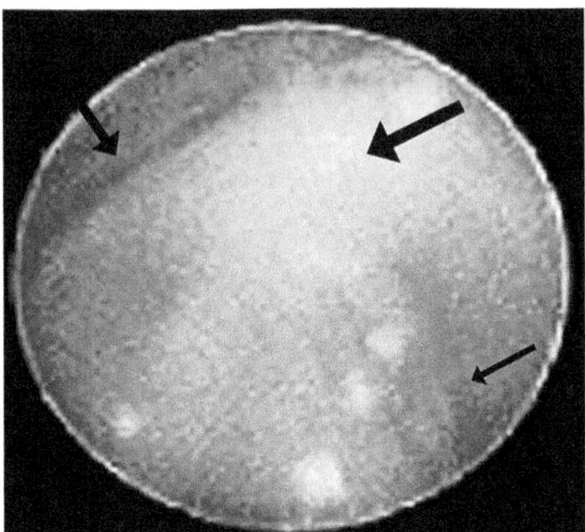

Fig. 4. Endoscopic view of the left anterior and mid vestibule looking medially through the OW approach, as described in the methods section; the 1.3-mm endoscope was used on this fixed cadaver TB specimen. Some of the recognizable landmarks are the line between the saccule and utricle (*small arrow*), the anterior vestibular artery and vein (*medium arrow*), and the opening of the vestibular aqueduct (*large arrow*).

an intracranial trajectory was necessary; use of a very flexible endoscope or laser fiber for this approach might be possible.

The use of 2 simultaneous entry points into the vestibule was explored in various ways. With the endoscope entering the OW and the forceps or laser fiber entering through an SCC, or vice versa, a coordinated approach was possible (**Fig. 7**). Nonparallel visualization of the instrument and anatomic structures allowed for precise aim of the laser fiber and manipulation and grasping by the forceps within the vestibule. In this TB study, it was possible to not only remove small clay tumors of the vestibule

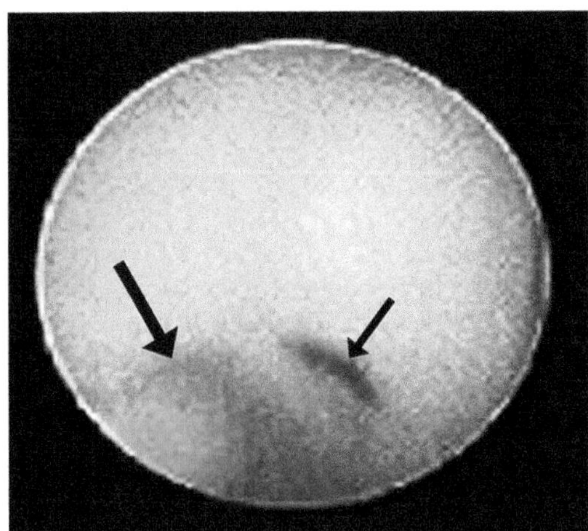

Fig. 5. A view of the left posterior vestibule in a fixed cadaver TB using the 0.75-mm endoscope. The E-OW approach was used. Looking medially, the common crus (*small arrow*), and the 200-μm laser fiber (*large arrow*) are seen.

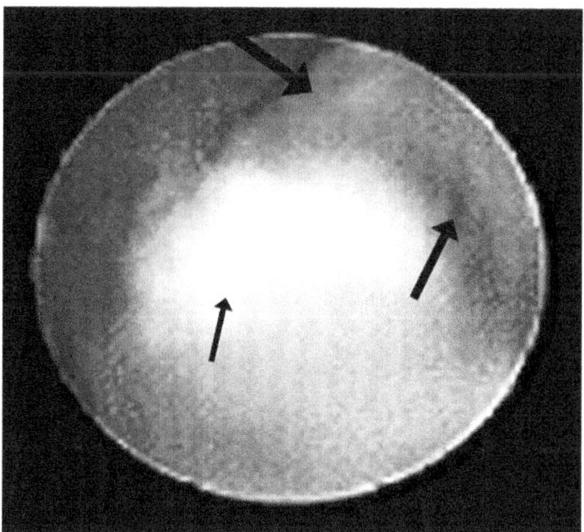

Fig. 6. A left cadaver TB showing the posterior vestibule using the 0.75-mm endoscope. A 200-μm laser fiber (*large arrow*) engaging a clay tumor mass (*small arrow*) just ahead of the common crus (*medium arrow*) is observed medially using the E-OW approach.

using the E-OW approach but also use second entry sites simultaneously. Vestibular tumor resection was performed while also preserving gross anatomic integrity of the cochlea and the anterior-most vestibule. Current endoscopic technology did not allow for an endoscope and the microforceps to be simultaneously placed through a single SCC. In addition, the laser produced gas bubbles, which impeded visualization and negatively affected nearby anatomic structures. The use of 2 simultaneous entry points was useful for visualization and instrument manipulation.

Under endoscopic guidance, the modiolus was entered using a 30-gauge needle below the osseous spiral lamina. Finger pressure was sufficient to submerge the

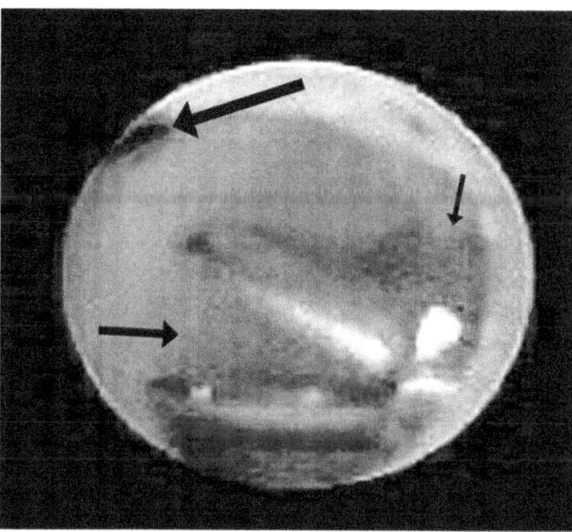

Fig. 7. A 0.75-mm endoscopic view of the vestibule in an anterior direction through the H-SCC of a dry right TB. A simultaneous double-entry site procedure was used for the forceps using an E-OW approach. The areas of the S-SCC ampullae (*large arrow*), utricle (*medium arrow*), and vestibular aqueduct (*small arrow*) are seen in this dry TB.

beveled needle tip into the modiolus as a preliminary maneuver for the injection of 0.02 mL of neurotrophin and cellular solution (see **Fig. 2**). The habenula perforata may have contributed to ease of insertion in some insertion attempts into the modiolus.

DISCUSSION

Literature reports of cochlear implant experience, surgery, and natural pathologies, all support the concept of preservation of inner ear function despite traumas of various kinds to the inner ear.

In relation to cochlear implants (CI), endoscopy was used to determine the patency of the scala tympani; however, as the reported cases were already deaf before endoscopy, the effects of the endoscopy on their cochlear function could not be studied, although the implants were successful.[1,3] It is known ,however, that vestibular function is well preserved in CI patients.[7] The experience with CI patients suggests that endoscopes, which have a shape similar to cochlear implants, could be used in the cochlea and still preserve vestibular function. Similarly, the experience of soft surgery and partial insertion techniques used during cochlear implantation under electro-acoustic stimulation (EAS) protocols has shown that entry into the cochlear basal turn does not necessarily further destroy hearing or vestibular function.[8,9] Studies on the hearing damage caused by minimal entry of an endoscope into the basal turn at the round window have been reported in guinea pigs using auditory brain stem responses (ABR) and distortion product otoacoustic emissions (DPOAE).[2] There was preservation of hearing, especially at a distance from the endoscope intrusion point. A United States patent was granted in 1995 for a complex flexible endoscope for specific use within the inner ear, but it has not yet become available.[10]

Large defects in the otic capsule do not always lead to complete loss of inner ear function. Otologic surgeons have reported on chronic cholesteatoma cases that had marked erosion into the SCCs or vestibule, and yet, had preservation of hearing function.[11–17] Preservation of hearing has also been reported after the acute trauma of translabyrinthine intracanalicular acoustic neuroma removal.[18] The author had similar experiences with vestibular and/or cochlear organ function preservation during schwannoma tumor removal from the cochlea, endoscopy of the SCCs for Meniere disease, cochlear and vestibule endoscopy during cochlear implantation, and stapedotomy of the fossula post fenestram. Thus, destruction of parts or all of either the cochlea or the vestibule by itself does not necessarily lead to complete loss of inner ear function. Endoscopic entry into the inner ear may enable a surgeon to cause minimal trauma to the ear and preserve function.

The current surgical treatment options for intralabyrinthine schwannomas are ablative and contrast with what a minimally invasive endoscopic alternative may offer. The 2 current options most used are the transotic and translabyrinthine approaches. The 2 main goals of the "trans" procedures are total removal of tumor and eradication of vertigo symptoms. In these surgical treatments, the inner ear is removed in the process of tumor resection. Although these procedures are very effective at meeting the surgical goals, use of the trans approaches will destroy all useful inner ear function.[19–21] An endoscopic procedure could be markedly less traumatic and offer the possibility of preservation of function. Preserving cochlear and vestibular function using endoscopic surgery may be applicable in some cases of intralabyrinthine schwannoma.

Endoscopy causes some degree of trauma, but may be tolerated in some instances. It is unknown where the demarcation line for viability of cochlear or vestibular function is when various parts of the labyrinth have been traumatized. How and when surgery can be performed within the inner ear and still preserve inner ear function is poorly understood. There may also be mechanisms, important to surgery of the ear, that limit the damage to one area of the inner ear from spreading to another area. Perhaps anatomically constricted points such as the ductus reunions and the utriculosaccular duct undergo collapse and closure under some situations and thereby prevent serial damage to inner ear structures distant from the trauma. Endoscopic manipulation of these constricted points may enable successful future outcomes. Overall, endoscopy could be used as a much gentler and less traumatic method than the present surgical approaches.

It appears from the TB laboratory studies and clinical experience that the location of a pathologic lesion may influence overall hearing and balance outcomes. The proximity of the lesion to adjacent functioning structures is of primary importance in attempting preservation of those structures. Depending on location, the use of endoscopes and micro instruments may be anatomically tolerated since the endoscopic surgical field is much more constricted compared with conventional trans-surgery. For tumors, the use of localized endoscopic surgery could achieve the preoperative goals of tumor removal and elimination of vertigo, and preserve part of the inner ear function. An example of the importance of location is an intracochlear schwannoma. It is situated such that endoscopic removal is atraumatic to the vestibular structures and could possibly even preserve uninvolved cochlear structures.

The posterior-most area of the vestibule and the SCCs are other possible locations for minimally invasive intralabyrinthine endoscopic surgery. From the case reports in the literature, it is known that some acute or chronic traumas to the posterior vestibule does not destroy hearing function. The anatomic structures preserved during endoscopic OW and E-OW surgeries may be sufficient to support function in patients. In the TB laboratory, the posterior vestibule has been endoscopically operated upon using the OW and the E-OW approaches. The posterior vestibule has been successfully entered by the E-OW approach clinically by the author to perform stapedectomy surgery for the biscuit footplate. As the posterior vestibule is relatively distant from the cochlea, a lesion can be removed and the cochlea left intact anatomically. Even if patients experienced lowered residual hearing after endoscopic surgery, other options such as an EAS implant, or a cochlear implant, would be applicable; trans cases would not have this option.

Lesions arising in the anterior vestibule may be the least approachable for purposes of retaining function. They lie close to, or adhere to, the cochlear basal turn and the vestibular structures. With surgical avulsion of the saccule and cochlear duct hook, any preservation of hearing function would be doubtful. The adjacent structures of the mid and posterior vestibule would probably be similarly traumatized during removal of a lesion from the anterior vestibule. With further study, the anatomic plane separating the saccule from the utricle may be of consequence in eventually achieving success in the anterior vestibule, especially if a consistent position of the saccular duct is determined (see **Fig. 3**). The saccular duct could be sealed to isolate cochlear from vestibular anatomy, possibly making this location more approachable.

The endoscope-guided entry into the modiolus by the 30-gauge needle was deemed successful in that entry was easy with finger pressure to submerge the beveled needle tip, and 0.02 mL was injected into the basal and middle turn modiolus and spiral ganglion.

A Trichotomy arises when considering lesion locations and intralabyrinthine preservation surgery (**Fig. 8**). The Trichotomy is mainly dependent on the anatomy that is unaffected by surgical removal of a lesion. If there is a cochlear lesion, then vestibular

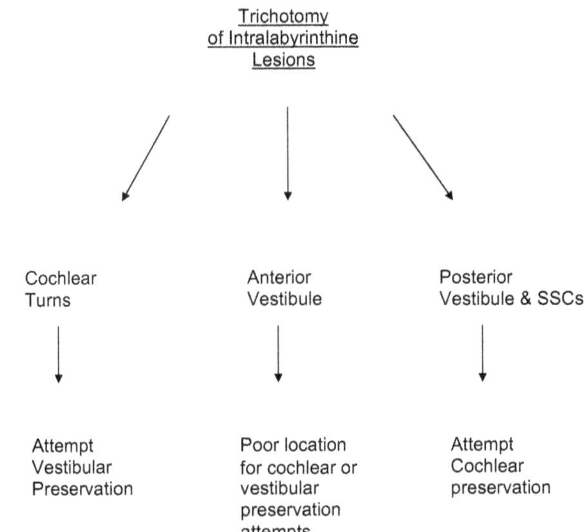

Fig. 8. TB studies revealed a Trichotomy for Intralabyrinthine Lesions. Some lesion locations are predicted to be especially favorable for conservation surgery of the inner ear.

function may be preserved. If there is a posterior vestibular lesion, then cochlear function may be saved. If there is an anterior vestibular lesion, then neither hearing nor vestibular function are likely to be saved.

The present TB laboratory and clinical case observations are very early experiences in understanding the consequences of endoscopic surgical treatment of the inner ear. To improve the endoscopic approaches and outcomes, many improvements will be needed. Major improvements in equipment (such as dedicated intralabyrinthine endoscopes, angled-view endoscopes, flexible endoscope tips, curved-tip laser fibers) and instruments, and specifically, micromanipulators would be necessary for practical attempts at working within the labyrinth. Better protocols for high-strength magnetic resonance imaging to better define normal and pathologic inner ear anatomy would be of great help to the surgeon. In addition, preoperative protective medications and antioxidants may help to prepare the ear to better withstand the shock of endoscopic surgery. Intralabyrinthine schwannoma is a pathology that particularly lends itself to endoscopic surgery; the soft technique can be used initially, progressing to an ablative procedure only if needed. Through further TB laboratory studies and selected endoscopic surgery experiences, a better insight into the workings of the labyrinth and the possibilities of surgery on the inner ear may be gained.

SUMMARY

Although daunting, intralabyrinthine conservation surgery may be a useful technique in some pathologies, such as selected intralabyrinthine schwannomas or endolymphatic hydrops. Endoscopic inner ear surgery offers the possibility of preservation of cochlear and vestibular anatomy and function, while expanding the scope of care that a surgeon can offer. The herein described new endoscopic techniques, such as the OW, E-OW, SCC, and the Simultaneous Double-Entry Site approaches offer possible ways to achieve successful intralabyrinthine surgery. From TB laboratory and clinical experiences, a prognostic Trichotomy for inner ear surgery is proposed.

Presently available equipment and technologies require more design specificity for the inner ear and are under development. Attempts to save remaining inner ear anatomy and function unaffected by a specific pathology are meaningful and can lead to improved postoperative patient function.

ACKNOWLEDGMENT

The author wishes to thank Mrs Rebecca S. Colson, administrative assistant, for her assistance with the preparation of this manuscript.

REFERENCES

1. Balkany TJ. Endoscopy of the cochlea during cochlear implantation. Ann Otol Rhinol Laryngol 1991;99:919–22.
2. Balkany TJ, Hodges AV, Whitehead M, et al. Cochlear endoscopy with preservation of hearing in guinea pigs. Otolaryngol Head Neck Surg 1994;111:439–45.
3. Gstottner W. Cochleoskopie. HNO 1997;45:179–80.
4. Monfared A, Blevins NH, Cheung ELM, et al. In vivo imaging of mammalian cochlear blood flow using fluorescence microendsocopy. Otol Neurotol 2006; 27:144–52.
5. Matsuoka AJ, Kondo T, Miyamoto RT, et al. Enhanced survival of bone-marrow-derived pluripotent stem cells in an animal model of auditory neuropathy. Laryngoscope 2007;117:1629–35.
6. Anson BJ, Donaldson JA. Surgical anatomy of the temporal bone. Philadelphia: WB Saunders Publishers; 1981. p. 346–9.
7. Buchman CA, Joy J, Hodges A, et al. Vestibular effects of cochlear implantation. Laryngoscope 2004;114:1–22.
8. Lehnhardt E. Intrakochleare plazierung der cochlear-implant-elektroden in soft surgery technique. HNO 1993;41:356–9.
9. von Illberg C, Kiefer J, Tillein J, et al. Electric-acoustic stimulation of the auditory system. ORL J Otorhinolaryngol Relat Spec 1999;61:334–40.
10. Arenberg IK, Flock ST, Waner M. Multi-function endoscope apparatus. US Patent 5,419,312, 1995.
11. Phelps PD. Preservation of hearing in the labyrinth invaded by cholesteatoma. J Laryngol Otol 1969;83:1111–4.
12. Bumstead RM, Sade J, Dolan KD, et al. Preservation of cochlear function after extensive labyrinthine destruction. Ann Otol Rhinol Laryngol 1977;86:131–7.
13. Jahrsdoefer RA, Johns ME, Cantrell RW. Labyrinthine trauma during ear surgery. Laryngoscope 1978;88:1589–95.
14. Thomsen J, Barford C, Fleckenstein P. Congenital cholesteatoma: preservation of cochlear function after extensive labyrinthine destruction. J Laryngol Otol 1980; 94:263–8.
15. Palva T, Johanson LG. Preservation of hearing after removal of the membranous canal with a cholesteatoma. Arch Otolaryngol Head Neck Surg 1986;112:982–5.
16. Kobayashi T, Sakurai T, Okitsu T, et al. Labyrinthine fistulae caused by cholesteatoma: improved bone conduction by treatment. Am J Otol 1989;10:5–10.
17. Sade-Sadowsky N. The damage to the membranous labyrinth during fenestration and its influence upon hearing. J Laryngol Otol 1955;69:753–6.
18. McElveen JT, Williams RH, Molter DW, et al. Hearing preservation using the modified translabyrinthine approach. Otolaryngol Head Neck Surg 1993;108:671–80.
19. Green JD, McKenzie JD. Diagnosis and management of intralabyrinthine schwannomas. Laryngoscope 1999;109:1626–31.

20. Kennedy RJ, Shelton C, Salzman KL, et al. Intralabyrinthine schwannomas: diagnosis, management and a new classification system. Otol Neurotol 2004;25:160–7.
21. Fitzgerald DC, Grundfast KM, Hecht DA, et al. Intralabyrinthine schwannomas. Am J Otol 1999;20:381–5.

Index

Note: Page numbers of article titles are in **boldface** type.

A

B

C

D

E

Otolaryngol Clin N Am 42 (2009) 1223–1229
doi:10.1016/S0030-6665(09)00169-8

oto.theclinics.com

M

N

O

P

R

S

Printed and bound by CPI Group (UK) Ltd, Croydon, CR0 4YY
03/10/2024
01040444-0005